Nonprescription Products:

Patient
Assessment
Handbook

NOTICE

The inclusion in this book of any drug in respect to which patent or trademark rights may exist shall not be deemed, and is not intended as a grant of or authority to exercise, any right or privilege protected by such patent or trademark. All such rights or trademarks are vested in the patent or trademark owner, and no other person may exercise the same without express permission, authority, or license secured from such patent or trademark owner.

The listing of selected brands is intended only for ease of reference. The listed brands are a representative sampling of drug products, not a comprehensive listing. The inclusion of a brand name does not mean the editors or publisher has any particular knowledge that the brand listed has properties different from other brands of the same drug, nor should its inclusion be interpreted as an endorsement by the editors or publisher. Similarly, the fact that a particular brand has not been included does not indicate the product has been judged to be in any way unsatisfactory or unacceptable.

The nature of drug information is that it is constantly evolving because of ongoing research and clinical experience and is often subject to interpretation. Although great care has been taken to ensure the accuracy of the information presented herein, the reader is advised that the authors, editors, reviewers, contributors, and publisher cannot be held responsible for the continued currency of the information or for any errors or omissions in this book or for any consequences arising therefrom. Readers are advised that decisions regarding drug therapy must be based on the independent judgment of the clinician, changing information about a drug (e.g., as reflected in the literature and manufacturer's most current product information), and changing medical practices.

Nonprescription Products:

Patient Assessment Handbook

Published by
American Pharmaceutical Association
Washington, DC

Pharmaceutical Editors: Lynn Limon, PharmD, Angela Cimmino, PharmD, Jonathan Lakamp, PharmD

Editorial Services: Linda R. Harteker, Daniel H. Albrant, PharmD, Terry A. Anderson

Managing Editor: Julian I. Graubart

Editorial Coordinator: Susan C. Kendall

Art and Production Director: Mary Jane Hickey

Graphics Production: Tina Offerjost

Proofreader: Rebecca Berg

Indexing Services: Mary E. Coe

Library of Congress Catalog Card Number: 96-079456
ISBN 0-917330-82-X

Printed in the United States of America

How to Order This Book

By phone: **800-878-0729** (802-862-0095 from outside the United States)
VISA®, MasterCard®, and American Express® cards accepted.

Table of Contents

PREFACE

As the self-care revolution spreads, pharmacists are relied upon increasingly to consult with patients on many different health problems. The preface to the *Handbook of Nonprescription Drugs,* on which this book is based, noted that self-care with nonprescription drug therapy is appropriate if pharmacists can

■ Assess patient risk factors;

■ Help in product selection;

■ Screen for allergies, adverse drug reactions, and side effects, and drug-drug or drug-disease interactions;

■ Monitor response to therapy;

■ Discourage use of fraudulent or quack remedies;

■ Assess the need for referral for medical services.

Our goal was to create a pocket-sized reference that pharmacists in ambulatory practice could use for assessment and triage of patients who have questions about nonprescription products and the medical conditions for which the products might be used. We hope that we have achieved our goal.

Lynn Limon, PharmD
Angela Cimmino, PharmD
Jonathan LaKamp, PharmD

ABOUT THIS BOOK

Nonprescription Products: Patient Assessment Handbook, is abstracted from the American Pharmaceutical Association's *Handbook of Nonprescription Drugs,* 11th edition. Whereas the much longer *Handbook* is a comprehensive textbook used in classrooms at virtually every U.S. school or college of pharmacy, this book is designed for the busy practitioner in virtually every ambulatory-care pharmacy.

At its core, this new reference provides (1) the key questions, by product category, that pharmacists may ask when assessing patients' nonprescription product needs and (2) practical patient counseling guidelines on the use of these products. In other words, this book aims to help practitioners heighten their role in self-care consultation.

Nonprescription Products: Patient Assessment Handbook does not purport to be a comprehensive reference on nonprescription pharmacotherapy. Omitted from this book, for example, are discussions on anatomy and physiology of the affected area and pathophysiology of the affected system. The chapters, however, are numbered the same as those in the *Handbook of Nonprescription Drugs,* facilitating lookups for detailed information when needed.

The book also cross-references the *Handbook of Nonprescription Drugs'* companion volume, *Nonprescription Products: Formulations & Features,* a tabular source of information on more than 3,500 brand-name products including diagnostic and monitoring devices.

ACKNOWLEDGMENTS

The American Pharmaceutical Association (APhA) gratefully acknowledges the contributions of the following organization and individuals whose efforts made possible the publication of *Nonprescription Products: Patient Assessment Handbook.*

The book was developed by APhA and supported by an unrestricted educational grant from Johnson & Johnson/Merck Consumer Pharmaceuticals Co.

James C. Appleby, BS Pharmacy, publisher of two APhA periodicals, the *Journal of the American Pharmaceutical Association* and *Pharmacy Today,* and assistant director of APhA's Professional Resources Division, conceived and developed the idea for the book.

Fifty-seven authors and coauthors with demonstrated expertise in nonprescription pharmacotherapy wrote the full-length chapters in the *Handbook of Nonprescription Drugs,* 11th edition, on which this manual is based. They are cited on the first page of each chapter.

The counsel of the following 12 persons composing the *Handbook of Nonprescription Drugs'* Advisory Panel is reflected in *Nonprescription Products: Patient Assessment Handbook:* Manju T. Beier, PharmD; William L. Blockstein, PhD (deceased); Carol A. Bugdalski, BS Pharmacy; Tom Dammer; Janet P. Engle, PharmD; Edward G. Feldmann, PhD; Jack E. Fincham, PhD; Daniel A. Hussar, PhD; Jerry D. Karbeling, BS Pharmacy; Howard Maibach, MD; and Milap C. Nahata, PharmD.

One hundred fifty-five peer reviewers, who were selected from many pharmacy practice settings and allied health professions, helped ensure that the chapter discussions of self-care and nonprescription pharmacotherapy embraced the perspectives of their respective practice settings or professions. Space does not allow listing them here; their names are found on pages ix-xvii of the *Handbook of Nonprescription Drugs.*

CHAPTER 1

Self-Care and Nonprescription Pharmacotherapy

Nonprescription drugs are powerful chemical entities that should be viewed just like prescription drugs with respect to their pharmacology, toxicology, contraindications (absolute and relative), precautions for use, adverse-effect profiles, drug interaction potential, and special considerations in dosage and administration. All the expertise that is focused on the safe, appropriate, and effective use of prescription drugs should also be applied to nonprescription pharmacotherapy.

A variety of clinical and economic factors are fostering growth of nonprescription drug therapy. The following factors are of particular significance.

- The public is becoming increasingly health conscious. Individuals want more control over their personal health care and want to self-medicate when appropriate.

- The reclassification of prescription drugs to nonprescription status has accelerated and is expected to continue.

- Managed care and cost-containment initiatives are eroding profit margins on legend drug dispensing. Profit margins on nonprescription drugs are often higher than those on prescription drugs.

- America is aging. Persons 65 years of age and older now comprise approximately 13% of the total population. These individuals consume 33% of all nonprescription drugs sold.

- Approximately 60% of all dosage units consumed (prescription and nonprescription) are nonprescription drugs. Well over 400 medical conditions are treatable with one or more nonprescription drugs as primary or major adjunctive therapy (Table 1).

- The pharmacist is the most accessible health professional, is the only health professional who receives formal university-based education and training in nonprescription drug pharmacotherapy, and is perceived very favorably by the public. Thus, pharmacists should differentiate themselves from other health care professionals by offering value-added informational services concerning the safe and effective use of medications.

The Self-Care Revolution

Many consumers today are taking an informed and active role in managing their own health care. They are increasingly self-medicating with nonprescription drugs. A host of factors may influence individual attitudes, values, and practices relative to self-care (Table 2). These attitudes, values, and practices vary from individual to individual. Patients should be viewed as individuals with unique backgrounds and needs.

The health problems most likely to be treated with a nonprescription drug have not changed substantially over the past decade. Headache leads the list, followed by the common cold, muscle aches and pains (including sprains and strains), dermatologic conditions (e.g., acne, cold sores, dandruff, dry skin, athlete's foot, jock itch), minor wounds (e.g., cuts, scratches), premenstrual and menstrual symptoms, upset stomach, and

---

Editor's Note: This chapter is adapted from Tim R. Covington, "Self-Care and Nonprescription Pharmacy," in Covington, T.R., ed., *Handbook of Nonprescription Drugs*, 11th edition, which is based, in part, on the 10th edition chapters "The Self-Care Movement," written by Gary A. Holt and Edwin L. Hall, and "FDA's Review of OTC Drugs," written by William E. Gilbertson. For a more extensive discussion of this topic, readers are encouraged to consult Chapter 1 of the *Handbook*.

TABLE 1   Selected medical conditions amenable to nonprescription drug therapy[a]

Abrasions	Cuts (superficial)	Jock itch
Aches and pains (general, mild to moderate)	Dandruff	Motion sickness
	Deficiency disorders (mineral, vitamin, enteral food supplements)	Myalgia
Acne		Nausea
Allergic rhinitis		Nutrition (infant)
Anemia	Dental care	Obesity
Arthralgia	Dermatitis (contact)	Ostomy care
Asthma	Diabetes mellitus	Otitis (external)
Athlete's foot	Diaper rash	Periodontal disease
Bacterial infection (topical, superficial, uncomplicated)	Diarrhea	Pharyngitis
	Dry skin	Pinworm infestation
Blisters	Dysmenorrhea	Premenstrual syndrome
Blood pressure monitoring	Dyspepsia	Prickly heat
Boils	Feminine hygiene	Psoriasis
Burns (minor, thermal)	Fever	Ringworm
Calluses	Flatulence	Seborrhea
Candidal vaginitis	Gastritis	Sinusitis
Canker sores	Gingivitis	Smoking cessation
Carbuncles	Hair loss	Sprains
Chapped skin	Halitosis	Strains
Cold sores	Head lice	Stye (hordeolum)
Colds (viral upper respiratory infections)	Headache	Sunburn
	Heartburn	Swimmer's ear
Congestion (chest, nasal)	Hemorrhoids	Teething
Conjunctivitis	Impetigo	Thrush
Constipation	Indigestion	Toothache
Contact lens care	Ingrown toenails	Vomiting
Contraception	Insect bites and stings	Warts (common and plantar)
Corns	Insomnia	Xerostomia
Cough	Jet lag	Wound care

[a]The pertinent nonprescription drug(s) for a particular condition may serve as primary or major adjunctive therapy.

sleeping problems. Self-medication with nonprescription drugs is often the initial level of care in a tiered system of health care. The average American experiences one potentially self-treatable health problem every 3–4 days.

The self-care revolution should encourage development of knowledge and skill in the promotion of wellness as well as in the treatment of medical conditions. Responsible use of nonprescription drugs is a large part of self-care. The large majority of patients respect these drugs, recognize their limitations, and follow labeling information carefully. Other consumers are uninformed or misinformed. Casual and inappropriate use of nonprescription drugs can lead to serious adverse consequences of both a direct (e.g., adverse drug reaction, drug-drug interaction) and indirect (e.g., delays in seeking appropriate medical attention) nature. Such practices should be discouraged and addressed through adequate package labeling and direct-to-consumer advertising that has a strong educational emphasis. Most important is patient education by pharmacists and other qualified health professionals.

TABLE 2 Selected attitudes, values, and practices likely to influence self-care behavior

Attitudes and beliefs

Appreciation of the value of wellness and prevention initiatives in managing illness

Willingness to accept a significant degree of personal responsibility for one's own health

Perception of the degree of seriousness of the medical condition one wishes to prevent or treat

Acceptance of traditional health care providers and the traditional health care delivery process

Willingness to communicate with legitimate, informed, mainstream health care providers

Tendency to be influenced by friends, relatives, alternative caregivers, and printed health information that is not mainstream

Demographics

Age

Family size

Gender

Socioeconomic position

Economics

Economic status (individual)

Cost of care (products and services)

Access to health care products and services

Availability of health care products and services

Education/Knowledge

Educational level

Baseline knowledge about the relevant medical condition(s)

Baseline knowledge about the relevant treatment regimen

Ability to comprehend verbal and written consumer health information, package labeling, and package insert information

Access to quality consumer health information through the lay press, media, and similar sources

Access to learned intermediaries who can assist in interpreting consumer health information and offer additional advice

Susceptibility to vague or misleading advertising or claims regarding alternative health care (e.g., acupuncture, chelation therapy, megavitamin therapy, naturalism)

The Pharmacist's Responsibility in Pharmaceutical Care

In the initial encounter with a patient seeking assistance with nonprescription drug use, the pharmacist should:

■ Assess, by interview and observation, the patient's physical complaints, symptoms, and medical condition;

■ Differentiate self-treatable conditions from those requiring medical intervention; and

■ Advise and counsel the patient on the proper course of action (i.e., no drug therapy, self-treatment with nonprescription products, or referral to a physician or other caregiver).

If self-treatment with nonprescription drugs is appropriate, the pharmacist can:

■ Assess patient risk factors (e.g., contraindications, warnings, precautions, comorbidity, age, organ function);

■ Assist in product selection;

■ Counsel the patient regarding proper drug use (e.g., dosage, administration technique, monitoring parameters);

■ Maintain a patient drug profile that includes nonprescription as well as prescription drugs;

■ Monitor drug therapy for:

>Drug allergies or hypersensitivities;
>Adverse drug reactions;
>Drug-drug interactions;
>Appropriate response to therapy; and
>Signs and symptoms of drug overuse or dependency;

■ Discourage the use of fraudulent remedies;

■ Assess the potential of nonprescription drugs to mask symptoms of a more serious condition; and

■ Prevent delays in seeking appropriate medical attention.

Such an approach is consistent with pharmaceutical care, which is defined as "the patient-focused provision of drug therapy and cognitive services for the purposes of achieving positive health outcomes and improved quality of life." Pharmaceutical care:

■ Produces safe, appropriate, effective, and economical drug use;

■ Maximizes the benefit of drug therapy;

■ Prevents, identifies, and resolves drug-related problems and therapeutic misadventures; and

■ Assists in promoting optimal therapeutic outcomes.

FDA Regulation of Nonprescription Drugs

The OTC Review

In 1972, the Food and Drug Administration (FDA) initiated a massive scientific review of the active ingredients in nonprescription drug products to ensure that they were safe and effective and bore fully informative labeling. This three-phase review process is often referred to as the over-the-counter (OTC) drug review. The FDA is also responsible for the reclassification of drugs from prescription to nonprescription status and the establishment of regulations for package labeling.

The OTC drug review generated substantial amounts of new data on nonprescription drugs, and additional data have been developed on many of the ingredients to demonstrate their safety and effectiveness. Ingredients that could not be shown to be both safe and effective for their intended uses have been and continue to be dropped from formulations.

Nonprescription Drug Labeling

Concerns about labeling center on three areas: comprehensibility, readability, and essential information.

Comprehensibility

FDA regulations require that nonprescription drug labeling contain terms that are likely to be understood by the average consumer, including the person of low comprehension, under customary conditions of purchase and use. Meeting this requirement is challenging, because a significant percentage of the population is below average in its ability to read, comprehend, discern, and act properly on label information.

Readability

The FDA and manufacturers of nonprescription drugs have been engaged in initiatives to increase drug label readability. Label standardization that is being considered addresses text, format, and the provision of essential information in the same order and in the same area of every drug label. One option being evaluated is the use of a "Drug Facts" box similar to the "Nutrition Facts" box on food labeling.

Essential Information

Essential information that should be displayed prominently on all nonprescription drug labeling consists of the following:

- Product name/ingredients;
- Product indications/claims;
- Package contents;
- Directions for use;
- Contraindications/warnings/precautions/adverse effects;
- Indications for seeking medical attention;
- Manufacturer's information;
- Expiration date and batch code; and
- Label flags.

Drug Reclassification: Prescription to Nonprescription

The FDA OTC drug review is responsible for the reclassification of many drugs from prescription to nonprescription status. In 1991, the FDA announced the establishment of the Nonprescription Drug Advisory Committee to review and evaluate the safety and effectiveness of nonprescription drug products and to provide a forum for the exchange of views regarding the prescription and nonprescription status of various drugs. This process has produced more than 50 reclassifications from prescription-only to nonprescription status over the past 20 years.

A Third Class of Drugs?

In 1995, the General Accounting Office (GAO) of the U.S. Congress completed a 3-year study of whether there were significant benefits or costs associated with a third class of drugs based on experience in 10 countries. The GAO report concluded that, at this time, no major improvements in nonprescription drug use are likely to result from restricting the sale of some nonprescription drugs to pharmacies or by pharmacists. Nonetheless, more and more groups are declaring that a third class of drugs is an idea whose time has come.

Nonprescription Drug Advertising

Although it can prohibit the sale of falsely advertised products, the FDA does not regulate or have authority over nonprescription drug advertising. Such authority rests with the Federal Trade Commission.

In the 1970s, the Federal Trade Commission Act was amended to prohibit advertisers, when describing the therapeutic benefits of nonprescription products, from using language not approved by the FDA for labeling. In 1973, the National Association of Broadcasters and the Nonprescription Drug Manufacturers Association developed guidelines for manufacturers to follow in creating television advertisements for nonprescription drugs. According to these guidelines, an advertisement should:

- Urge the consumer to read and follow label directions carefully;
- Emphasize uses, results, and advantages of the product advertised;
- If it references scientific or consumer studies, present actual research performed and interpret results honestly and accurately;
- Not contain unsubstantiated claims of product effectiveness;
- Not reference doctors, hospitals, or nurses unless such representations can be supported by independently conducted research;
- Not be presented in a manner that suggests prevention or cure of a serious condition that must be treated by a licensed practitioner;
- Not dramatize the ingestion of a medication unless it is illustrating proper medication administration; and
- Not present negative or unfair reflections on competing nonprescription products unless those reflections can be scientifically supported and presented in a manner such that consumers can perceive differences in the uses.

Print advertising should be held to the same integrity standards as the electronic media. Health professionals and consumers should become "students" of advertising messages. Pharmacists are well qualified and positioned to protect and serve the public interest as an objective, informed source of nonprescription drug information.

CHAPTER 2

Patient Assessment and Consultation

Nonprescription drugs allow patients to manage many medical problems rapidly, economically, and conveniently without unnecessary visits to a physician. Appropriate use of a nonprescription product, like that of any other medication, requires certain restrictions and limitations. Labeling alone may be inadequate; the patient often needs professional assistance in selecting and properly using nonprescription drugs. Unfortunately, many patients are unaware of the need for such assistance. A clear indication of this attitude is the large number of nonprescription products purchased in supermarkets and convenience stores, where pharmacist assistance is not available.

To serve patients better, pharmacies need to maximize the personal service of the pharmacist. Patient inquiries should always be referred to the pharmacist, who must promote the value of a pharmacist's guidance in selecting and monitoring nonprescription drug treatment.

Pharmaceutical Care

Pharmaceutical care entails designing, implementing, and monitoring a therapeutic plan, in cooperation with the patient and other health professionals, to produce specific therapeutic outcomes. Each time a patient presents a therapeutic request (e.g., a question about self-care or drug therapy, a request for a new prescription), the pharmacist systematically works with the patient and other health care providers to identify any actual or potential drug therapy problems and to review and determine the best response to all the patient's drug-related needs. Table 1 presents an overview of the pharmacist's assessment questions.

Assessing Drug Therapy Problems

The identification of drug therapy problems is a primary responsibility of the pharmacist. To fulfill it, the pharmacist must establish an efficient method of gathering pertinent information. The single most important piece of information is an accurate account of all medications that the patient is using. One way to do this is to print out the patient's medication profile for the previous 6–12 months and to review this list with the patient. The list is supplemented by a discussion of the patient's use of physician samples, medications obtained from other pharmacies, and self-care remedies. The next step is to tie the use of each of these medications to the patient's medical conditions. Table 2 presents the categories of drug therapy problems and their causes.

Improving Patient Compliance

Noncompliance significantly increases morbidity, hospitalizations, and health care

---

Editor's Note: This chapter is adapted from Wendy Klein-Schwartz and Brian J. Isetts, "Patient Assessment and Consultation," in Covington, T.R., ed., *Handbook of Nonprescription Drugs,* 11th edition, which is based, in part, on the 10th edition chapter "Patient Assessment and Consultation," written by Wendy Klein-Schwartz and J. Michael Hoopes; and on the 9th edition minichapters "Nonprescription Drug Use in Children," written by Mark W. Veerman and Miriam L. Marcadis, and "Nonprescription Drugs and the Elderly" written by Peter P. Lamy. For a more extensive discussion of this topic, readers are encouraged to consult Chapter 2 of the *Handbook.*

TABLE 1 Pharmacist's assessment questions

1. Does the patient need this drug regimen?
   Does the patient have a medical condition? (Misusing drug unintentionally? Addicted? Using for recreation?)
   Does this condition call for this drug regimen? (Avoidable adverse drug reaction? Nondrug therapy indicated? Duplicate therapy?)

2. Is this drug/form the most effective and safe?
   For the medical condition? (Consider condition onset time, potency, acute/chronic use, oral/topical use, potential adverse reactions)
   For the patient? (Consider age, sex, pregnancy/lactation, race)
   With other diseases? (Consider patient's other disease states)
   With the patient's history? (Refractory condition? Allergic/intolerant?)
   Considering cost?

3. Is this dosage the most effective and safe?
   Too low? (Consider weight, patient class, disease states)
   Too high or changing too fast? (Consider weight, patient class, disease states)

4. If side effects are unavoidable, does the patient need additional drug therapy to alleviate them?

5. Will storage or administration impair the drug's efficacy or safety? (Consider lost potency, timing of doses, incorrect dosing technique)

6. Will any drug interactions impair efficacy or safety?
   Drug–drug interactions? (Consider prescription and nonprescription drugs, samples, social drugs)
   Drug–food interactions? (Consider food affecting drug, drug affecting nutrition)
   Drug–laboratory interactions?

7. Will the patient follow this drug regimen?
   Is the regimen available to the patient? (Drug unavailable? Unaffordable?)
   Is the patient physically able to follow the regimen? (Cannot swallow/administer drug?)
   Is the patient mentally able/willing to follow the regimen? (Cannot remember? Does not know how? Not motivated? Dislikes form/dosing?)

8. Does the patient need any additional drug regimen? For untreated condition? Synergism? Prophylaxis?

9. Does the patient need any nondrug therapy or information?
   (Consider other products, referral to health professional or support group, information about disease state)

Reprinted from Tomechko MA, Strand LM, Morley PC, et al. Q and A from the pharmaceutical care project in Minnesota. *Am Pharm.* 1995; NS35(4): 34.

TABLE 2 Categories of drug therapy problems and their causes

Assessment	Drug therapy problems	Causes
Indication	Unnecessary drug therapy	No medical indication; addiction or recreational drug use; nondrug therapy more appropriate; duplicate therapy; treatment for avoidable adverse reaction.
Effectiveness	Wrong drug	Dosage form inappropriate; contraindications present; condition refractory to drug; drug not indicated for condition; more effective medication available; drug interaction.
	Dosage too low	Dose incorrect; frequency inappropriate; duration inappropriate; storage incorrect; administration incorrect; drug interaction.
Safety	Adverse drug reaction	Unsafe drug for patient; allergic reaction; incorrect administration; drug interaction; dosage increase or decrease too fast; undesirable effect.
	Dosage too high	Dose incorrect; frequency inappropriate, duration inappropriate; drug interaction.
Compliance	Inappropriate compliance	Drug product not available; patient cannot afford drug product; patient cannot swallow/administer drug; patient does not understand instructions; patient prefers not to take medication.
Untreated indication	Needs additional drug therapy	Untreated condition; synergistic therapy; prophylactic therapy.
	None known	—

Reprinted from Tomechko MA, Strand LM, Morley PC, et al. Q and A from the pharmaceutical care project in Minnesota. *Am Pharm.* 1995; NS35(4): 35.

expenditures. Factors affecting compliant behavior include patient satisfaction and motivation. By ensuring that medication decisions are based on the patient's own lifestyle, environment, values, and attitudes, as well as on an understanding of associated risks, pharmacists can have a strong influence on patient compliance.

Counseling Patients

The pharmacist is often the patient's first contact with the health care system. He or she can assess the situation and recommend a course of action. This may include recommending a nonprescription drug, dissuading the patient from buying medication when drug therapy is not indicated, recommending nondrug treatment, or referring the patient to another health care practitioner.

Communication

When a pharmacist responds to a patient's request, the ensuing interaction can be referred to as a therapeutic dialogue. The goal of this interaction is to establish a therapeutic relationship. A therapeutic relationship is a partnership between the patient and the pharmacist characterized by trust and a reciprocal commitment to work together to prevent drug therapy problems and to identify and solve such problems when they occur. This relationship allows the pharmacist to gather detailed, and sometimes intimate, information from the patient.

Principles of Good Communication

An effective patient–pharmacist relationship will be established if the pharmacist is a capable, empathetic source of information. The pharmacist's attitude toward the patient will influence the quality of communication; for this reason, the pharmacist must avoid biases that may be based on the patient's level of education, socioeconomic or cultural background, interests, or attitude. The patient must be assured that any information discussed with the pharmacist will be strictly confidential.

Because people may resent being told what they already know, the pharmacist should first determine the patient's level of knowledge. When interacting with patients, the pharmacist should use words that a layperson can understand.

Effective Questioning

Two types of questions are generally used: open- and closed-ended. Open-ended questions—e.g., "Would you please tell me more about your symptoms?"—are essential because they provide more information than questions that can be answered with a simple yes or no. To be sure that a patient understands dosage instructions, the pharmacist could ask, "So that I know that I haven't forgotten to tell you anything, would you please tell me how you're supposed to take this medicine?"

Closed-ended questions—e.g., "How long have you had this pain?"—help the pharmacist gather specific information or clarify information obtained through open-ended questions. Closed-ended questions are sometimes a helpful means of summarizing or redirecting a dialogue.

Effective Listening

The pharmacist must focus on the patient and exclude distracting elements such as the telephone and computer monitor. The pharmacist often must clarify the details of the patient's problem and be receptive to the patient's responses. The pharmacist should respond with empathy, perhaps by paraphrasing the patient's words or by reflecting on what was said in terms of the patient's own experience. This technique is sometimes called "active listening." For instance, after listening to a complaint of pain, the pharmacist might say, "You have a sharp, stabbing pain in your wrist, is that right?" and end with a statement such as "That must be very uncomfortable." The pharmacist should reinforce correct decisions the patient has made. The pharmacist should be nonjudgmental and should communicate warmth, feeling, and interest.

Nonverbal Communication

Body language, such as posture and facial expression, communicates strong, direct messages. An open body posture—facing the patient with arms and legs uncrossed—indicates a willingness to communicate and listen. It is important to maintain an appropriate distance from the patient; the pharmacist should be close enough for confidential communication to occur without making the patient uncomfortable. If the patient backs away or moves closer, the pharmacist should maintain the new distance that the patient has established. It is important for the pharmacist to maintain eye contact with the patient and control his or her facial expressions to avoid showing negative reactions such as disapproval or shock.

The patient's nonverbal communication is equally important. If a patient has a closed body posture—arms crossed, legs crossed, body turned away from the pharmacist—the pharmacist may need to find out why the patient is uncomfortable and try to allay those concerns. The pharmacist should watch the patient for signs of anxiety, nervousness, and even physical symptoms such as pain.

Physical Barriers to Communication

Discussions between the patient and the pharmacist should be as private as possible. High counters, glass separators, and elevated platforms inhibit communication; the pharmacist should try to be at the same eye level as the patient. Ideally, a private area of the pharmacy should be designated for patient consultation.

Communication Techniques for Special Populations

Special techniques may be required with some patients. If a hearing-impaired patient reads lips, the pharmacist should be close to and directly in front of the patient and should maintain eye contact while speaking. The pharmacist should speak slowly and distinctly in a low-pitched, moderately toned voice. A quiet, well-lit environment is essential. The pharmacist should use visual reinforcement, such as pointing to the part of the body that hurts or to the directions on the container. Writing down the information may be necessary. Before depending on written communication, the pharmacist must be sure that the patient is literate.

When counseling a blind patient, a pharmacist should first identify him- or herself as a pharmacist. The pharmacist should depend on tone of voice and verbal feedback to convey empathy and interest in the patient's problem. If touching seems appropriate, the pharmacist should first ask the blind person if it would be acceptable.

The Patient Interview

Counseling patients about self-treatment carries with it a great professional responsibility. Such interaction may be initiated by a question posed by the patient or pharmacist (Figure 1).

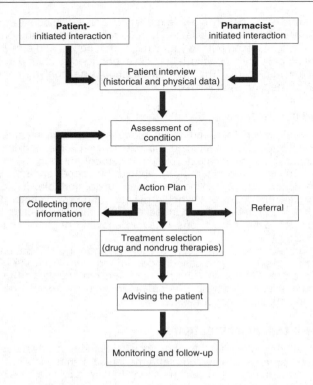

FIGURE 1 Patient-pharmacist consultation process.

Information Gathering

The most important piece of information is an accurate account of each medication the patient is using. One way to obtain this information is to print out the patient's medication profile every time the patient presents with a new prescription, nonprescription drug, or general medication question. An alternative method is to place a computer monitor in the private counseling area and to conduct a joint review the patient's current medications.

The pharmacist may then say, "I would like to review each medication you are taking to make sure that the medication that we select (or is prescribed) for you fits with your current regimen. Here is a list of the medications you have received at our pharmacy. Let's see which ones you are currently taking as well as what other medications you may be using."

Next, the pharmacist should tie all medications the patient is currently taking to each of the patient's medical conditions. At this point, information on the patient's drug allergies and the medical histories of his or her relatives may be gathered.

The pharmacist need not try to obtain all relevant information in one encounter. The follow-up step of care continues the initial assessment process and allows the pharmacist to obtain additional information. With practice, the pharmacist learns to use every patient encounter to gather whatever additional information is needed.

Historical Data

A broad overview enables the pharmacist to identify the condition that the patient seeks to treat and to make the most appropriate recommendation. The pharmacist can ask the following questions:

- Can you describe the problem?
- When did the problem start?
- How long does it last? Does it come and go, or is it continuous?
- Does the problem limit your daily activities (e.g., sleeping, eating, working, walking, etc.)?
- Is this a new problem, or is it the recurrence or worsening of an old one?
- Are there other problems that occur concurrently?
- Does any food, drug, or physical activity make the problem worse?
- Does anything relieve the problem? What has relieved it in the past?
- What has been done to treat the problem?

The next step in the process is to gather patient-specific data. The pharmacist should selectively elicit the following information:

- Who is the patient? Is the patient the person in the pharmacy or someone else?
- How old is the patient?
- Is the patient male or female? If the patient is female, is she pregnant or breast-feeding?
- Does the patient have any other medical problems that may alter the expected effects of a given nonprescription drug or be aggravated by the drug's effects? Is the complaint related to a chronic disease?
- Does the patient have any allergies?
- Is the patient on a special diet? Does the patient have any special nutritional requirements?
- Is the patient using any prescription, nonprescription, or social drugs (e.g., vitamins or food supplements, caffeine, nicotine, alcohol, or marijuana)? How long has the patient been taking these drugs?
- Has the patient experienced adverse drug reactions in the past?

Throughout the encounter, the pharmacist is formulating a hypothesis based on the identification of actual or potential drug therapy problems. The pharmacist should determine whether the patient has misinterpreted the condition, done any harm by waiting to seek advice, or worsened the condition by previous self-treatment.

Observed Physical Data

Physical data include pulse rate, heart sounds, respiration rate, age, and weight. Depending on the pharmacist's training and skills, physical data are collected by all or some of the following techniques: observation or inspection, palpation or manipulations, percussion, and auscultation.

Although some pharmacists use hands-on techniques to obtain physical data, most obtain this information through observation. Many clues to a patient's general health and to the seriousness of a condition can come from simple observation. For example, the degree of discomfort caused by pain may be judged from a patient's facial expressions or lack of use of a particular limb. Toxicity from an infection may be manifested by lethargy and pallor. The pharmacist would need to inspect the patient's skin before offering advice about a skin rash, which may result from a simple contact phenomenon or may suggest systemic disease.

Assessment of Condition

Assessment is the evaluation of all the data—historical and physical—collected from the patient to determine the etiology and severity of the medical condition. Determining etiology and severity is essential for reaching appropriate conclusions about treatment and the need for referral. Many times the etiology and severity of a condition cannot be determined conclusively because certain data may not be accessible. In such situations, referral may be required.

Certain groups of patients are at greater risk for complications and require more careful evaluation. They include elderly patients, infants and children, patients with certain chronic diseases such as diabetes or renal or heart disease, patients with multiple medical conditions and those who are taking multiple medications, recently hospitalized patients, and patients treated by several physicians.

Action Plan

After collecting all the available information and assessing the patient's condition, the pharmacist must formulate an action plan. A well-considered plan can help ensure proper management of the patient, even if all the desired information is not in hand. A sound action plan requires paying careful attention to five areas:

- Collecting more information;
- Selecting physician referral;
- Selecting self-treatment;
- Advising the patient on self-treatment; and
- Maintaining follow-up contact.

Collecting More Information

Obtaining more information may entail talking to the patient's parent or another adult. In some situations, communication with the patient's physician may be necessary. This occurs, for example, when the pharmacist must obtain data on preexisting medical conditions.

Selecting Physician Referral

When the pharmacist has enough information to assess the condition, he or she must decide whether to refer the patient to a physician or advise self-treatment. If the plan involves physician referral, the pharmacist must consider the type of treatment center to which the patient will be referred (physician's office or emergency care facility) as well as the urgency for treatment.

Physician referral is indicated in any of the following situations:

- The symptoms are too severe to be endured by the patient without definitive diagnosis and treatment.
- The symptoms are minor but have persisted and do not appear to be due to an easily identifiable cause.
- The symptoms have returned repeatedly for no readily recognizable cause.
- The pharmacist is in doubt about the patient's medical condition.

Selecting Self-Treatment

In advising self-treatment, the pharmacist must consider several factors. First, a measurable and achievable therapeutic objective must be identified. With this determined, a therapeutic modality—either drug or nondrug—may then be recommended. For example, the objective in a patient who has a productive cough but is having difficulty producing sputum would be to increase sputum production. Thus, an expectorant would be the agent of choice. Selecting a specific treatment requires reviewing drug variables (dosage forms, ingredients, side effects, adverse reactions, relative effectiveness, and price) and matching them with patient variables (age, gender, drug history, other physiologic problems, and ability to pay). Should self-treatment without drugs be indicated, selection of the nondrug modality would similarly be modified based on patient variables.

To measure the success of treatment, the pharmacist should set indices based on the therapeutic objective, the toxic or adverse effects of the treatment, the nature and severity of the condition, and the ability of the patient to understand the condition and its treatment. The objectives in treating sinusitis with decongestants, for example, are to facilitate drainage and relieve symptoms such as headache. Achievement of the first objective can be determined by observing or asking about the nature of nasal discharge (quantity, color, and viscosity); achievement of the second, simply by asking about the headache. Indices of toxicity are those symptoms indicative of an excessive dose or an untoward reaction. Indices that suggest the problem may be worsening and may require special attention should be identified. Indices relating to patient understanding of the condition and its treatment include determination of the appropriateness of the patient's questions to the pharmacist as well as his or her response to the pharmacist's queries. The patient's compliance with the treatment plan can also be considered.

Advising the Patient on Self-Treatment

The next step in the action plan is to advise the patient on self-treatment. The pharmacist should give advice in the following areas:

■ Reasons for self-treatment;
■ Description of the drug and/or treatment;
■ Administration of the drug and/or treatment;
■ Side effects and precautions; and
■ General treatment guidelines.

In advising the patient about the suggested treatment plan, the pharmacist should summarize the patient's condition, explain the significance of the symptoms, and outline the reasons for treatment. The therapeutic objective(s) should be clearly explained. The pharmacist should be prepared to present alternative treatments, with their relative merits. The pharmacist should then discuss the nonprescription drug(s) selected and describe the therapeutic action of the ingredients (e.g., decongestants, antihistamines, or laxatives) and the effect the product(s) will have on the patient's symptoms and condition. Finally, the pharmacist should tell the patient about the available dosage forms and the availability of any generic product. All oral information should be conveyed in lay terms.

Medication administration guidelines should be explained clearly. Covering a few of the most important points is better than overwhelming a patient with information. It is important to include information about length of treatment.

The patient should be told about the most common side effects or adverse reactions associated with a drug and instructed on how to manage them. Special warnings about activities, other drugs, foods, or beverages that should be avoided, as well as about medical conditions that may be complicated by use of the drug, should be discussed. Information should be written down if it is extensive or complex.

The pharmacist should offer the patient general guidelines about managing the condition. These guidelines might include lifestyle changes, additional products or services, and information sources. The pharmacist should provide a list of signs and symptoms that indicate whether the drug is working or causing adverse effects and when a physician's advice is needed. Finally, the patient should be told of the normal response time to the treatment, the time required to resolve the condition, and what to do if response is delayed.

Maintaining Follow-up Contact

The patient should be encouraged to check back if the condition does not improve within a specific period of time or if problems with the medication develop. Follow-up helps the pharmacist determine the utility of the information provided and allows the pharmacist to assess whether his or her communication skills require modification. It also assures the patient that the pharmacist cares.

Pharmaceutical Care for High-Risk and Special Groups

Four groups of patients—the very young, elderly persons, pregnant women, and nursing mothers—often experience a higher incidence of drug therapy problems than other patients. Awareness of their physiologic state, possible pathologic conditions, and special social context is necessary for the proper assessment of their medical conditions and recommendation of treatment.

Pediatric Patients

In considering nonprescription drugs for the pediatric age group, certain relatively predictable differences between pediatric and adult age groups should be noted. These include, but are not limited to, physiologic differences, pharmacokinetic and pharma-codynamic properties of administered drugs, and special administration procedures (e.g., dose, route of administration, dosage form, palatability).

When considering nonprescription drug therapy, it is essential to differentiate pediatric age periods, as follows:

- *Preterm neonate (premature)*: gestational age of less than 38 weeks;
- *Full-term neonate:* gestational age of 38–42 weeks;
- *Newborn:* first postnatal month of life;
- *Infant (baby):* 1–12 months of age;
- *Toddler (young child):* 1–5 years of age;
- *Older child:* 6–12 years of age; and
- *Adolescent:* 13–18 years of age.

Package labeling often encourages medical evaluation in children under the age of 1 or 2 years. Some package labeling provides dosage guidelines specific to age groups.

Physiologic Differences

Pediatric patients are at risk for drug therapy problems because their body and organ functions are in a continuous state of development. While both hepatic metabolism and renal elimination of drugs are usually slower in neonates and young infants, they rise rapidly over the first year of life. Children metabolize some drugs more rapidly than adults do. Illness in children is potentially more serious because their physiologic state is less tolerant of changes. Children are also very susceptible to fluid loss, so fever, vomiting, or diarrhea represent greater potential risks to them.

Effects of Altered Drug Pharmacokinetics

The pharmacokinetic properties of drugs (e.g., absorption, distribution, metabolism, elimination) in pediatric patients may be quite different from those in adults. These properties may also vary substantially among pediatric age groups.

Absorption. The gastrointestinal (GI) absorption of drugs is influenced by many factors, including gastric pH, gastric emptying time, motility of the GI tract, enzymatic activity, blood flow/perfusion of the GI mucosa, permeability and maturation of the mucosal membrane, and concurrent disease process. Significant changes in these factors occur during the first few years of life.

Distribution. Several differences in pediatric age groups affect the distribution of drugs when compared with that in adults. They include differences in the percentage of total body water to total body weight, percentage of body fat, and rates of plasma protein binding.

Metabolism. Drugs are metabolized primarily in the liver. The activity of the processes involved in metabolism remains low in the neonate, and each hepatic metabolic process matures at a different rate. Once the metabolic function of the liver matures, it may actually exceed the adult capacity to metabolize drugs on a milligram-per-kilogram-per-day basis. This increased capacity probably occurs because the liver weighs proportionately more in children than in adults.

Excretion/Elimination. Excretion or elimination is primarily the function of the kidneys; this process also undergoes significant age-related changes. At birth, the glomerular filtration rate (GFR) is approximately 30% or less than that of adults. The GFR increases significantly in the first 2 weeks of life and reaches adult values by 1 year of age. Renal tubular secretion and reabsorption mature at a rate slightly slower than the GFR.

Other Potential Drug Therapy Problems

The pharmacist should be sensitive to the potential for drug therapy problems among children. For some illnesses, such as diarrhea, nondrug therapy is often more appropriate than therapy with nonprescription antidiarrheal drugs. In some situations, specific drugs are contraindicated; for example, aspirin should not be administered to young children with certain viral illnesses because of its association with Reye's syndrome. (See Chapter 4.) For younger children, solid dosage forms are inappropriate, and the pharmacist will need to guide parents to liquid medications or chewable tablets.

Inaccurate Dosing. Inaccurate dosing is another potential problem. Labeling on nonprescription drugs generally uses age-based guidelines for determining dosages; however, many products do not provide dosage information for children under 6 years of age. Because nonprescription medications have a wide therapeutic index (the ratio of the toxic dose to the therapeutic dose), safe doses may generally be determined by weight. For some drugs, children require larger milligram-per-kilogram doses than adults do because children metabolize these drugs more rapidly. Average weights for children at different ages are presented in Table 3.

Improper Administration. Liquids are relatively easy to administer, and the dose can be titrated to the patient's weight; therefore, they are often used in pediatrics. Because elixirs and syrups can have a high alcohol and sugar content, respectively, these liquid forms may be less desirable than suspensions and solutions. A suspension may also mask the disagreeable taste of a drug.

To ensure accurate dosing, the American Academy of Pediatrics Committee on Drugs recommends the use of a medication cup, cylindrical dosing spoon, oral dropper, and oral

TABLE 3 Average pediatric weight by age grouping

| | Average weight | |
Age	Pounds	Kilograms[a]
Birth	7.3	3.3
6 mo	17.0	7.7
1 y	21.6	9.8
15 mo	23.0	10.5
2 y	27.0	12.3
3 y	32.0	14.5
4 y	36.4	16.5
5 y	41.0	18.6
6 y	46.0	20.9
7 y	52.0	23.6
8 y	57.2	26.0
9 y	62.0	28.2
10 y	68.0	30.9

[a]1 kg equals 2.2 lb.

Reprinted from Nykamp D. Nonprescription medications in the pediatric population. *Am Pharm.* 1995 Apr; 35: 10–29.

syringe. Medication cups are fairly accurate for volumes of exact multiples of 5 mL (i.e., 5 mL, 10 mL, 15 mL). With higher-viscosity liquids, the oral syringe is preferable because it completely expels the dose. Potent liquid medications should always be administered with an oral syringe. Drawing up the dose in the syringe requires dexterity. The pharmacist should explain to parents how to use and read it.

Precision oral dosing devices help by reducing underdoses and eliminating adverse drug effects from potential overdoses. These devices may also enhance acceptance of medication by infants and children. Parents may need instructions on using these devices, as well as on giving medications to reluctant or struggling children.

Tablets or capsules can usually be swallowed by a child over 4 years of age. Tablets that are not sustained-release or enteric-coated formulations may be crushed; most capsules may be opened and the contents sprinkled on small amounts of food (e.g., applesauce, jelly, or pudding). Table 4 presents selected guidelines for administering oral medications to pediatric patients.

Adverse Effects. Side effects may be different in children than in adults. For example, antihistamines and central nervous system (CNS) depressants may cause excitation.

Noncompliance. Noncompliance may occur when children refuse to take the medication. It can also occur when parents do not understand instructions or do not pass them on to day care providers. In these cases, written directions are essential.

Assessment and Counseling

Assessment and counseling for pediatric patients usually involve the parents. For younger children, the pharmacist can work with the parents to recommend treatment and assess drug therapy problems. The pharmacist can involve the older child in the counseling process.

TABLE 4   Selected medication administration guidelines for oral medications

Infants

- Use a calibrated dropper or an oral syringe.
- Support the infant's head while holding the baby in the lap.
- Give small amounts of medication to prevent choking.
- If desired, crush nonenteric-coated or slow-release tablets to a powder and sprinkle them on small amounts of food.
- Provide physical comforting while administering medications to help calm the infant.

Toddlers

- Allow the child to choose a position in which to take the medication.
- If necessary, disguise the taste of the medication with a small volume of flavored drink or small amounts of food. A rinse with a flavored drink or water will help remove an unpleasant aftertaste.
- Use simple commands in the toddler's jargon to obtain cooperation.
- Allow the toddler to choose which medications (if multiple) to take first.
- Provide verbal and tactile responses to promote cooperation.
- Allow the toddler to become familiar with the oral dosing device.

Preschool children

- If possible, place a tablet or capsule near the back of the tongue and provide water or a flavored liquid to aid the swallowing of the medication.
- If the child's teeth are loose, do not use chewable tablets.
- Use a straw to administer medications that could stain teeth.
- Use a follow-up rinse with a flavored drink to help minimize any aftertaste.
- Allow the child to help make decisions about dosage formulation, place of administration, which medication to take first, and the type of flavored drink to use.

Geriatric Patients

Pharmacokinetic, pharmacodynamic, and various nonpharmacologic factors predispose the elderly to problems with nonprescription drugs. Elderly patients may confuse their problems with age-associated problems and therefore misreport their symptoms. In addition, elderly patients are often reluctant to share health information.

Effects of Physiologic Aging

Aging is associated with physiologic changes that predispose patients to disease. Subtle changes in mental status, such as confusion, may be anticipated in elderly patients in whom illness has caused anxiety over their health status. In addition, the elderly often suffer from impaired vision (e.g., difficulty reading and differentiating colors) and hearing loss. Pharmacists should take such impairments into consideration and, for example, provide instructions in large, high-contrast, dark print.

Aging alters the absorption, distribution, metabolism, and elimination of certain drugs, increasing the susceptibility of the elderly patient to drug therapy problems. Such pharmacokinetic changes can result in an unexpected accumulation of these drugs to toxic levels. Finally, the aging process, as well as many chronic diseases, can alter a patient's nutritional status. The patient's nutritional status and weight are important because they can also alter the pharmacokinetics and pharmacodynamics of drugs.

Effects of Altered Drug Pharmacokinetics

Absorption. Pharmacokinetic changes are caused not only by advancing age but also by the effects of disease states and multiple drug use. For example, coexisting diseases may alter the absorption of some drugs.

Distribution. As the ratio of lean body weight to lipid tissue changes with age—the volume of distribution (Vd) of water-soluble drugs decreases, possibly promoting more intense action of these drugs. Extracellular and other body fluids also decrease with age, thereby decreasing the Vd of water-soluble drugs. Alpha$_1$-acid glycoprotein, a plasma protein, increases with age in healthy elderly patients, whereas albumin levels decrease. Therefore, drugs that are highly protein bound should show altered distribution patterns in elderly patients.

Metabolism. It is generally agreed that elderly patients probably have diminished capacity to metabolize drugs and that it is primarily the oxidative drug-metabolizing mechanism that changes with age.

Excretion/Elimination. Renal function declines with age but to a variable degree and at a variable rate. The GFR declines with age. The decline is more rapid in men than in women. Altered physiologic processes, resistance, and hypotension, may also reduce the GFR. The renal function of older people is more vulnerable to insults imposed by drug therapy and overall stress.

Effects of Altered Drug Pharmacodynamics

The pharmacodynamics (e.g., the hypoglycemic effect, the extent and duration of pain relief, and the effect of a drug on heart rate) are of major interest in the pharmacologic management of chronic diseases in the elderly. Pharmacodynamics govern the duration of a given concentration of a drug at its site of action. Pharmacodynamics change with age (and disease), but it is difficult to differentiate between normal aging effects and pathophysiologic effects and their influence on pharmacodynamics.

Reduced Physiologic Reserve. The elderly are more susceptible to decompensation under stress because of the loss of physiologic reserve. Older people are less able to regulate blood glucose levels, pulse rate, blood pressure, and oxygen consumption. Therefore, it is not unreasonable to assume that drugs can bring about unanticipated adverse effects on an elderly patient's functional reserve.

Altered Hemostatic and Thermoregulatory Mechanisms. There is evidence that the efficiency of postural stability is reduced with advancing age. Any drugs that affect this homeostatic mechanism (e.g., antihistamines that affect the CNS) can decrease the body's ability to maintain balance, possibly leading to a greater incidence of falls and fractures. The efficiency of the thermoregulatory mechanism, which controls body temperature, decreases with advancing age.

Altered Drug-Receptor Interactions. Most drugs bind to receptors to initiate their action. Age-related altered drug action may also be related to altered drug-receptor interactions. There may be receptor changes with age in certain parts of the body but not in others. Receptors, in adapting to drug therapy, may also become supersensitive or desensitized.

Drug-receptor response may be increased or decreased in the elderly. It has been suggested for some time that the elderly appear to be more "sensitive" to some drugs.

Altered Neurologic Function. With advanced age, there is increased conduction time, decreased cerebral blood flow, and possibly increased permeability of the blood-brain barrier. The elderly have an enhanced CNS sensitivity to drugs, prompting a reduced dose requirement (perhaps by as much as 50%) for some drugs.

Increased brain sensitivity and other changes, such as decreased coordination, prolongation of reaction time, and impairment of short-term memory, manifest as increased frequency of confusion, frequency of urinary incontinence, and number of falls. Drug therapy may exaggerate all these changes.

Control of bowel and bladder function is lessened with advancing age. The impact of nonprescription drugs on these functions is often increased when such drugs are added to an already-existing therapeutic regimen.

Altered Cardiovascular Function. The action of cardiac drugs in the elderly is assumed to differ from that in younger people because measurements start from a different point. Peak cardiac output at exercise also declines with age. Adaptation of the aging heart to stress is diminished because of a delayed and reduced reaction of the sympathetic nervous system. The heart manifests an increased sensitivity to the toxic effects of some drugs (e.g., digoxin).

Changes in the cardiovascular system also involve reductions in blood vessel elasticity, leading to increased arterial blood pressure. The elderly generally present with a relatively reduced fluid volume. These hemodynamic and fluid volume changes are expected to change the response of the elderly to drugs.

The elderly are more likely than younger people to become symptomatically orthostatic, even without drugs. Therefore, all drugs that could cause orthostatic hypotension, particularly if used in combination, should be used cautiously in the elderly.

Altered Endocrine Function. The reduced availability of hormones results in diminished endocrine regulatory mechanisms with age as well as deficiencies in hormonal feedback mechanisms.

Alterations in pancreatic and adrenal hormone levels result in decreased glucose tolerance and an increased susceptibility to drug-induced hypoglycemia. In women, reduced estrogen levels have been correlated with a greater incidence of osteoporosis. Decreased thyroid levels make the elderly more sensitive to the action of digitalis and increase the risk of drug-induced hypothermia.

Altered Immunologic Function. Age-related changes in immune function reflect several different alterations. All these factors combine to decrease cellular immune competence. Infections are more prevalent in the elderly; however, the infections common in older people (influenza, pneumococcal pneumonia) are not usually associated with immune deficiency, rather they are caused by opportunistic organisms.

Elderly patients who take prescribed or self-prescribed nonsteroidal anti-inflammatory drugs (NSAIDs) may be at heightened risk of gastric and duodenal ulceration.

Altered GI Function. Muscular atrophy, thinning of gastric mucosa, infiltration of the submucosa with elastic fibers, and reduced intestinal blood flow accompany the aging process. Tension or anxiety influence stomach motility and secretory function. Chronic gastritis, irritable colon, heartburn, ulcerlike distress, and nausea can result.

Gastric secretion declines with age. Slowing of gastric emptying follows a reduction in gastric acid secretion; gastric emptying is also negatively affected by stress, lack of ambulation, gastric ulcer, intestinal obstruction, myocardial infarct, and diabetes mellitus.

Some drugs (e.g., antacids, anticholinergics, isoniazid, lithium, narcotic analgesics) delay gastric emptying. A delay in gastric emptying permits gastrotoxic agents a longer residence time, and, therefore, more opportunity to exert their toxic effect.

NSAID-Induced Adverse Effects. As people age, their use of NSAIDs increases, and the adverse effects of these drugs also increase disproportionately. The potential gastrotoxicity of these drugs may be enhanced by their simultaneous administration with other gastrotoxic drugs, coffee, or alcohol. Through inhibition of the protective effects of GI prostaglandins and via local noxious effects, salicylates and other NSAIDs can cause superficial gastric and duodenal erosions and ulcer formation, which could then result in GI bleeding and perforations. All NSAIDs can interfere with platelet function and prolong bleeding time. Elderly patients may be especially susceptible to NSAID-associated peptic ulcer disease.

NSAIDs can exacerbate the severity of renal disease by blocking interrenal cyclo-oxygenase (reduction of renal prostaglandin secretion). This risk is increased in volume-depleted elderly.

Other Potential Drug Therapy Problems

Duplicate Therapy. Many elderly people have serious and multiple diseases that can be aggravated by concurrent therapy. Concomitant illness or certain drugs may contraindicate the use of other drugs. It is important to consider whether an elderly patient is requesting a nonprescription drug to treat an adverse reaction from another medication.

Appropriate Dosing/Dosage Forms. Normal drug doses may be too high in the elderly because of impaired hepatic and renal function. This would necessitate lowering the dose or increasing the dosing interval. Further, elderly patients may experience difficulty with some dosage forms (e.g., swallowing large tablets, using inhalers) because of physical impairment.

Poor Compliance. Poor compliance in the elderly may result from difficulty swallowing or administering the drug. It may also result from an inability to afford the drug.

The Pregnant Patient

Drug therapy during pregnancy may be necessary to treat medical conditions or it may be considered to manage common complaints of pregnancy such as vomiting or constipation. Because most drugs cross the placenta to some extent, a mother who takes a drug might expose her fetus to it. The desire to ease the mother's discomfort must be balanced with concern for the developing fetus.

Potential Problems

Teratogenic Effects. Several factors are important in determining whether a drug taken by a pregnant woman will adversely affect the fetus. Two of the most important are the stage of pregnancy and the ability of the drug to pass from maternal to fetal circulation via the placenta. The first trimester, when organogenesis occurs, is the period of greatest teratogenic susceptibility. Exposure at other periods of gestation may be no less important, however, because the exact critical period depends on the specific drug in question.

Drug therapy problems are also important considerations in the pregnant patient. Although dosage guidelines for some prescription drugs are different for the pregnant patient than for other patients, there is no information on dosage adjustments for nonprescription drugs. Unnecessary drug therapy should be avoided. Use of cigarettes and alcohol should also be limited since they have been associated with increased risk to the fetus.

In the pregnant patient, the primary concern is related to the safety of the drug. All practitioners should be familiar with the A-B-C-D-X system for evaluating the safety of drugs in pregnancy (Table 5). Often the issue is not whether there is a more effective drug available but whether there is a safer drug available. For example, aspirin should be avoided during pregnancy, especially during the last trimester. Acetaminophen, taken in standard therapeutic doses, is the nonprescription drug of choice for antipyresis and analgesia. Naproxen, a NSAID, can be taken early in pregnancy; however, it should not be used late in pregnancy.

Noncompliance. Nausea and vomiting associated with the pregnancy may make it difficult for the pregnant patient to comply with taking oral medications.

Management of the Pregnant Patient

The pharmacist can aid the self-treating pregnant woman in deciding which drug or nondrug treatments she should consider and when self-treatment may be harmful to her or her unborn child.

The pharmacist must be alert to the possibility of pregnancy in any woman of childbearing age who has key symptoms of early pregnancy, such as nausea, vomiting, and frequent urination. Any woman who fits this description should be warned not to take a drug that might be of questionable safety if she is pregnant.

The pharmacist should advise the pregnant patient to avoid using drugs, in general, at any stage of pregnancy unless it is deemed essential by her physician. The pharmacist should also explain that safety and effectiveness of homeopathic and herbal remedies in pregnancy have not been established.

The pharmacist should advise the pregnant patient to increase her reliance on nondrug modalities. For example, the first approach to nausea and vomiting should be to eat small, frequent meals and to avoid foods, smells, or situations that cause vomiting. Next, taking an effervescent glucose or buffered carbohydrate solution may be effective. Only if these

---

TABLE 5   FDA categories for evaluating the safety of drugs during pregnancy

A: Adequate studies in pregnant women have not demonstrated a risk to the fetus in the first trimester of pregnancy, and there is no evidence of risk in later trimesters.

B: Animal studies have not demonstrated a risk to the fetus, but there are no adequate studies in pregnant women . . . or . . . Animal studies have shown an adverse effect, but adequate studies in pregnant women have not demonstrated a risk to the fetus during the first trimester of pregnancy, and there is no evidence of risk in later trimesters.

C: Animal studies have shown an adverse effect on the fetus, but there are no adequate studies in humans; the benefits from the use of the drug in pregnant women may be acceptable despite its potential risks . . . or . . . There are no animal reproduction studies and no adequate studies in humans.

D: There is evidence of human fetal risk, but the potential benefits from the use of the drug in pregnant women may be acceptable despite its potential risks.

X: Studies in animals or humans demonstrate fetal abnormalities, or adverse reaction reports indicate evidence of fetal risk. The risk of use in a pregnant woman clearly outweighs any possible benefit.

measures are ineffective should an antihistamine or antiemetic be considered. Physician consultation may be indicated at this point.

Finally, the pharmacist should refer the patient to a physician for problems that carry increased risk of poor outcomes in pregnancy (e.g., high blood pressure, vaginal bleeding, urinary tract infection, rapid weight gain, edema).

The Nursing Mother

When taken in therapeutic dosages, most nonprescription drugs are not present in breast milk in sufficient amounts to cause significant harm to the infant. However, several drugs are contraindicated for use while breast-feeding, and several others should be used cautiously by nursing mothers. The American Academy of Pediatrics Committee on Drugs published a statement on drugs in human milk. Of the nonprescription drugs included in the statement, aspirin and other salicylates are the only ones that were considered to have had significant effects on some nursing infants and that nursing mothers should take with caution. Nonprescription drugs that are usually considered compatible with breast-feeding include:

- *Analgesics:* acetaminophen, ibuprofen, naproxen, and ketoprofen;
- *Antacids;*
- *Antidiarrheals:* kaolin-pectin and attapulgite;
- *Antihistamines:* brompheniramine, chlorpheniramine, diphenhydramine, and triprolidine;
- *Antisecretory agents:* cimetidine, famotidine, ranitidine, and nizatidine;
- *Cough preparations:* dextromethorphan;
- *Decongestants:* phenylephrine, phenylpropanolamine, and pseudoephedrine;
- *Fluoride;*
- *Laxatives:* bran type, bulk-forming type, docusate, glycerin suppositories, magnesium hydroxide, and senna; and
- *Vitamins.*

There are also many nonprescription drugs for which data on their transfer into breast milk and their possible clinical effects are not available.

When advising a nursing mother, the pharmacist should decide if a drug is really necessary, recommend the safest drug (e.g., acetaminophen instead of aspirin) if one is necessary, and advise the mother to take the medication just after a breast-feeding or just before the infant's lengthy sleep periods.

Chapter 3

In-Home Testing and Monitoring Products

Questions to ask in patient assessment and counseling

Fecal Occult Blood Test Kits

- Have you ever suffered from any bowel disorder? Have you or anyone in your family had colorectal cancer? Have any family members suffered from stomach or colon problems (e.g., ulcers or hemorrhoids)?
- Are you currently experiencing hemorrhoidal or menstrual bleeding?
- What nonprescription or prescription medications are you taking?
- Do you have any visual limitations?

Ovulation Prediction Test Kits

- Do you have any chronic medical conditions?
- Are you consulting or have you consulted a doctor who specializes in fertility problems?
- Are your periods regular?
- Have you ever used a product like this? If so, which one?
- Do you have any visual limitations?

Pregnancy Test Kits

- How late is your period?
- Do you have any chronic medical conditions?
- What nonprescription or prescription medications are you taking?
- Have you ever used a pregnancy test? If so, which one?
- Do you have any visual limitations?

Cholesterol Test Kits

- Do you have any conditions that cause excessive bleeding from a finger prick?
- Do you have any chronic medical conditions?
- What nonprescription or prescription medications are you taking?
- Have you used this product before?

Home Blood Pressure Monitoring Devices

- Do you or any family members have a history of high blood pressure?
- Are you taking any medications to control high blood pressure?
- Have you been instructed on the use of a blood pressure monitor?

Editor's Note: This chapter is adapted from Wendy P. Munroe and Marcus D. Wilson, "In-Home Testing and Monitoring Products," in Covington, T.R., ed., *Handbook of Nonprescription Drugs,* 11th edition, which is based, in part, on a chapter with the same title that appeared in the 10th edition but was written by Susan M. Meyer. Products used in the self-monitoring of asthma and diabetes are presented in chapters 9 and 18, respectively. For a more extensive discussion of this topic, readers are encouraged to consult Chapter 3 of the *Handbook.*

■ *Have you monitored your blood pressure in the past? If so, what type of device did you use?*

■ *Do you have difficulty with your hearing or vision?*

Selection and Use of Home Diagnostic Kits

Home testing and monitoring kits are designed to serve two basic purposes: early disease detection and disease therapy monitoring. To be effective, the kits must be properly used. Pharmacists can play an important role in helping patients select and use the kits appropriately and understand their limitations.

General Principles of Use

Patients should follow these general guidelines for using home test kits:

■ Check the test kit expiration date and follow the manufacturer's instructions for storage.

■ Read the instructions entirely before attempting to perform a test. Note the time of day the test is to be conducted, the length of time required, and any necessary equipment.

■ Follow the instructions exactly and in sequence. Use a timing device that measures seconds.

■ Make sure you are capable of interpreting results. Many test results are based on color changes. If you are color-blind or have any other visual impairment, have a family member or friend help you read the results.

■ It is important that patients understand these products are self-*testing,* not self-*diagnosing.* Positive test results should be reported to a physician immediately for definitive diagnosis and management. Negative test results should be questioned if the patient is experiencing definite symptoms of a suspected condition.

Product Selection Guidelines

In selecting a product, the major variables to consider are the test's complexity, ease of reading results, presence of a control, and cost.

Complexity of the Test Procedure

Since human error plays such an important part in the ultimate value of these products, simplicity of use deserves major consideration. Each step and manipulation required is a potential source of error. Simple tests are generally more desirable.

Ease of Reading Results

In most home test kits, the result is indicated by a change in color. With some products, this color change is easily discernible (e.g., the appearance of a plus sign or a check mark). Other products require that the user recognize subtle variations in shade. The latter results are more open to misinterpretation.

Presence of a Control

When possible, patients should select a test that includes a control to ensure that the test has been performed correctly.

Cost

Many products provide more than one test per kit. When considering cost, patients should determine the cost per test *unit.*

Fecal Occult Blood Kits

Fecal occult blood testing products can be used as an adjunct to invasive tests to detect any gastrointestinal bleeding. They are designed to detect occult blood in feces with a colorimetric assay for hemoglobin. The best-known use of these tests is for colorectal cancer screening.

The reagent is sandwiched between two layers of biodegradable paper and is placed in the toilet bowl following a bowel movement. These kits are based on the premise that a significant amount of fecal blood will remain on the surface of the toilet bowl water after a bowel movement.

Two nonprescription products, ColoCARE and EZ Detect, are available (see product table "Fecal Occult Blood Test Kits" in *Nonprescription Products: Formulations & Features*). The differences between the two are minor. The main advantage of EZ Detect is that it imposes no dietary restrictions because the results are not affected by red meat or vitamin C. With ColoCARE, vitamin C in excess of 250 mg per day may interfere with the peroxidase action of hemoglobin, causing false-negative results. ColoCARE contains three pads for testing three consecutive bowel movements. The EZ Detect kit contains five test pads and a positive control chemical package.

Factors that Affect Results

- Medications that may cause gastritis may also cause sufficient bleeding to produce false-positive results; thus, they should be avoided for at least 2–3 days before and during the test period.
- Aspirin, nonsteroidal anti-inflammatory drugs, steroids, reserpine, and rectally administered medications should be avoided immediately before and during the testing period.
- Patients should be advised to consult their physicians before discontinuing any prescribed medications.
- Toilet-bowl cleaners may produce false-positive results. Before using these tests, patients should flush the toilet twice to remove any chemicals and cleansers from the bowl.
- Patients should avoid consuming raw or rare cooked red meat 2–3 days before and during the test period.
- Vitamin C in excess of 250 mg per day may cause false-negative results with ColoCARE.

Patient Counseling

The pharmacist should stress the following points:

- Follow the package instructions carefully.
- Do not perform the test during times of known bleeding, as when experiencing hemorrhoidal or menstrual bleeding.
- Increase dietary fiber intake for several days before testing. Roughage increases the accuracy of the test by stimulating bleeding from lesions that might not otherwise bleed.
- Perform the test on three consecutive bowel movements. Complete all three tests, even if the first two produce negative results.

The pharmacist should emphasize that a positive test result may indicate any medical condition that causes a loss of blood through the gastrointestinal system (e.g., hemorrhoids, peptic ulcers, colitis, diverticulitis, polyps, esophageal varices). The primary value of these tests is to alert patients and physicians that a thorough workup may be needed. The kits are *not* intended to replace other diagnostic procedures.

Ovulation Prediction and Pregnancy Test Kits

A complete discussion of the female reproductive cycle appears on pages 35–36 of the *Handbook*.

Basal Thermometry

Resting basal body temperature is usually below normal during the first part of the 28-day female reproductive cycle. After ovulation, basal body temperature rises to a level closer to normal.

Women who use this method of ovulation prediction take their temperature (orally, rectally, or vaginally) with a basal thermometer each morning before arising. These temperature measurements are then plotted on a graph. A rise in temperature is a signal that ovulation has occurred. When the increase occurs, women seeking to become pregnant should have intercourse as soon as possible.

Choosing a Test

The only equipment necessary for basal body temperature monitoring is a basal thermometer. Although basal thermometry is a relatively simple method of ovulation prediction, recording and interpreting temperature data can be confusing. Some women may have difficulty reading mercury thermometers accurately. Because the temperature increase that follows ovulation is small ($0.4°–1.0°F$ [$0.2°–0.6°C$]), women who have trouble reading a thermometer may miss the increase altogether.

The Bioself Fertility Indicator uses computer technology to avoid these potential problems and provides a digital temperature reading in just 2 minutes. The device can also store temperature readings in its memory for 120 consecutive days. It may be used to take oral, vaginal, or rectal temperature. A built-in alarm reminds users when to obtain a measurement.

Factors that Affect Results

- Emotions, movements, and infections can influence the basal metabolic temperature.
- Eating, drinking, talking, and smoking should be postponed until after each measurement is obtained.

Patient Counseling

Patients who opt to use basal thermometry as a method of predicting ovulation should be advised of the following:

- Choose one method for temperature measurement (i.e., rectal, oral, or vaginal) and use it consistently.
- Take the temperatures just before arising each morning after at least 5 hours of sleep.
- Try to take the temperature at approximately the same time each day.
- If conception does not occur, refer to the product instructions for further information regarding use of the Bioself Fertility Indicator. The device allows the user to store information that may be shared with a fertility specialist.

Ovulation Prediction Kits

Ovulation prediction kits are marketed to women who are having trouble conceiving and need to pinpoint ovulation. These tests indicate the increase in luteinizing hormone (LH) that appears in the serum approximately 20–48 hours before ovulation. Approximately 8–12 hours after it appears, the LH surge is detectable in the urine.

The LH surge is revealed by a difference in color or color intensity from that noted on the previous day of testing. The intensity of the color is directly proportional to the amount of LH in the urine sample.

Choosing a Test

The kits vary in the complexity of the procedure, the length of time needed to complete the test, and the number of individual tests provided. With the simplest kits, a woman urinates onto a test stick and reads the result in 3 minutes. The more complicated products require a series of precisely timed manipulations involving test tubes and droppers. The more steps that are involved, the greater is the potential for human error.

Factors that Affect Results

■ Medications used to promote ovulation (e.g., menotropins) may cause a false-positive result.

■ Conditions associated with high levels of LH, such as menopause and polycystic ovary syndrome, may cause false-positive results.

■ A false-positive result may be obtained if the user is already pregnant.

If the patient has recently discontinued using oral contraceptives, the start of ovulation may be delayed for one to two cycles. Thus, it would not be appropriate for this individual to use an in-home ovulation prediction test kit until fertilization has been attempted unsuccessfully for several months following discontinuation of the oral contraceptives.

Patient Counseling

The pharmacist should stress the following points about ovulation prediction tests:

■ Follow all package instructions carefully.

■ Begin testing 2–3 days before ovulation is expected. The kit contains directions to help the woman determine when to begin testing.

■ Collect the sample in the morning, if possible. The LH surge usually begins early in the day, and the urine concentration is relatively consistent at this time.

■ Test the sample immediately after collection. If this is not feasible, store the urine under refrigeration for the length of time specified in the directions. The sample must reach room temperature by standing 20–30 minutes before the testing procedure is begun. Do not redisperse any sediment that may be present in the sample.

■ Look for the first significant increase in color intensity, which indicates that the LH surge has occurred and that ovulation will occur within a day or two. Once ovulation occurs, the ovum remains viable for fertilization for 12–24 hours. The optimal days for fertilization are the 2 days before ovulation, the day of ovulation, and the day after ovulation. For the greatest chance of achieving pregnancy, intercourse should take place within the 24 hours after the LH surge.

■ Discontinue testing once the LH surge is detected. Remaining tests can be used later, if necessary.

If the LH surge is not detected, one of the following possibilities may have occurred: (1) the test may not have been performed properly, (2) the woman may not have ovulated, or (3) the test may have been used too late in the cycle. The woman should carefully review the testing procedure and consider testing for a longer period in the next cycle to increase her chances of detecting the LH surge.

It is generally recommended that these products not be used for longer than 3 months. If a woman has not conceived within this time, she should consult her physician.

Home Pregnancy Tests

Home pregnancy tests are designed to detect the presence of human chorionic gonadotrophin (HCG) in the urine. HCG is detectable in the urine within 1–2 weeks after conception and is considered a diagnostic indicator of pregnancy.

If correctly used, these tests have a reported accuracy of more than 95%.

Choosing a Test

The available products vary in the complexity of the testing procedure and the length of time needed to complete the test. With the simplest kits, a woman urinates onto a test stick and can read the result in 3 minutes. The more steps involved, the greater the potential for human error.

Factors that Affect Results

- False-negative results may occur if these tests are performed too soon after conception.
- False-negative results may occur if the urine sample was refrigerated and not allowed to return to room temperature.

Patient Counseling

The pharmacist should advise patients to pay special attention to the following points:

- Follow the package instructions carefully.
- Wait after menses is due before performing the test. Performing the test too early may produce false-negative results. Most tests may be used as early as the day of a missed menstrual period.
- Collect a sample from the first morning urine. The levels of HCG, if present, will be concentrated at that time. Some tests allow the use of a sample collected at any time, as long as the woman restricts her fluid intake 4–6 hours prior to urine collection.
- Use the urine collection device provided in the kit.
- Test the urine sample immediately after collection. If this is not possible, store the urine in the refrigerator and allow it to reach room temperature before testing. Do not redisperse any sediment that may be present in the sample.

If the test result is positive, the woman should assume she is pregnant and see her family physician or an obstetrician as soon as possible. If the test result is negative, the woman should review the procedure and make sure she performed the test correctly. If she did not wait the number of days recommended by the manufacturer, she should wait the prescribed time and test again if menses has not begun. If the results of the second test are negative and menses still has not begun, she should seek the advice of a physician.

Home Cholesterol Test Kit

The Advanced Care Cholesterol Test is the only marketed nonprescription test kit that enables patients to measure their total blood cholesterol at home. The test kit includes one test cassette, a single-use lancet, one gauze pad, one adhesive bandage, an instruction booklet, a question-and-answer booklet, and a chart for interpreting the test results. Appropriately used, the test is 97% accurate, a standard that is comparable to laboratory results.

The test device is a palm-sized, single-use, noninstrumented, plastic cassette that is read like a thermometer. Cholesterol from a blood sample obtained through a finger prick is converted into hydrogen peroxide through two chemical reactions involving cholesterol esterase and cholesterol oxidase. The peroxide reacts with horseradish peroxidase and a dye to produce the color that rises along the test's measurement scale. Two separate indicator spots change color to show that the test is functioning properly. One spot also indicates that the test has been completed and it is time to read the scale. Table 1 summarizes test instructions.

Factors that Affect Results

- Good finger-pricking technique is necessary.
- Two or three hanging drops of blood are needed; excessive squeezing of the finger will affect the quality of the blood sample.
- If sufficient blood cannot be obtained from the first finger prick, a second finger should be used.
- A low cholesterol value may result if the blood sample is too small or if it takes longer than 5 minutes to collect the necessary amount of blood.
- Doses of 500 mg or more of vitamin C or standard doses (i.e., 325–1000 mg) of acetaminophen should be avoided for 4 hours before the test.
- Patients with hemophilia or individuals who take anticoagulants should not take this test.

Patient Counseling

The pharmacist should advise patients to pay special attention to the following points:

- Follow all package instructions carefully.
- Keep the cassettes at room temperature.
- Dispose of used cassettes, which are considered potentially biohazardous, appropriately.
- Any consumer who obtains a result of 200 mg/dL or greater should see a physician for a repeat measurement, lipid profile, and medical workup.

TABLE 1 Instructions for Advanced Care Cholesterol Test

- Wash hands carefully.
- Lance the fingertip.
- Wipe away the first sign of blood with a gauze pad.
- Gently squeeze the fingertip to obtain a large, hanging drop of blood.
- Touch the drop to the bottom of the sample well of the test cassette.
- Add more drops until the black fill line is covered.
- After 2–4 minutes, pull the clear plastic tab on the right side of the cassette until it clicks into place and a red line appears.
- After 10–12 minutes, when the "END" indicators turns green, measure the height of the purple column against the scale printed on the cassette.
- Interpret this number using the paper result chart included in the kit.

Home Blood Pressure Monitoring Devices

How Blood Pressure Monitoring Devices Work

There are two types of indirect measurement of blood pressure: auscultatory (measurement of sound) and oscillometric (measurement of vibration). Currently, there are three categories of monitors for home use: mercury column, aneroid, and digital. The detection device, which is usually indicated on the cuff with a tab or other marking, is placed directly over the brachial artery. The brachial artery can be found by palpating 1–2 inches above and just to the inside of the antecubital space. As cuff pressure increases, the brachial artery is compressed and blood flow is obstructed. As cuff pressure is gradually released, blood flow is reestablished and Korotkoff's sounds can be heard in different phases. Phase I, which corresponds to systolic pressure, can be identified when at least two consecutive "beats" are heard as cuff pressure is decreased. The nature of the sounds changes over the next three phases. Diastolic pressure is identified as phase V, the disappearance of sound.

Using the appropriate size cuff is essential for accurate measurement of blood pressure (Table 2). For wrist cuffs, instructions on cuff placement should be followed closely: careful attention must be paid to the level of the wrist in relation to the heart. Because these devices are also highly sensitive to changes in wrist level, it is best to support the arm on a table with a pillow to raise the wrist to the appropriate level. Many clinicians feel that the finger cuffs currently on the market lack sufficient accuracy and reliability to warrant their routine use.

Choosing a Device

The choice of device is based on individual characteristics such as the patient's ability and willingness to learn, physical handicaps, economic status, and preference.

Mercury Column Devices

The reference standard in blood pressure measurement remains the mercury column blood pressure (BP) meter. These devices typically come with a cuff and an inflation bulb. The tubing from the cuff is attached to a column of mercury encased in a glass gauge. The stethoscope is usually sold separately.

TABLE 2 Arm circumferences for determining appropriate cuff size

Arm circumference (adult)[a]	Cuff size
<31 cm	Regular adult cuff
31–40 cm	Large adult cuff
>40 cm	Thigh cuff[b]

[a]Arm circumference should be calculated by measuring around the midpoint of the upper arm. Remeasure the patient's arm periodically, especially if he or she has recently gained or lost significant weight.

[b]For those patients needing a thigh cuff, a wrist monitor should be considered.

Source:
Soghikian K, Casper S, Fireman B, et al. Home blood pressure monitoring. Effect on use of medical services and medical care costs. *Med Care.* 1992; 30: 855–5.

Egmond J, Lenders J, Weernick E, et al. Accuracy and reproducibility of 30 devices for self-measurement of arterial blood pressure. *Am J Hypertens.* 1993; 6: 873–9.

Although mercury BP meters are the most accurate and reliable of the devices, their routine use for home measurement is discouraged because they are cumbersome and pose the risk of mercury toxicity should the glass tubing break.

Aneroid Devices

Next to the mercury column BP meters, the aneroid devices are the most accurate and reliable monitors. They are light, portable, and affordable, and they pose no risk from mercury toxicity. They also include several features that make patient teaching much easier. First, many devices now come with a stethoscope attached to the cuff; this keeps the patient from having to hold the bell of the stethoscope in place. Second, a D-ring on the cuff allows a single user to place the cuff on the arm easily. A few manufacturers offer a gauge that is attached to the inflation bulb; again, this makes it easier to manipulate the equipment since there are fewer pieces to control.

The device includes a gauge that indicates the need for recalibration. While these monitors are considered the option of choice for home use, they require careful patient instruction and follow-up. Good eyesight and hearing are necessary. For patients with reduced visual capacity, there are gauges available with large print on the face of the gauge.

Digital Devices

Digital devices include semiautomatic (manually inflating), fully automatic (auto-inflating), wrist, and finger blood pressure monitors. Such features as printouts, a pulse monitor, a digital clock, automated inflation and deflation, memory, a large display, a D-ring for the cuff, and a preformed cuff differentiate many of the devices. These features add significantly to the price.

A major drawback to the digital monitors is that the user cannot determine if the device is out of calibration. In addition, many devices on the market lack extensive accuracy and reliability data and are often found to be inadequate for routine use. For these reasons, many clinicians recommend the aneroid devices.

Factors that Affect Results

■ Blood pressure ranges are based on readings taken from patients in a resting state. Any deviation from this may produce artificial results.

■ Proper cuff size is essential (Table 2). For example, using a cuff that is too small can overestimate the patient's blood pressure by 20–30 mm Hg.

■ Holding the arm higher or lower than heart level while the blood pressure is being measured can significantly alter readings.

Patient Counseling

Specific instructions that should be given to each patient are as follows:

■ Avoid smoking and do not drink caffeine-containing beverages for at least 30 minutes before measuring your blood pressure.

■ Wait 10–15 minutes after a bath and 30 minutes after eating before measuring your blood pressure.

■ Take time to relax before measuring your blood pressure; if you feel pressured, results may be elevated.

■ Make sure the room is at a comfortable temperature.

- Sit in a comfortable chair, with your back supported and feet straight ahead and flat on the floor.
- Place your arm on a table.
- Remove restrictive clothing from the arm.
- Place the cuff on the arm. The cuff should be snug but not tight enough to restrict blood flow.
- Rest for at least 5 minutes in this position.
- Measure the blood pressure.
- Record the results. Include the time and date of the measurement.
- Do not self-adjust blood pressure medications on the basis of home measurements unless your physician has specifically instructed you to do so.

CHAPTER 4

Internal Analgesic and Antipyretic Products

Questions to ask in patient assessment and counseling

Pain Characteristics

- *Where is the pain? Is it in one place, or does it spread to other parts of the body?*
- *On a scale of zero to 10, with zero being no pain and 10 being pain as bad as you can imagine, what is your level of pain now?*
- *What words best describe your pain (e.g., sharp, dull, aching, burning, electrical, stabbing)? Is it constant, or does it come and go? Did it develop suddenly or gradually?*
- *How long have you had this pain? Has it changed or remained constant?*
- *Have you ever had pain like this before? If so, what caused it? What helped it?*
- *Is any part of your body red and swollen? Have you recently been injured?*
- *Does the pain occur at any particular time of the day? What makes it worse or better? Is it relieved by changing your body position?*
- *Do you have any other symptoms (e.g., visual disturbances, numbness, weakness, a tingling sensation, dizziness, unusual drowsiness, nausea, vomiting, fever, mental confusion, unusual sensitivity to light or sounds)?*

Drug Therapy for Pain

- *Have you had this pain before? If so, what medications did you take to relieve it?*
- *Have you already taken any medications for the pain? What are they? How much did you take? For how long? How effective were they?*
- *Do aspirin or other pain relievers upset your stomach?*
- *Have you ever had an allergic reaction to aspirin or any other medication for pain, swelling, or fever?*
- *Have you ever had an allergic reaction to foods, dyes, or food additives?*
- *Have you ever had hives or a recurrent skin rash?*
- *Have you ever had an ulcer or stomach problem?*
- *Have you ever had asthma, nasal polyps, or a breathing problem?*
- *Do you now have or have you ever had asthma, allergies, ulcers, gout, high blood pressure, heart failure, kidney disease, or a blood-clotting disorder?*
- *Are you taking medication for gout, arthritis, asthma, high blood pressure, or diabetes?*
- *Are you taking any drug that may thin your blood? Have you taken any such drug within the last week?*
- *What other prescription or nonprescription drugs are you now taking?*

Editor's Note: This chapter is adapted from Arthur G. Lipman, "Internal Analgesics and Antipyretic Products," in Covington, T.R., ed., *Handbook of Nonprescription Drugs*, 11th edition, which is based, in part, on the 10th edition chapters "Internal Analgesic Products," written by W. Kent Van Tyle and "Antipyretic Drug Products," written by Thomas E. Lackner. For a more extensive discussion of this topic, readers are encouraged to consult Chapter 4 of the *Handbook*.

- *(If the patient is under 15 years of age) Has your child had recent symptoms of influenza or chickenpox?*

- *(If the patient is a woman of child-bearing age) Are you pregnant? Are you breast-feeding? If you are pregnant, do you plan to breast-feed?*

Fever

- *How long have you had this fever? (If the patient is a child) How long has your child had a fever?*

- *How high is your [your child's] fever?*

- *How did you measure the temperature (i.e., by the oral, armpit, rectal, or ear canal method)?*

- *Do you [Does your child] have any other symptoms?*

- *What medication or other treatment have you used to treat the fever?*

- *Have you ever had a convulsion, seizure, or brain disorder?*

Patients come to pharmacies for analgesics more often than they do for any other type of nonprescription medication. Fever is among the most common symptoms for which parents seek nonprescription drugs to treat their children.

Pain

Definition, Classification, and Management

The International Association for the Study of Pain describes pain as an unpleasant sensory and emotional experience associated with actual or potential tissue damage or described in terms of such damage. This definition recognizes that pain can have physical, affective, and learned components; it is not necessarily a result of physical injury.

The Integrated Approach to the Management of Pain, the 1986 report of the National Institutes of Health, concluded that pain should be considered as three distinct entities: acute pain, chronic pain associated with malignant disease, and chronic pain not associated with malignant disease.

Types of Pain

Table 1 outlines the characteristics of the three types of pain. Because each type of pain is managed differently, the pharmacist must determine the type of pain involved before deciding to recommend therapy or refer the patient for further evaluation.

Acute Pain.   Acute pain is what most people think of when they describe pain. Acute pain is an immediate reaction to noxious stimuli such as mechanical (e.g., fracture, muscle sprain) or thermal injury. Analgesics often prevent acute pain from worsening.

Chronic Malignant Pain.   Chronic pain associated with malignant disease includes the pain of cancer or any advanced, progressive disorder. Examples of such disorders are multiple sclerosis, amyotrophic lateral sclerosis (Lou Gehrig's disease), acquired immunodeficiency syndrome (AIDS), end-stage renal or hepatic failure with pain, and painful end-stage respiratory disease. The principles of managing chronic malignant pain are also appropriate for diseases causing intermittent pain (e.g., sickle-cell disease).

Chronic Nonmalignant Pain.   Chronic pain not associated with malignant disease is the most complex, most misunderstood, and least well managed of the three categories of

TABLE 1 Categories of pain

	Acute	Chronic pain of nonmalignant origin	Chronic pain of malignant origin
Duration	Hours to days	Months to years	Unpredictable
Associated pathology	Present	Often none	Usually present
Prognosis	Predictable	Unpredictable	Increasing pain with possibility of disfigurement and fear of dying
Associated problems	Uncommon	Depression, anxiety, secondary gain issues	Many, especially fear of loss of control
Nerve conduction	Rapid	Slow	Slow
Autonomic nervous system involvement	Present	Generally absent	Present or absent
Biological value	High	Low or absent	Low
Social effects	Minimal	Profound	Variable— usually marked
Treatment	Primarily analgesics	Multimodal: often largely behavioral, drugs usually play a minor role	Multimodal: drugs usually play a major role

pain. This type of pain is related to a progressive, debilitating process. Nonprescription analgesics may be useful adjuncts for some chronic nonmalignant pain, but they drugs are of limited value in most such syndromes.

Pain Management
Acute pain and chronic malignant pain are often indications for aggressive drug therapy. These types of pain are often undertreated, leading to unnecessary suffering. Whenever pain is due to tissue damage, it is preferable for patients to take analgesic medications on a regular schedule to help prevent the recurrence.

Conversely, chronic nonmalignant pain is often inappropriately treated with analgesic and other central nervous system (CNS) depressant drugs that are not effective as primary treatment modalities. This can produce adverse effects, dependence, psychologic complications, and worsening pain. Rehabilitation and behavioral treatments are the principal treatment modalities for these types of pain.

Nonprescription or prescription medications should not be used in lieu of referral of these patients for evaluation by a pain treatment team. Such teams increasingly include pharmacists.

Selected Pain-Associated Conditions Responsive to Nonprescription Analgesics

Headache

Headaches are the most common pain complaint. There are several types of headaches (Table 2).

Other Types of Headaches. Mixed vascular-muscle contraction headaches may also occur. One type usually causes the other. Treatment of the underlying type of headache often suffices. Other headaches amenable to nonprescription drug treatment may be caused by fever or "hangover." The latter respond to acetaminophen or nonsteroidal anti-inflammatory drugs (NSAIDs); however, the condition does not fully resolve for several hours. Nonprescription stimulants such as caffeine may provide some relief in headaches related to fatigue. Headaches can be caused by eye strain or infection; they may also be a manifestation of anxiety or depression. Nonprescription medications are usually not effective in treating these types of headaches.

Myalgia

Diffuse muscle pain tends to be dull, constant, and aching. It can result from systemic infections, strenuous exercise, tension, or poor posture and body mechanics. Diffuse muscle soreness and aching may be the initial symptom of rheumatoid arthritis (RA).

Muscle pain usually responds well to nonprescription analgesics and adjunctive treatment with heat or massage. Analgesics should be started soon after the injury and taken on a regular schedule and in sufficient doses. Remobilization of the affected area soon after the injury is essential. If muscle pain becomes chronic, the painful area may require application of ice or vapo-coolant sprays, or injections of local anesthetics to facilitate remobilization with physical therapy.

Periarticular Pain

Injury or inflammation of the tissues surrounding a joint can cause pain. The pain can be elicited by maneuvers that stress the structure but not the associated joint. Periarticular pain tends to be nocturnal and often involves the shoulder, elbow, or knee. It responds well to nonprescription analgesics and limitation of motion in the affected joint.

Arthralgia

Joint pain often involves inflammation of the synovial membrane (synovitis). Cartilage loss with associated synovitis can be the result of mechanical stress and wear or of erosive processes.

Degenerative Joint Disease. The primary complaint of persons with degenerative joint disease (DJD) is joint stiffness and aching in weight-bearing joints. Joint stiffness lasts only a few minutes following initiation of joint motion. Earlier stages of DJD respond well to nonprescription analgesics. Acetaminophen is an analgesic of choice. For acute flares when inflammation exacerbates the problem, NSAIDs and local heat are often beneficial. Progressive disease, especially of weight-bearing joints, requires orthopedic management.

Rheumatoid Arthritis. Rheumatoid arthritis (RA) may begin with a prodrome of fatigue, weakness, joint stiffness, arthralgia, and myalgia. Multiple joints of the hands, wrists, and feet show symmetrical involvement. Involved joints become warm, red, and swollen, and range of motion is limited. RA is a progressive disease. Duration of morning stiffness can be used to assess severity. Managing RA normally requires more than nonprescription analgesics, although NSAIDs are a mainstay of therapy. RA is best managed with a

TABLE 2 Comparison of selected types of headaches

	Muscle contraction (tension) headache	Vascular/Migraine	Sinus headache
Presentation/ Symptomatology	Bilateral, diffuse pain often over the top of the head and extending to the rear and base of the skull.	Recurrent, hemicranial, throbbing headache. Nausea, vomiting, photophobia, phono-phobia, lightheadedness, and vertigo are common. **Classic** migraines begin with an aura (neurologic symptoms such as one-sided weakness, difficulty speaking, or flashing lights or blind spots in the visual field). **Common** migraines begin immediately with throbbing pain.	Usually localized to the periorbital area or forehead. Pain tends to occur upon wakening and may subside grad-ually after the patient has been upright for awhile. Stooping or blowing the nose often intensifies the pain.
Possible causes	Can result from tight muscles in the upper back, neck, or scalp, or from myofacial "trigger points" in the muscles of the cervical area, occiput, or scalp.	Possibly due to distention or dilation of intracranial arteries or traction or displacement of large intracranial veins or their meningeal cover-ings. Women experience migraines up to five times more than men: these headaches may be associated with certain phases of the menstrual cycle.	Occurs when infection or blockage of the paranasal sinuses causes inflamma-tion or distention of the sinus walls.
Duration	Up to several days	Aura: up to 30 minutes Other symptoms: several days	Several days or more. Persistent sinus pain or discharge sug-gests possible bacterial infection and requires referral for medical evaluation.
Onset	Gradual	Acute	Gradual
Management	**Acute:** responds well to nonprescription analgesics. **Chronic:** often requires physical therapy and relaxation exercises.	NSAIDs or acetamino-phen can effectively control pain in some patients if dosed appropriately and taken soon enough after onset of symptoms.	Nonprescription analgesics and decongestants are often useful in facilitating drainage of the sinuses and relieving pain.

multimodal approach that includes education, physical therapy, nutritional counseling, and medications. Pharmacists should ensure that patients receive referral for appropriate care.

Assessment of Pain

Assessment should include inquiry about the etiology, duration, location, and severity of pain as well as factors that relieve and exacerbate it. Nonprescription analgesics are often appropriate for managing acute pain if it is not too severe and the complaints are not suggestive of a serious underlying disorder. Patients with pain that has lasted longer than is expected from the underlying cause or with pain of more than 2 weeks' duration should usually be referred for medical evaluation.

Asking whether the pain is mild, moderate, or severe often leads to inconsistent reports. Simple, validated rating scales should be used. The two most common methods are the verbal numerical rating scale and the visual analog scale (VAS). When using the VAS, the pharmacist should ask the patient to rank his or her present pain on a scale of zero to 10, with zero being no pain and 10 being the most severe pain imaginable. The VAS allows the pharmacist to note the patient's pain by making a mark at the appropriate place on a 10-cm line. To quantify the pain, the pharmacist measures the line with a metric ruler and records the pain level on a scale of 1 to 10 (Figure 1). Other scales are available for pain rating in children, adolescents, non-English speakers, and other special populations.

Fever

Fever is defined as a body temperature that is higher than the normal core temperature of 98.6°F (37°C). Patients' ability to perceive fever varies. Fever may sometimes be ignored because of more unpleasant concomitant symptoms.

In the course of a single day, body temperature can vary by as much as 1.8°F (1°C) in adults and as much as 2.5°F (1.4°C) in children. Normal temperature values are shown in Table 3.

Most fevers are self-limited and nonthreatening; however, fever can cause a great deal of discomfort and, in some cases, may indicate serious underlying pathology (e.g., an acute, infectious process) for which prompt medical evaluation is indicated. The principal reason for treating fever is to alleviate discomfort. Treatment should target the underlying cause whenever possible. Serious complications of fever are uncommon, and overly aggressive fever management may be more dangerous than the fever itself.

Etiology of Fever

Fever is usually caused by a microbiological agent, often a virus for which specific anti-infective therapy is not available. Fever may also be induced by certain drugs or physiologic processes, or be of unknown origin.

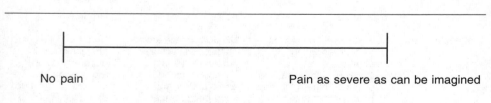

No pain   Pain as severe as can be imagined

FIGURE 1 Example of a visual analog scale.

TABLE 3   Normal body temperatures

Method	Normal temperature
Rectal temperature	101.8°F (38.8°C)
Oral temperature	100° F (37.8°C)
Axillary (armpit) temperature	99°F (37.2°C)

Microbe-Induced Fever

Most febrile episodes are due to infection by exogenous pyrogens, including viruses, bacteria, fungi, yeasts, and protozoa. Fever from exogenous pyrogens is often less marked in elderly patients than in younger individuals. Consequently, infection may not be easily recognized in older patients if fever is the primary assessment criterion.

Pathology-Induced Fever

Noninfectious pathologic causes of fever include malignancies, tissue damage (e.g., myocardial infarct [MI], surgery), metabolic disorders (e.g., hyperthyroidism, gout), antigen-antibody reactions, and dehydration.

TABLE 4   Selected agents responsible for episodes of drug-induced fever

Cardiovascular
Methyldopa
Quinidine
Procainamide
Hydralazine
Nifedipine

Antimicrobial
Penicillin G
Ampicillin
Methicillin
Cloxacillin
Cephalothin
Cephapirin
Cefamandole
Tetracycline
Lincomycin
Sulfonamide
Sulfamethoxazole–
  trimethoprim
Streptomycin[a]
Vancomycin
Colistin

Isoniazid
Para-aminosalicylic acid
Nitrofurantoin
Mebendazole

Antineoplastic
Bleomycin
Daunorubicin
Procarbazine
Cytarabine
Streptozocin
6-Mercaptopurine
L-Asparaginase
Chlorambucil
Hydroxyurea

Central nervous system
Phenytoin
Carbamazepine
Chlorpromazine
Nomifensine
Haloperidol
Triamterene

Benztropine[a]
Thioridazine
Trifluoperazine[a]
Amphetamine

Anti-inflammatory
Ibuprofen
Tolmetin
Aspirin

Other
Iodide
Cimetidine
Levamisole
Metroclopramide
Clofibrate
Allopurinol
Folate
Prostaglandin E_2
Ritodrine
Interferon
Propylthiouracil

[a]Fever seen during drug overdose.

Adapted with permission from Mackowiak PA, LeMaistre CF. *Ann Intern Med.* 1987; 106: 729.

Drug-Induced Fever

Many drugs may induce fever (Table 4). Failure to discontinue the offending agent can result in substantial morbidity and even mortality. Drug-induced fever often goes unrecognized because consistent signs and symptoms are lacking.

Drug-induced fever is distinguished by

■ Fever during or shortly after treatment with a drug previously reported to cause fever or other allergic symptoms;

■ Fever accompanied by other manifestations of allergy; and

■ Temperature elevation despite patient improvement.

Diurnal temperature variations are often minimal in patients with drug-induced fever.

Management involves discontinuation of the suspected drug whenever possible. If feasible, all medications should be temporarily discontinued. If the fever is drug induced, the patient's temperature will generally decrease within 24–48 hours. Each medication may then be restarted, one at a time, while monitoring for fever recurrence. If an implicated drug cannot be discontinued, systemic corticosteroids may be given to suppress fever and minimize other allergic symptoms.

Fever in persons taking neuroleptic medications (e.g., phenothiazines, butyrophenones, thioxanthenes) could be secondary to neuroleptic malignant syndrome, a potentially life-threatening condition. When this syndrome is suspected, the neuroleptic medication should be discontinued and a physician contacted immediately.

Complications of Fever

Serious complications of fever are rare. Harmful effects (e.g., dehydration, delirium, seizures, coma, irreversible neurologic or muscle damage) are most likely to occur at temperatures above 106°F (41.1°C). However, even lower body temperature elevations may be life-threatening in patients with certain conditions and in pediatric patients.

Febrile seizures are seizures associated with fever in the absence of another cause. Most initial febrile seizures occur in children under 3 years of age. Seizures occurring after that age are usually unrelated to fever. Simple febrile seizures generally last no longer than 15 minutes, have no features characteristic of focal origin, and do not recur during a single febrile episode. Complex febrile seizures in children are repetitive during the course of a single febrile episode, generally last longer than 15 minutes, and exhibit signs characteristic of a focal origin. Although both the magnitude and rate of temperature increase appear to be critical determinants in precipitating febrile seizures, the temperature at which a particular child will seize is unpredictable.

Antipyretics rarely will prevent febrile seizures in children predisposed to them. For such therapy, valproate or diazepam is now considered the drug of choice.

Status epilepticus, which is characterized by recurrent or repetitive seizures without intervening periods of normal consciousness, occurs in 1%–2% of children who experience a febrile seizure. It can result in permanent brain damage, renal failure, cardiorespiratory arrest, and death. Any person experiencing such seizures requires immediate medical attention.

Measurement of Body Temperature

Body temperature may be measured at rectal, axillary, oral, or tympanic (ear canal) sites. The rectal method is more consistently accurate than other readings. During the course of an illness, the same thermometer should be used because the readings from different thermometers may vary. Regardless of the site or method used, thorough hand washing should precede and follow all temperature measurements.

Types of Thermometers

Mercury-in-glass and electronic thermometers are commonly used for temperature measurement. Both are accurate when used as directed. The advantages of mercury-in-glass thermometers over electronic thermometers are patient familiarity, low cost, light weight, and compact size. However, mercury-in-glass thermometers can break, rendering them useless and potentially dangerous.

Glass thermometers intended for oral use have a long, thin bulb. In contrast, the bulb of the rectal thermometer is short and thick, permitting insertion in the rectum with little risk of breakage. Although a rectal thermometer can be used for oral temperature measurement, an oral thermometer should never be inserted into the rectum because oral thermometers may break and injure rectal tissue. The same thermometer should never be used both rectally and orally because effective disinfection is difficult. Glass thermometers should be stored in a cool location and out of direct sunlight.

Electronic thermometers are available for oral, rectal, and axillary temperature measurement. These instruments may require about 30 seconds for equilibration. They register quickly. Disposable covers eliminate the need for disinfection following use. The digital display makes these thermometers easier to read than glass thermometers. Electronic thermometers can be used for children as young as 3 years of age.

Body temperature can be determined by tympanic membrane blood temperature measurement with the electronic thermometer. The tip of the instrument, placed in the ear canal, measures body temperature by sensing infrared radiation from the blood vessels in the eardrum. Instructions on inserting the thermometer should be followed carefully. The measurement takes only 1 second, is simple and accurate, and can be performed even on a sleeping child.

Technique for Temperature Measurement

Oral Measurement. How to Use a Mercury-in-Glass Thermometer to Measure Oral Temperature

- Inspect the thermometer for cracks or imperfections.
- Disinfect the thermometer by drawing it through a swab moistened with an antiseptic such as alcohol or a povidone-iodine solution.
- Rinse the thermometer with cool water. Hot water will make the mercury rise and give a falsely high reading.
- Rotate the thermometer slightly below eye level to confirm that the displayed temperature is below 96°F (35.6°C).
- If the temperature level is not below 96°F, shake the thermometer in a rapid, downward, snapping motion until the mercury column falls below this level. Pharmacists should demonstrate the correct shaking method when counseling patients about glass thermometers.
- Place the thermometer under the tongue, positioned slightly to one side of the mouth. Leave in place for 3–4 minutes.
- Have the patient close the lips around the thermometer to hold it in place and prevent air from flowing over it.
- Remove the thermometer from the mouth. Remove saliva from the thermometer by wiping from the stem toward the bulb.
- Hold the thermometer at or slightly below eye level. Read and record the temperature.
- Shake the mercury column down to below 96°F as previously described.

How to Use an Electronic Thermometer to Measure Oral Temperature

- Remove the probe from the thermometer base in which it is stored.
- Verify the temperature set-point.
- Insert the thermometer probe into a probe sheath.
- Place the thermometer probe sheath under the tongue, positioned slightly to one side of the mouth.
- Remove the thermometer from the mouth after the electronic display indicates that the temperature has been measured.
- Discard the contaminated sheath.
- Read and record the temperature display.
- Return the probe to the thermometer base.

To ensure reliable measurement, the patient should neither engage in vigorous physical activity nor heat or cool the oral cavity artificially by smoking or by drinking hot or cold beverages for at least 5 minutes (preferably 20 minutes) before temperature is measured. Oral temperature should not be taken when an individual is mouth breathing or hyperventilating, has recently had oral surgery, is not fully alert, or is uncooperative, lethargic, or confused. Oral thermometers are not appropriate for use in most children under 3 years because young children usually find it difficult to maintain a tight seal around the oral thermometer.

Rectal Measurement. If rectal temperature is measured in an adult, the patient should lie on one side with the legs flexed to about a 45-degree angle from the abdomen, and the bulb should be inserted ½–2 inches into the rectum. This is done by holding the thermometer ½–2 inches from the bulb and inserting it until the finger touches the anus. To facilitate passage of the thermometer through the anal sphincter, the patient should be told to take a deep breath; this helps to divert the patient's attention. If the patient has hemorrhoids, insertion of a thermometer into the rectum should be particularly gentle.

How to Use a Mercury-in-Glass Rectal Thermometer in a Child

- Disinfect and calibrate the rectal (security bulb) thermometer in the same manner as an oral glass thermometer.
- Lubricate the thermometer with a water-soluble lubricant.
- Place the infant or child face down on the lap.
- Separate the buttocks with the thumb and forefinger of one hand. Insert the thermometer gently in a direction pointing toward the child's umbilicus with the other hand.
- Insert the thermometer to the length of the bulb in infants and approximately 1 inch in young children.
- Hold the thermometer in place (in a straight line along its angle of insertion) for at least 3 minutes.
- Remove the thermometer. Clean it by wiping from the stem toward the bulb.
- Hold the thermometer at or slightly below eye level. Read and record the temperature.
- Disinfect the thermometer in the manner described for the oral thermometer.
- Remove any remaining lubricant from the anus.

Risks associated with taking rectal temperature include injury from broken glass, retention of the thermometer, rectal or intestinal perforation, and peritonitis. The patient should never be left unattended while the rectal thermometer remains in place because a positional change may cause the thermometer to be expelled or broken. Rectal temperature measurement is relatively contraindicated in patients who are neutropenic, have had recent rectal surgery or injury, or have rectal pathology (e.g. obstructive hemorrhoids), as well as in newborns who are more susceptible to mucosal perforation.

Axillary Measurement. Axillary temperature measurement is recommended for adults who are not candidates for oral or rectal temperature measurement (e.g., somnolent individuals recovering from rectal surgery or persons with severe diarrhea). Axillary temperature measurement may also be preferred in children 3 months to 5 years of age because intrusive rectal procedures can be very frightening to preschool children, children with diarrhea, or infants with severe diaper rash. Rectal temperature measurement is preferred for infants under 3 months of age.

Most oral thermometers can also be used to measure axillary temperature. This is accomplished by placing the thermometer in the armpit and holding the arm pressed against the body for at least 10 minutes or as long as the thermometer instructions indicate.

How to Measure Temperature via the Ear Canal

- Set the thermometer to display a tympanic temperature equivalent if the thermometer has this capability.
- Place a clean lens cover over the insertion end of the thermometer.
- Wait until the digital instruction panel indicates that the instrument is ready for use.
- Place the thermometer into the ear canal. Point the lens toward the patient's eye.
- Press the button for the amount of time indicated in the instructions (usually 1 second).
- Remove the thermometer from the ear.
- Read the display panel immediately and record the reading.
- Discard the disposable lens cover.

This technique varies somewhat for infants and older patients. The instrument provides an error message if measurement is not correctly performed.

Treatment of Fever

The argument that fever is an adaptive response and that elevated body temperature may be beneficial is often overstated. Given this fact, patient discomfort associated with fever alone may be an indication for antipyretic therapy. Arguments against such treatment include:

- The generally benign and self-limited course of fever;
- The possible elimination of a diagnostic or prognostic sign;
- The attenuation of enhanced host defenses (i.e., possible therapeutic effect of fever); and
- The untoward effects of antipyretic drugs.

There is no correlation between the magnitude or pattern of temperature elevation (e.g., persistent, intermittent, recurrent, or prolonged) and the underlying etiology or severity of the disease.

Treatment of fever with oral antipyretic agents is indicated if the oral temperature in an adult exceeds 102°F (38.9°C). When a lower temperature and its associated discomfort are present, nonpharmacologic or pharmacologic intervention may be used. All nonprescription antipyretic agents are also analgesics, and the discomfort associated with a fever of less than 102°F may be the primary indication for any of the nonprescription analgesic/antipyretic medications (i.e., acetaminophen, aspirin, ibuprofen, naproxen sodium, ketoprofen).

Because infants younger than 3 months are at greater risk of serious outcomes from fever than are older children, they should be evaluated by a physician when their temperature rises above 100°F. For infants older than 3 months, a rectal temperature that is above 104°F is cause for contacting a physician immediately and withholding antipyretic medication pending the physician's directive.

A physician should be contacted at the first sign of fever in a child predisposed to seizures. In such individuals, antipyretic medication should be administered every 4 hours with one dose given during the night, and therapy should be continued for at least 24 hours.

If a fever-induced seizure occurs, sponging with lukewarm water should be initiated and the physician notified immediately. Nonpharmacologic treatment should consist of providing light clothing, removing blankets, maintaining room temperature at 78°F (25.6°C), and supplying sufficient fluid intake to replenish insensible losses.

If the body temperature exceeds 104°F (40°C), body sponging with tepid water can be started to facilitate heat dissipation. Body sponging is not routinely recommended for children with a temperature under 104°F because this procedure is usually uncomfortable and often causes the child to shiver, which could raise the temperature even higher. Ice-water baths or spongings with hydroalcoholic solutions (e.g., isopropyl or ethyl alcohol) are not recommended.

Fluid intake in febrile children should be increased by at least 1 oz of fluids per hour (e.g., soft drinks, fruit juice, water, or other fluids), unless oral fluids are contraindicated.

Nonprescription Analgesic/Antipyretic Agents

The nonprescription analgesic/antipyretic agents available in the United States are the salicylates (i.e., aspirin, choline salicylate, magnesium salicylate, and sodium salicylate), acetaminophen, ibuprofen, naproxen sodium, and ketoprofen.

The selection of an analgesic/antipyretic medication should be based on the agent's clinical effectiveness, the incidence and severity of adverse effects associated with its use, its absolute and relative contraindications, the convenience of its administration, and the cost of therapy. Under most circumstances, these drugs are equally effective and have similar times to onset of effect and similar times to peak antipyretic activity. Their antipyretic durations of action are also similar, but naproxen sodium may have a slightly longer analgesic duration. Because of the causal relationship between salicylates and Reye's syndrome in children under 15 years of age who have influenza or herpes zoster-varicella virus infections, aspirin is rarely used as a pediatric antipyretic in the United States today.

Acetaminophen and the NSAIDs are effective analgesics and contribute to the relief of numerous symptoms that often accompany fever. The onset of antipyretic activity after an oral dose of one of these agents occurs within 30 minutes to 1 hour. Maximum temperature reduction is evident between 2 and 3 hours after the dose, and antipyretic effects are generally sustained for 4–6 hours. Because the average maximum reduction in temperature is only 2–3°F (1.1°–1.7°C), "normalization" of temperature should not necessarily be a goal of therapy; the most important objective is to relieve patient discomfort. The adult dosages of commonly used nonprescription analgesics and antipyretics are listed in Tables 5 and 6.

Salicylates

Salicylates are effective in treating mild to moderate pain and fever from a variety of etiologies. These agents are most commonly used for musculoskeletal indications. They

TABLE 5 Dosages of nonprescription analgesic/antipyretic agents commonly used for pain or inflammation

| Agent | Dosage (maximum) | |
	Analgesic	Anti-inflammatory
Acetaminophen	650–1,000 mg, 3–4 times/ day (4,000 mg/day)	—
Aspirin	650–1,000 mg every 4 h (4,000 mg/day)	2,400–3,900 mg/day for 5–7 days
Ibuprofen	200–400 mg every 4–6 h (1,200 mg/day)	400–800 mg, 3–4 times/day[a] (3,200 mg in 2 wk)
Naproxen sodium	220 mg every 6–8 h (660 mg/day)	275–550 mg, 2 times/day[a] (1,650 mg/day for 2 wk)
Ketoprofen	12.5–25 mg every 6–8 h (75 mg/day)	50–75 mg, 3–4 times/day[a,b] (300 mg/day)

[a]Dosage exceeds that recommended in nonprescription product labeling.
[b]Dosage should be reduced in elderly and renally impaired patients.
Information extracted from Whelton A. Renal effects of over-the-counter analgesics. *J Clin Pharmacol.* 1995;35: 453–63.

TABLE 6 Adult dosages of nonprescription salicylates

Agent	Dosage forms	Usual adult dosage
Aspirin	Tablets, effervescent, enteric coated, buffered; suppositories; chewing gum	650–975 mg (three 325-mg doses) or 1,000 mg (two 500-mg doses) every 4–6 h, not to exceed 4,000 mg/day
Choline salicylate	Oral solution (870 mg/5 mL)	870 mg every 3–4 h, not to exceed 6 daily doses
Magnesium salicylate	Tablets (325 and 500 mg)	650 mg every 4 h or 1,000 mg, 3 times/day
Sodium salicylate	Tablets, enteric coated (325 and 650 mg)	650 mg every 4 h

are usually ineffective in pain of visceral origin. Sodium salicylate and magnesium salicylate offer no advantages over aspirin except that patients allergic to aspirin may be able to tolerate these forms.

Dosage

Recommended pediatric antipyretic doses are listed in Table 7. Aspirin dosages in the range of 4–6 g per day are often needed to produce anti-inflammatory effects. Anti-inflammatory efficacy often will not occur unless the drug is used at the high end of the acceptable dosage range. Therefore, many clinicians now recommend NSAIDs in inflammatory disorders.

Overdose

Symptoms of chronic salicylate intoxication include headache, dizziness, ringing in the ears, difficulty in hearing, dimness of vision, mental confusion, lassitude, drowsiness, sweating, thirst, hyperventilation, nausea, vomiting, and occasional diarrhea. All are reversible upon lowering the plasma concentration to a therapeutic range.

Symptoms of acute salicylate intoxication include lethargy, tinnitus, tachypnea and pulmonary edema, convulsions, coma, nausea, vomiting, hemorrhage, and dehydration.

Emergency management of acute salicylate intoxication is directed toward preventing the absorption of salicylate from the gastrointestinal (GI) tract. Emergency medical personnel and poison control centers commonly advocate using ipecac syrup at home to empty the stomach for mild to moderate unintentional ingestions by children under 6 years of age.

Adults and children over 12 years of age should be given 30 mL of ipecac syrup followed by 8 oz of water, clear liquids, or noncarbonated beverages, and should be ambulated to

TABLE 7 Recommended pediatric antipyretic doses

Body weight	Age (y)	Single dose (mg)[a]
Acetaminophen		
(10–15 mg/kg)	<2	Physician directed
	2–3	160
	4–5	240
	6–8	320
	9–10	400
	11–12	480
	Adult	650
Aspirin		
(10–15 mg/kg)	<2	Physician directed
	2–3	162
	4–5	243
	6–8	324
	9–10	405
	11–12	486
	Adult	650

[a]Individual doses may be repeated every 4–6 hours as needed, up to four to five daily doses. Do not exceed five doses in 24 hours.

stimulate emesis. If emesis does not occur in 20–30 minutes, the process should be repeated. For children 1–12 years of age, the recommended dose of ipecac syrup is 15 mL (1 tbsp or 3 tsp) followed by 8 oz of water, clear liquids, or noncarbonated beverages. The dose should be repeated if vomiting does not occur within 20–30 minutes. In children under 1 year of age, vomiting should be induced only under medical supervision.

Administering ipecac syrup or other oral liquids to a person who is convulsing or not completely conscious is absolutely contraindicated.

Pharmacokinetics of Aspirin and Other Salicylates

Because enteric-coated aspirin is absorbed only from the small intestine, its absorption is markedly slowed by food, which increases the gastric emptying time. Buffered aspirin products are absorbed more rapidly than nonbuffered products, but this has little therapeutic significance in terms of onset of drug effect. Rectal absorption of salicylate is slow and unreliable.

There is no difference in the amount of gastric damage produced by buffered and nonbuffered products; however, enteric coating eliminates the local gastric irritation produced by aspirin. Equivalent doses of plain, buffered, or enteric-coated aspirin produce essentially the same plasma levels of salicylate; however, the time to peak is delayed with the enteric-coated product. Thus, for patients requiring rapid pain relief, enteric-coated aspirin is inappropriate. For patients requiring prolonged aspirin therapy, enteric-coated aspirin may be preferred because it produces less gastric mucosal injury than plain or buffered aspirin.

Sustained-release aspirin products may produce less GI irritation than regular aspirin. However, aspirin-induced reversible deafness has been reported to occur to a much greater extent with high-dose sustained-release aspirin than with equivalent daily doses of plain aspirin.

Effervescent aspirin solutions (e.g., Alka-Seltzer) are rapidly absorbed; however, there is no evidence that such products produce more rapid or effective analgesia than oral solid dosage forms of salicylates. Effervescent aspirin solutions contain large amounts of sodium and must be avoided by patients requiring restricted sodium intake.

Therapeutic Considerations

Impaired Platelet Aggregation and Hematologic Effects. The acetyl moiety makes aspirin a more effective anti-inflammatory agent than other salicylates. However, that moiety also acetylates platelets, causing irreversible inhibition of platelet aggregation. This effect provides a unique advantage in preventing blood clots, but it can also increase risks of bleeding. A single 650-mg dose of aspirin can double the bleeding time. Aspirin therapy should be discontinued at least 48 hours before surgery and should not be used to relieve the pain of tonsillectomy, dental extraction, or other surgical procedures except under the close supervision of a physician or dentist. Aspirin is contraindicated in patients with hypoprothrombinemia, vitamin K deficiency, hemophilia, history of any bleeding disorder, or history of peptic ulcer disease (PUD).

Acetaminophen does not affect platelet aggregation or bleeding time. When peripheral anti-inflammatory activity is not needed and aspirin's effect on hemostasis is a concern, acetaminophen is an appropriate analgesic for self-medication. Most other NSAIDs impair platelet aggregation while the drugs are at analgesic serum levels, but these effects resolve as the drug is cleared from the serum. The prescription salicylate compounds salsalate and choline magnesium trisalicylate are reasonable alternatives when a peripheral anti-inflammatory agent is indicated. Sodium salicylate does not affect platelets, but it does increase prothrombin time.

Effect on Uric Acid Elimination.   Salicylates can affect uric acid secretion and reabsorption by the renal tubules. The effect on plasma uric acid is dose related. All salicylates should be avoided in patients with a history of gout or hyperuricemia.

Gastrointestinal Irritation and Bleeding.   Aspirin produces local GI damage by penetrating the protective mucous and bicarbonate layers of the gastric mucosa and permitting the back diffusion of acid, causing cellular and vascular erosion. There are two distinct mechanisms by which this occurs. Gastritis is a local effect that can occur without risk of ulceration. Conversely, ulceration is due to systemic activity and it can be asymptomatic until it is advanced.

GI blood loss with aspirin is dose dependent. Normal subjects with no aspirin exposure lose approximately 0.5 mL of blood per day in the stool. Moderate aspirin intake increases this amount to 2–6 mL per day. Chronic GI bleeding of this magnitude can deplete total body iron and produce iron-deficiency anemia. Aspirin use should be discontinued for at least 3 days prior to a test for fecal occult blood.

In a small percentage of patients, aspirin use can produce massive GI bleeding (acute hemorrhagic gastritis). Elderly patients, patients with a history of gastric ulceration or bleeding, and those with alcoholic liver disease are at increased risk for acute hemorrhagic gastritis with aspirin use and therefore should avoid aspirin. Patients who take aspirin should be advised that ingesting aspirin with alcohol appears to increase the incidence of GI bleeding.

Aspirin Allergy.   Many patients report that they are allergic to aspirin because they have experienced gastritis or heartburn following its use. These are common side effects, not allergy or hypersensitivity, and they are not contraindications to future trials of aspirin. True aspirin allergy is uncommon. Manifestations include hives (urticaria), edema, difficulty in breathing, bronchospasm, rhinitis, or shock; these adverse effects usually occur within 3 hours of aspirin ingestion. Aspirin allergy is usually allergy to acetylated salicylates, not to all salicylates; therefore, nonacetylated salicylates may be used by many patients who are allergic to aspirin.

Patients intolerant to aspirin may also cross-react with other chemicals or drugs. The cross-reaction rates for acetaminophen and ibuprofen in documented aspirin-intolerant patients are 6% and 97%, respectively. High cross-reaction rates in aspirin-intolerant patients are also reported with some prescription NSAIDs. Patients with a history of aspirin intolerance should be advised to avoid all aspirin- and NSAID-containing products and to use acetaminophen.

Even though the cross-reaction rate for acetaminophen is low, aspirin-intolerant patients may exhibit urticarial or bronchospastic symptoms with this drug. Other nonprescription analgesics that have a low risk of cross-reactivity include sodium salicylate and choline salicylate.

Pregnancy/Lactation.   Aspirin consumption during pregnancy may produce adverse maternal effects including anemia, antepartum or postpartum hemorrhage, and prolonged gestation and labor. Aspirin ingestion on a regular basis during pregnancy may increase the risk for complicated deliveries. The Food and Drug Administration (FDA) requires drug products that contain aspirin to carry labels that warn against using the drugs during the last 3 months of pregnancy unless the patient is directed to do so by a physician.

Aspirin and other salicylates are excreted into breast milk in low concentrations.

Women should be advised to avoid aspirin during pregnancy, especially during the last trimester, and when breast-feeding. At these times, acetaminophen is the preferred analgesic for self-medication.

Reye's Syndrome. Reye's syndrome is an acute, potentially fatal illness occurring almost exclusively in children under 15 years of age. It is characterized by vomiting, progressive CNS damage, signs of hepatic injury, and hypoglycemia. The onset usually follows a viral infection with influenza (type A or B) or varicella-zoster (i.e., chickenpox).

Although the cause of Reye's syndrome is unknown, viral and toxic agents, especially salicylates, have been associated with it. Since 1988, the FDA has required that a Reye's syndrome warning be added to the labels of nonprescription aspirin and aspirin-containing products. In 1993, the FDA proposed that the warning be extended to all nonprescription products containing bismuth subsalicylate except those marketed solely for diarrhea.

A strong association has been confirmed between the use of salicylate during an antecedent viral infection and the subsequent development of Reye's syndrome. Thus, it is imperative that pharmacists warn against giving products containing aspirin or nonaspirin salicylates to children and teenagers who have influenza or chickenpox. In such cases, acetaminophen is the preferred nonprescription analgesic/antipyretic. A simple viral upper respiratory infection (e.g., a common cold) is not a contraindication to aspirin use; however, symptoms of this type of infection may mimic some of those seen in influenza and chickenpox. Therefore, many clinicians recommend a conservative approach of aspirin avoidance when symptoms resembling influenza are present. The use of aspirin as a pediatric antipyretic has all but ceased in the United States, as have reports of Reye's syndrome.

Drug Interactions

Aspirin, the other nonprescription salicylates, acetaminophen, ibuprofen, naproxen sodium, and ketoprofen interact with several other important drugs and drug classes. Adverse effects are additive with other agents or diseases that cause similar disorders. Patients at increased risk of toxicity from NSAIDs include individuals with marked renal or hepatic impairment (i.e., uremia, cirrhosis, hepatitis); patients with metabolic disorders (i.e., hypoxia, hypothyroidism); patients with unstable disease (i.e., cardiac arrhythmias, intractable epilepsy, brittle diabetes); patients with status asthmaticus; and elderly patients in general because of the increased incidence of multiple system disorders. Clinically important drug interactions that have been reported with aspirin and other nonprescription analgesic/antipyretic drugs are listed in Table 8.

Nonacetylated Salicylates

Choline Salicylate. Choline salicylate (Arthropan) is an oral liquid salicylate preparation. A 5-mL dose of choline salicylate (174 mg/mL, or 870 mg) is equivalent to 650 mg of aspirin in salicylate content. For patients who find the fishy odor of the liquid product unacceptable, choline salicylate oral solution may be mixed with liquid just before administration. Comparative analgesic/anti-inflammatory efficacy studies are not available for choline salicylate. The product was found to be less effective than either aspirin or acetaminophen as an antipyretic in children.

Magnesium Salicylate. Magnesium salicylate is available as the tetrahydrate (Arthriten, Backache). The salicylate content of 377 mg of magnesium salicylate tetrahydrate is equivalent to that of 325 mg of sodium salicylate. Patients with compromised renal function must avoid using magnesium salicylate because of the potential for decreased renal excretion and the systemic magnesium toxicity. Aspirin and magnesium sulfate both taken in 500 mg doses four times daily, were found equally effective in relieving the pain of degenerative arthritis.

TABLE 8 Clinically important drug interactions with nonprescription analgesic/antipyretic agents

OTC analgesic/antipyretic	Drug	Potential interaction	Management/Preventive measures
Ibuprofen, high-dose salicylates	Phenytoin	Phenytoin displaced from serum protein-binding sites if phenytoin metabolism is saturated or folate levels are low	Monitor unbound phenytoin levels; adjust dose, if indicated; ensure that patient has sufficient folate
Aspirin	Valproic acid	Oxidation of valproate inhibited; up to 30% reduction in clearance	Avoid concurrent use; use naproxen instead of aspirin (no interaction)
Acetaminophen	Zidovudine	Incidence of bone marrow suppression may be increased; interaction is usually not significant	Avoid concurrent use in patients with AIDS and AIDS-related complex
NSAIDs (several)	Digoxin	Renal clearance inhibited	Monitor digoxin levels; adjust doses as indicated
NSAIDs (several)	Aminoglycosides	Renal clearance inhibited	Monitor antibiotic levels; adjust doses as indicated
NSAIDS (several)	Antihypertensive agents; beta-blockers, ACE inhibitors, vasodilators, diuretics	Antihypertensive effect antagonized; hyperkalemia may occur with potassium-sparing diuretics and ACE inhibitors	Monitor blood pressure and cardiac function; monitor potassium levels
NSAIDs	Oral anticoagulants	Risk of bleeding increased, especially GI bleeding,	Avoid concurrent use, if possible; risk is lowest with salsalate and choline magnesium trisalicylate
NSAIDs (some)	Lithium	Renal clearance inhibited	Monitor lithium levels; adjust doses as indicated; interaction less likely with aspirin than with ibuprofen or naproxen
NSAIDs	Alcohol	Risk of GI bleeding increased	Avoid concurrent use, if possible; minimize alcohol intake when using NSAID
NSAIDs (several)	Methotrexate	Methotrexate clearance decreased	Avoid NSAIDs with high-dose methotrexate therapy; monitor levels with concurrent treatment
Naproxen	Probenecid	Naproxen clearance inhibited	Monitor for adverse effects
Naproxen	Aluminum hydroxide	Naproxen absorption decreased	Increase naproxen dose as needed
Salicylates	Antacids in high doses	Salicylate levels possibly reduced 25%	Determine if salicylate doses should be increased
Salicylates (moderate to high doses)	Sulfonylureas	Hypoglycemic activity increased	Avoid concurrent use, if possible; monitor blood glucose levels when changing salicylate dose
Salicylates	Corticosteroids	Salicylate clearance possibly increased with long-term, high-dose salicylate therapy	Monitor salicylate levels when changing steroid dose; adjust salicylate dose, if indicated

Note: NSAIDs include the salicylates.

Sodium Salicylate. Due to the fact that the maximum 4-g dose of sodium salicylate contains 560 mg (25 mEq) of sodium, patients on strict sodium restriction should avoid sodium salicylate.

Divided oral doses of enteric-coated aspirin and enteric-coated sodium salicylate, 4.8 g per day, have been shown to be equally effective in the treatment of rheumatoid arthritis. Both drugs have produced similar degrees of pain relief, increased grip strength, reduced joint tenderness, and decreased digital joint circumference. Patients allergic to aspirin may be able to tolerate sodium salicylate. However, sodium salicylate is less effective than an equal dose of aspirin in reducing pain or fever.

Comparison of Aspirin and Nonacetylated Salicylates

When doses containing equivalent amounts of salicylate are given, it appears that aspirin and the nonacetylated salicylates are equally well absorbed and produce similar plasma salicylate levels. However, choline salicylate oral solution produces peak plasma salicylate levels sooner than the oral solid dosage forms.

Because aspirin's effect on platelet aggregation with a prolongation of bleeding time requires the participation of the acetyl moiety, nonacetylated salicylates do not affect platelet aggregation or bleeding time significantly. With the exception of this difference, the nonacetylated salicylates have the same contraindications and interactions as aspirin because all other salicylate effects result from the production of salicylic acid. However, nonacetylated salicylates are weaker prostaglandin synthesis inhibitors than aspirin and, as such, appear to cause less GI erosion and bleeding, fewer renal complications, and a low level of cross-reactivity in aspirin-intolerant patients.

Acetaminophen

Indications

Acetaminophen is an effective analgesic and antipyretic. Unlike salicylates, acetaminophen produces analgesia through a central rather than a peripheral effect on the nervous system. Acetaminophen is effective in relieving mild to moderate pain of nonvisceral origin. It has no clinically significant anti-inflammatory activity.

Dosage

Table 7 lists recommended oral pediatric doses. Rectal bioavailability of acetaminophen is approximately 50%–60% of that achieved with oral administration. Equal doses of acetaminophen and aspirin administered by the same route produce equivalent degrees of analgesia.

Acetaminophen is available for oral administration in various liquid and solid dosage forms, including rectal suppositories and capsules. The capsules contain tasteless granules that can be emptied onto a teaspoon containing a small amount of drink or soft food. Patients and parents should not add the contents of the capsules to a glass of liquid because large numbers of granules may adhere to the side of the glass. Mixing with a hot beverage can result in a bitter taste.

Overdose

Symptoms of an acute overdose of acetaminophen may be slow to appear and may not reflect the seriousness of the exposure. Early symptoms of acetaminophen intoxication include nausea, vomiting, drowsiness, confusion, and abdominal pain. Clinical manifestations of hepatotoxicity begin 2–4 days after the acute ingestion of acetaminophen. In nonfatal cases, the hepatic damage is reversible. The most serious adverse effect of acute overdose with acetaminophen is a dose-dependent, potentially fatal hepatic necrosis.

Renal tubular necrosis and hypoglycemic coma may also occur. In adults, hepatotoxicity may occur after ingestion of a single dose of 10–15 g (150–250 mg/kg) of acetaminophen; doses of 20–25 g or more are potentially fatal.

Because of the potential seriousness of acetaminophen overdose, all cases should be referred to a poison control center or other medical personnel experienced in managing such cases. Immediate first-aid management of acute acetaminophen poisoning includes the induction of vomiting with ipecac syrup. If activated charcoal is administered in-home, this information must be made known to emergency medical personnel administering N-acetylcysteine so that appropriate dose adjustments can be made. Dosing recommendations for both ipecac syrup and activated charcoal are included in Chapter 16.

Therapeutic Considerations for Use

Acetaminophen sometimes is underdosed, especially in young patients. This occurs when parents reuse the 0.8-mL dropper provided with infant drops (80 mg/0.8 mL) to measure a dose of an equivalent volume of acetaminophen elixir in a concentration of 160 mg/5 mL, incorrectly assuming the same strength. In addition, recalculation of the pediatric dose according to present age and body weight is appropriate at the time of each treatment course.

Acetaminophen crosses the placenta but is considered safe for use during pregnancy. It appears in breast milk, producing a milk to maternal plasma ratio of 0.50:1.0. The only adverse effect reported in nursing infants exposed to acetaminophen through breast milk is a rarely occurring maculopapular rash.

Acetaminophen is potentially hepatotoxic in doses exceeding 4 g per day. Patients with preexisting liver disease who are taking other potentially hepatotoxic drugs, who do not eat regularly, and who ingest alcohol more than occasionally are at increased risk for acetaminophen-induced hepatotoxicity. Patients should be advised to avoid alcohol and fasting, if possible, when taking acetaminophen.

Drug Interactions

Clinically important drug interactions of acetaminophen are listed in Table 8. Acetaminophen produces no therapeutically significant drug interactions with the possible exception of zidovudine (AZT).

Evidence suggests, however, that short-term use of acetaminophen (less than 7 days) does not increase the risk of myelosuppression and neutropenia in AIDS patients receiving zidovudine. Given that these patients cannot take aspirin because of its anti-platelet effect, the short-term or intermittent use of acetaminophen is the recommended nonprescription analgesic for self-medication.

Ibuprofen

Indications

Ibuprofen has analgesic, antipyretic, and anti-inflammatory activity; it is also useful in managing mild to moderate pain of nonvisceral origin and dysmenorrhea.

Dosage

On a milligram-to-milligram basis, ibuprofen is approximately 3.5 times more potent than aspirin as an analgesic, and the analgesic effect may last up to 6 hours.

The oral 100 mg/5 mL ibuprofen suspension (Children's Motrin) is indicated for children aged 2–11 years as an antipyretic and for relief of minor aches and pains due to colds, influenza, sore throat, headaches, and toothaches. The duration of action may be as long as 8 hours. Dosage information appears in Table 9.

TABLE 9 Recommended analgesic/antipyretic dosages

Agent	Age	Dosage (maximum)
Ibuprofen	6 mo–12 y	7.5 mg/kg (30 mg/kg/day)
	>12 y	200–400 mg every 4–6 h (1,200 mg/day)
Naproxen sodium	<12 y	Not recommended
	12–65 y	220–440 mg every 8–12 h (660 mg/day)
	>65 y	220 mg every 12 h (440 mg/day)
Ketoprofen	<16 y	Not recommended
	>16 y	12.5 mg every 6–8 h; may take second dose after 1 h, if needed (75 mg/day)

In numerous clinical trials, ibuprofen has been shown to be superior to aspirin, nonacetylated salicylates, and acetaminophen for the symptomatic relief of primary dysmenorrhea.

Overdose

Overdose of ibuprofen usually produces minimal symptoms of toxicity and is rarely fatal. Common symptoms of overdose include nausea, vomiting, abdominal pain, lethargy, stupor, coma, nystagmus, dizziness, and lightheadedness. Hypotension, bradycardia, tachycardia, dyspnea, and painful breathing were also reported. In one study, 43% of ibuprofen-overdose patients were asymptomatic. Unless contraindicated by convulsions or unconsciousness, appropriate first-aid treatment of ibuprofen overdose includes the induction of vomiting with ipecac syrup or activated charcoal (see Chapter 16).

Therapeutic Considerations for Use

The most frequent adverse effects of ibuprofen involve the GI tract and include dyspepsia, heartburn, nausea, anorexia, and epigastric pain. Ibuprofen produces less GI bleeding than aspirin.

In dosages of 600–1800 mg per day, ibuprofen increased bleeding time by inhibiting platelet aggregation; however, this effect is reversible within 24 hours after medication is discontinued. Ibuprofen does not significantly affect whole blood clotting time or prothrombin time. Patients self-medicating with ibuprofen should be cautioned against the concurrent use of alcohol. Ibuprofen should not be recommended for self-medication to patients who are concurrently taking anticoagulants.

Ibuprofen may decrease renal blood flow and glomerular filtration rate. This may increase blood urea nitrogen and serum creatinine values, often with concomitant sodium and water retention. This effect is of greatest clinical importance in patients with preexisting renal impairment or congestive heart failure. As a result, patients with a history of impaired renal function, congestive heart failure, or diseases that compromise renal hemodynamics should not self-medicate with ibuprofen.

Ibuprofen is contraindicated in patients with a history of intolerance to aspirin or to any other NSAID in documented aspirin-intolerant patients. Patients with a history of asthma may experience a worsening of their bronchospastic symptoms with ibuprofen.

There is no evidence that ibuprofen is teratogenic in either humans or animals. However, because prostaglandin inhibitors can cause delayed parturition, postpartum bleeding, and closure of the ductus arteriosus, ibuprofen is contraindicated during the third trimester of pregnancy. In lactating women taking up to 2.4 g of ibuprofen per day, there is no measurable excretion of ibuprofen into breast milk.

The safety of ibuprofen in children has been demonstrated by a practitioner-based, randomized clinical trial that compared it with acetaminophen.

Drug Interactions

Clinically important drug interactions of ibuprofen are listed in Table 8.

Naproxen Sodium

Naproxen sodium (Aleve) was approved for use as a nonprescription analgesic, anti-inflammatory agent, and antipyretic in 1994. This NSAID is very similar to nonprescription ibuprofen. Naproxen sodium has a similar onset of activity but its duration of action may be somewhat longer.

Indications

The labeled indications for the nonprescription form of the drug are relief of minor pain associated with headache, the common cold, toothache, muscle ache, backache, arthritis, and muscle cramps as well as the reduction of fever.

Dosage

Children under 12 years of age should use the drug only under a physician's supervision. Naproxen is compatible with breast-feeding.

Overdose

The presentation and management of a naproxen sodium overdose should be similar to an ibuprofen overdose.

Drug Interactions

Clinically important drug interactions of naproxen are listed in Table 8. Naproxen sodium has a similar drug interaction profile to that of ibuprofen.

Ketoprofen

Ketoprofen (Orudis KT, Actron) was approved for nonprescription use as an analgesic and antipyretic in 1995.

Indications

Like ibuprofen and naproxen sodium, ketoprofen is a propionic acid derivative NSAID; therefore, its indications (analgesia, anti-inflammatory activity, and antipyresis) and pharmacologic activity are the same as these two agents.

Dosage

One 12.5-mg tablet of ketoprofen appears to be equivalent to one 200-mg tablet of ibuprofen.

Adverse Effects

Adverse effects related to ketoprofen are also similar to those of the other propionic acid derivative NSAIDs; these effects include gastric mucosal damage, inhibition of platelet aggregation, and renal effects. At normal nonprescription doses, adverse effects are rare.

No evidence of teratogenicity or toxicity to embryos has been uncovered in studies of pregnant animals given high doses of ketoprofen. There is also no evidence of adverse effects on fertility. The product labeling recommends that this drug not be used by nursing mothers.

Drug Interactions

A life-threatening interaction of ketoprofen and methotrexate has been reported.

Comparative Efficacy of Nonprescription Analgesics/Antipyretics

Aspirin versus Acetaminophen

Numerous controlled studies have demonstrated the equivalent analgesic efficacy of aspirin and acetaminophen on a milligram-for-milligram basis in various pain models, including postoperative pain, cancer pain, episiotomy pain, and oral surgery pain. Acetaminophen (1 g) has been shown to be superior to aspirin (650 mg) in the control of pain secondary to dental surgery or episiotomy.

Aspirin versus Ibuprofen

Ibuprofen has been shown to be at least as effective as aspirin in treating various types of pain, including dental extraction pain, dysmenorrhea, and episiotomy pain.

Controlled clinical trials have shown that ibuprofen is as effective as, but not superior to, aspirin in the treatment of rheumatoid arthritis. Both drugs reduced morning stiffness and improved grip strength to an equivalent degree. However, aspirin appeared superior to ibuprofen in the reduction of joint size. It is noteworthy that the daily aspirin dose approached the maximum for safe use while the ibuprofen dose was relatively low.

Ibuprofen versus Acetaminophen

Numerous comparisons of oral ibuprofen and acetaminophen in various pain models suggest that 100–200 mg of ibuprofen is approximately equianalgesic to 650 mg of acetaminophen. Ibuprofen has a clear superiority, however, in pain conditions associated with inflammation. Some studies have found ibuprofen superior to acetaminophen for pain associated with migraine headache, episiotomy, and oral surgery. Ibuprofen produced significantly greater temperature reductions during the first 4 hours of treatment in children than acetaminophen; this difference was not sustained over time.

Naproxen versus Ibuprofen

One 200-mg nonprescription naproxen sodium tablet appears to be very similar in indications and efficacy to one 200-mg ibuprofen tablet. Some RA patients do report better response to one NSAID than to another for reasons that are unclear.

Combination Products Containing Caffeine or Antihistamines

Many nonprescription analgesics are available as combination products containing aspirin, ibuprofen, or acetaminophen as primary ingredients plus caffeine or an antihistamine. The adjuvant ingredients are claimed to enhance the analgesic efficacy of the product.

A growing body of clinical literature supports the enhancement of analgesia by the inclusion of either caffeine or an antihistamine with a nonprescription analgesic. Combination dosage forms containing a decongestant and either acetaminophen or an NSAID are also available. Such combinations appear logical for use in sinus headaches or other indications in which both analgesia and decongestion are needed.

CHAPTER 5

External Analgesic Products

Questions to ask in patient assessment and counseling

- Where is the pain? How long has it been present? When did it first appear? How often does it occur? Have you experienced it before?
- Can you relate the pain to any specific event, such as an accident, overwork, or a sports-related activity?
- Is the pain in a joint or the muscle? If the pain is in a joint, is the joint red, swollen, or warm to the touch?
- Is the pain worse when you get up? Does it tend to subside as the day goes on?
- Does the pain move to other areas of the body?
- Has any specific treatment been helpful in relieving the pain?
- Do you have a fever or any flu symptoms?

Types of Muscular Pain

Overuse Injuries

There are three major categories of this so-called "overuse" syndrome: tendinitis, bursitis, and occupational repetition strain.

Tendinitis

Tendinitis, which results from a strain or injury of tendons, is often seen at times of maximum physical effort, such as during athletic competition. Although tendinitis in the shoulder area is a major cause of pain, athletes often suffer injury of tendons in other areas of the body, including the biceps, patella, and iliotibial band. Achilles' tendinitis may be the most common sports injury.

Many factors contribute to producing an overuse injury such as tendinitis. In industry, they include poorly designed equipment, awkward working positions, lack of job variation, long work hours, and inadequate breaks. In athletics, contributing factors can include the athlete's age, poor technique, and improper conditioning; exercise of prolonged intensity or duration; and poorly designed equipment or clothing.

The Food and Drug Administration (FDA) has received reports of 25 cases of tendon rupture associated with fluoroquinolone antibiotics. Updated labeling for all commercially available fluoroquinolones includes a recommendation to discontinue treatment with these agents at the first sign of tendon pain or inflammation and to refrain from exercise until the diagnosis of tendinitis can be excluded.

Bursitis

Bursae are sacs formed by two layers of synovial tissue located at sites of friction between tendon and bone or skin and bone. Repetitive trauma from friction of the overlying tendon

---

Editor's Note: This chapter is adapted from Arthur I. Jacknowitz, "External Analgesic Products," in Covington, T.R., ed., *Handbook of Nonprescription Drugs,* 11th edition. For a more extensive discussion of this topic, readers are encouraged to consult Chapter 5 of the *Handbook.*

or from external pressure may cause the bursa to become inflamed, with resultant fluid buildup in the bursal wall. This condition, termed bursitis, is a common cause of localized pain, tenderness, and swelling. Pain may be acute or chronic; in the latter case, an infectious cause should be suspected. Most cases of bursitis are due to overuse. This is particularly true in sports that involve repetitive motions, such as swimming, gymnastics, skiing, and weight lifting. Runners commonly are afflicted with bursitis of the knees, hips, ankles, and feet.

Bursitis often results in limited motion of adjacent joints. Symptoms of bursitis that mimic arthritic pain can be distinguished by a physical examination.

Occupational Repetition Strain

Occupational repetition strain injuries involve the upper limbs, shoulder girdle, and neck. They are caused by an overload on particular muscles due to awkward working postures or repeated use. Assembly-line workers and typists are likely candidates for this type of strain injury.

Soft-Tissue Injury

These terms—sprain, bruise, and strain—are used to characterize injury to soft tissue.

- A sprain is a partial or complete rupture of a ligament.
- A bruise is a rupture of tissue resulting in a hematoma.
- A strain is a partial tear of muscles.

Sprains occur when a joint is forced beyond its normal range of motion (e.g., a hyperextended knee) or forced in a plane through which little or no motion actually exists (e.g., a lateral ankle sprain). Most strains, on the other hand, occur during forceful muscle action. The injury might occur soon after an activity has begun, such as coming out of the blocks at the start of a race. When these injuries occur, the muscles become sore, and movement becomes difficult.

Arthritis

Arthritic pain may be caused by rheumatoid arthritis, which may involve almost all peripheral joints, tendons, bursae, and the cervical spine; or by osteoarthritis, which involves degeneration of cartilage with secondary changes in joints. Although both types are chronic systemic diseases, local treatment of painful joints, coupled with rest, may give temporary symptomatic relief.

Lower Back Pain

This regional musculoskeletal disorder is due primarily to a sedentary lifestyle, as well as to poor posture, improper shoes, excess weight, poor mattresses and sleeping posture, and improper technique in lifting heavy objects.

Other causes of backache include congenital anomalies, osteoarthritis, spinal tuberculosis, and referred pain from diseased kidneys, pancreas, liver, or prostate. Emotional factors, including tension, anxiety, and other manifestations of psychosocial stress, have also been postulated to correlate with lower back pain.

Other Types of Muscular Pain

Acute, temporary stiffness and muscle pain can result from cold, dampness, rapid temperature changes, and air currents. In some cases, visceral stimuli resulting from cardiovascular disease or gastrointestinal complaints are felt as referred pain in the skeletal muscles of the shoulder. These episodes tend to be sudden in onset but self-limiting. Elimination of the cause and symptomatic treatment generally provide relief.

Patient Assessment

To assess the patient's condition accurately before recommending a nonprescription counterirritant preparation, the pharmacist should ask the patient questions such as those that appear at the beginning of this chapter. Analysis of the patient's responses may involve the following considerations:

- Duration. Conditions amenable to nonprescription treatment are self-limiting. Prolonged use of external analgesics can increase the sensitivity to and decrease the effectiveness of these products. Pain that has been apparent for longer than 7 days may indicate a more serious underlying condition.

- Cause. Muscular or joint pain can be brought on by overexertion. Such pain is a valid indication for nonprescription external analgesics.

- Location and severity. If the pain is mild, it may be appropriate to recommend a nonprescription product. However, if the patient has difficulty locating the origin of the pain, it may be referred pain. For example, pain in the lumbar area may be referred from pelvic viscera and may be an early manifestation of disease in these organs. If the pain is in a joint and the joint is red, swollen, warm, and tender, there may be a fracture, a rupture of ligaments or tendons, or arthritic involvement. Nonprescription products would delay an accurate diagnosis. Nonprescription treatment should not be recommended if the pain is severe.

- Previous diagnosis of arthritis. If the patient is under medical supervision for arthritis, it may be appropriate to recommend only a counterirritant preparation as adjunctive treatment. The topical analgesic helps the patient over intermittent painful episodes, thus reducing his or her intake of oral analgesics, which may pose a greater risk of adverse reactions.

- Concurrent prescription or nonprescription medication. Knowledge of the patient's medication history enables the pharmacist to recommend an appropriate external analgesic while minimizing the risk of both duplication of therapy and drug–drug interactions.

If the pharmacist determines that the condition is minor and that there are no serious underlying conditions, it may be appropriate to recommend a nonprescription preparation. If the symptoms persist or are not relieved by the preparation within 7 days or if the symptoms clear up and occur again within a few days, the medication should be discontinued and a physician should be consulted. The pharmacist should also arrange a follow-up consultation.

Treatment

Mechanism of Action

External analgesics are topically applied substances that may have local analgesic, anesthetic, antipruritic, or counterirritant effects.

Topical counterirritants are applied to the intact skin to relieve pain. They differ from the other three types of agents in that they relieve pain indirectly by stimulating cutaneous receptors to induce sensations such as cold, warmth, and sometimes itching. Some counterirritant agents, when present in low concentrations, depress cutaneous receptors in a manner similar to local anesthetics, analgesics, and antipruritics.

Patients should be told not to use heating pads or other heating devices in conjunction with all topically applied external counterirritants and not to apply these products immediately after strenuous exercise, especially during hot, humid weather.

There is no evidence that the risk of adverse reactions to counterirritants increases when the application site is lightly bandaged. However, there is an increased risk of irritation, redness, or blistering with tight bandaging or occlusive dressing.

The action of counterirritants in relieving pain has a strong psychologic component. These agents may exert a placebo effect through pleasant aromatic odors or the sensation of warmth or coolness they produce on the skin.

Pharmacologic Agents

Ingredients of Proven Safety and Effectiveness

The FDA has recognized the following ingredients as safe and effective (Category I) counterirritants for use in adults and children over the age of 2 years. Table 1 classifies the counterirritants by their relative potencies.

Allyl Isothiocyanate. Allyl isothiocyanate, also known as volatile oil of mustard, is derived from powdered seeds of the black mustard plant and other species of mustard. In high concentrations, it is absorbed from intact skin as well as from all mucous membranes. Because penetration into the skin is rapid, ulceration may occur if the agent is not removed soon after application.

Allyl isothiocyanate is considered to be safe and effective for topical nonprescription use in concentrations of 0.5%–5.0%. It should be applied to the affected areas no more than three or four times a day; this dosage is for adults and children over 2 years of age.

TABLE 1 Classification of nonprescription counterirritant external analgesics

Group	Characteristics	Ingredients	Concentration (%)
A	Induce redness and irritation; are more potent than other commonly used counter-irritants	Allyl isothiocyanate Ammonia water Methyl salicylate Turpentine oil	0.5–5.0 1.0–2.5 10–60 6–50
B	Produce cooling sensation; have strong organoleptic properties	Camphor Menthol	3–11 1.25–16
C	Cause vasodilation	Histamine dihydrochloride Methyl nicotinate	0.025–0.1 0.25–1.0
D	Incite irritation without rubefaction; are equal in potency to Group A ingredients	Capsicum Capsicum oleoresin Capsaicin	0.025–0.25 0.025–0.25 0.025–0.25

Adapted from *Federal Register.* 1979; 44: 69874.

Stronger Ammonia Water. Stronger ammonia water, also known as strong ammonia solution, stronger ammonium hydroxide solution, and Spirit of Hartshorn, is an aqueous solution of ammonia containing 27%–30% by weight of ammonia. This product should be handled with care, and the vapors should not be inhaled. To be safe and effective for topical use by adults and children over 2 years of age, the product must be diluted. The concentration used is a 1.0%–2.5% solution of available ammonia, which should be applied to the affected area no more than three or four times a day.

Methyl Salicylate. Methyl salicylate is the most widely used counterirritant. At very low concentrations (0.04%), methyl salicylate is used in oral preparations for its pleasant flavor and aroma. It has been used as a flavoring agent in candies, cough drops, lozenges, chewing gum, toothpastes, and mouthwashes. Ingestion of more than small amounts of the substance is hazardous because of its high salicylate content. Regulations require the use of child-resistant containers for liquid preparations containing more than 5% methyl salicylate.

The recommended topical dosage of methyl salicylate for adults and children over 2 years of age is a 10%–60% concentration applied to the affected area no more than three or four times a day. Because percutaneous absorption can occur, this product should be used with caution in individuals who are sensitive to aspirin or who suffer from severe asthma or nasal polyps, conditions associated with aspirin sensitivity.

Turpentine Oil. Turpentine oil has a long history of safety and efficacy. It is both a primary irritant and a sensitizer. As an irritant, it usually acts by defatting the skin, causing dryness and fissuring. It is often used as a cleanser for removing paints and waxes, and it can cause hand eczema by irritating sensitive skin.

The recommended dosage for adults and children over 2 years of age is a 6%–50% concentration applied to the affected area no more than three or four times a day. Application of turpentine liniments to the skin in greater amounts may cause local burning and irritation, gastrointestinal upset, and respiratory symptoms in susceptible individuals. Several human fatalities from the ingestion of turpentine oil have been reported.

Menthol. Menthol may be used safely in small quantities as a flavoring agent and has found wide acceptance in candy, chewing gum, cigarettes, cough drops, toothpaste, nasal sprays, and liqueurs. Menthol has also been used extensively in inhalant preparations for the relief of nasal congestion. Menthol is usually combined with other ingredients with antipruritic or analgesic properties, such as camphor.

When menthol is used in topical preparations in concentrations of 0.1%–1.0%, it depresses sensory cutaneous receptors and acts as an antipruritic. When used in higher concentrations of 1.25%–16.0%, it acts as a counterirritant: applied to the skin, menthol stimulates the nerves that perceive cold while depressing the nerves that perceive pain.

Menthol causes sensitization in certain individuals although the sensitization index is low. The fatal dose of menthol in humans is approximately 2 g. This may be an underestimate, since in acute studies, menthol appears to be a substance of very low toxicity.

The recommended dosage for menthol when used as a counterirritant for adults and children over 2 years of age is a 1.25%–16.0% concentration applied to the affected area no more than three or four times a day.

Camphor. In concentrations of 0.1%–3.0%, camphor depresses cutaneous receptors and is used as a topical analgesic, anesthetic, and antipruritic. In concentrations exceeding 3%, particularly when combined with other counterirritant ingredients, camphor stimulates the nerve endings in the skin and induces relief of pain and discomfort by masking moderate-to-severe deeper visceral pain with a milder pain arising from the skin at the same level of innervation. Applied vigorously, it produces a rubefacient reaction.

Topical camphor products should be applied no more than three or four times a day. The recommended concentration for external use as a counterirritant for adults and children over 2 years of age is 3%–11%. Higher concentrations are not more effective and can cause more serious adverse reactions if accidentally ingested. In 1994, the American Academy of Pediatrics Committee on Drugs advised parents to be aware of these products and their potential danger and recommended modalities that do not contain camphor should be used.

Histamine Dihydrochloride.   Histamine dihydrochloride in a 0.025%–0.10% concentration is considered to be a safe and effective counterirritant when applied no more than three or four times a day. Aqueous vehicles seem to be superior to ointments for percutaneous absorption.

Methyl Nicotinate.   Methyl nicotinate, used in a 0.25%–1.0% concentration, is a safe and effective counterirritant when applied no more than three or four times a day. Methyl nicotinate is not indicated in children under the age of 2 years. Although nicotinic acid is inactive topically, this ester possesses a marked power of diffusion and readily penetrates the cutaneous barrier. Indomethacin, ibuprofen, and aspirin significantly depress the skin's vascular response to methyl nicotinate. Susceptible persons who apply methyl nicotinate over large areas may experience a drop in blood pressure and pulse rate and syncope due to generalized vascular dilation.

Capsicum Preparations.   Capsicum preparations (capsaicin, capsicum, and capsicum oleoresin) are derived from the fruit of various species of plants of the nightshade family. When applied to normal skin, capsaicin elicits a transient feeling of warmth. Capsicum preparations do not cause blistering or reddening of the skin, even in high concentrations, because they do not act on capillaries or other blood vessels.

The recommended dosage for adults and children over 2 years of age is a concentration of capsicum preparation that yields 0.025%–0.25% capsaicin, applied to the affected area no more than three or four times a day. The duration of action is 4–6 hours. Pain relief is usually noted within 14 days after therapy has begun, but will occasionally be delayed by as much as 4–6 weeks. Because of variations between lots of capsicum, the concentration range for this drug cannot be expressed as a percentage and must be calculated for each lot.

Combination Products.   Two or more safe and effective active ingredients may be combined when each active ingredient contributes to the claimed effect and the combination does not decrease the safety or effectiveness of any individual active ingredient. Table 1 lists the individual ingredients in each of the four groups of these products and classifies them according to their relative potency and acceptable concentration ranges. Many products combine active ingredients from one group of counterirritants with one, two, or three other active ingredients, provided that each active ingredient is from a different group.

Ingredients of Unproven Effectiveness and/or Safety

Eucalyptus Oil.   In a recent report, the FDA has advised that eucalyptus oil has not been shown to be generally recognized as safe and effective for its intended use and that it should be eliminated from nonprescription counterirritant products.

Trolamine Salicylate.   Trolamine salicylate (formerly known as triethanolamine salicylate), although a salicylate salt, is not a counterirritant analgesic. Although the FDA's review of the data indicated that trolamine salicylate studies did not show any significant differences between active drug and placebo, several subsequent reports suggest that trolamine may be effective in alleviating neuralgia caused by unaccustomed strenuous exercise.

Dosage Forms

The nonprescription counterirritant preparations are usually available as liniments, gels, lotions, sprays, creams, and ointments. Specific considerations relating to each of these forms are as follows.

Liniments. Liniments with an alcoholic or hydroalcoholic vehicle are useful when rubefacient or counterirritant action is desired; oleaginous liniments are used primarily when massage is desired. Oleaginous liniments are less irritating to the skin than alcoholic liniments. Liniments should not be applied to skin that is broken or bruised.

Gels. A greater sensation of warmth is experienced with a gel than with equal quantities of the same product as a lotion or ointment. Patients should be advised against using excessive amounts of gels or rubbing them vigorously into the skin because increased penetration may cause an unpleasant burning sensation.

Lotions. Depending on the ingredients, lotions may be alcoholic or aqueous. They are often emulsions. Their fluidity allows for rapid and uniform application over a wide surface area and makes them especially suited for application to hairy body areas.

Ointments. These semisolid dosage forms are particularly desirable for counterirritation because the agents are applied with massage.

Clinical Considerations. Dosage forms referred to as "greaseless" are oil-in-water formulations that may be removed with water and are usually preferred for daytime use.

There is little agreement on how long the preparations should be left in contact with the skin for optimal results. A practical guideline is that preparations should be used no more than three or four times a day. Although it is desirable to protect clothing from stains by covering the application site, the covering should not be tightly applied. Tight bandages increase the risks of irritation, redness, and blistering.

Nondrug Measures

There are simple physical methods of inducing counterirritation. Perhaps the most frequently used method is heat applied by means of a heat lamp, hot water bottle, heating pad, or moist steam pack. Heat helps restore the elastic property of collagen. Heat also acts selectively on free nerve endings in the tissue and on peripheral nerve fibers to increase the pain threshold. This results in an analgesic effect. Heat should be applied with extreme caution, if at all, in conjunction with a counterirritant preparation.

Massaging the painful area is another method of producing counterirritation. Massage increases the flow of blood and lymph in the skin and underlying structures. Many clinicians have found that massage is therapeutically beneficial in select situations and use it extensively.

Patient Counseling

Precautions

Pharmacists should provide the following important information to patients using counterirritant preparations:

- This product is for external use only. If you accidentally swallow some of the product, contact a poison information center or physician immediately.

- Do not use this product near the eyes or apply it to mucous membranes.

- Do not apply this product to open wounds or to broken, damaged, or sunburned skin.

- Discontinue use of this product if your condition worsens or improves only briefly. If symptoms persist for more than 7 days or if the pain is constant and felt in any position, consult a physician.

- Do not apply this product more than three or four times a day, except on the advice and under the supervision of a physician.

- Massage only a small amount into the affected area of your skin.

- Avoid excessive exposure to sunlight or sunlamps after using this product. Do not use a hot water bottle or electric heating pad concurrently with this product. Do not apply this product before a sauna or professional massage.

- If you apply a covering over this product, do not bandage it tightly.

- Wash your hands thoroughly after applying this product. If arthritic hand joints are the site, wait 30 minutes after application before washing them.

- Do not handle or insert contact lenses following application without washing your hands.

- Do not apply this product on children under 2 years of age, except on the advice and under the supervision of a physician.

- Keep this and all other medications out of the reach of children.

Adverse Effects

Some individuals overreact to the irritant properties of counterirritants and develop rashes and blisters. In addition to irritation, counterirritants also may produce sensitization, in which case immune complexes are involved. It may be difficult to distinguish between direct topical irritation and topical sensitization. Skin in sensitive areas (e.g., behind the knees) may be particularly susceptible to irritation.

Drug Interactions

Concern has recently arisen concerning interaction between external analgesics and the anticoagulant warfarin. Such interactions may be prevented by the following precautions:

- Know all the drugs the patient is taking;

- Restrict drugs to those that are genuinely indicated and keep therapy as simple as possible;

- Educate the patient on the importance of not changing or adding to the medication, whether prescription or nonprescription, without first consulting a physician or pharmacist;

- Avoid occasional use of drugs known to cause clinically important interactions; and

- Keep changes in drug therapy to a minimum and monitor coagulation status closely for a number of weeks after any changes.

Chapter 6

Vaginal and Menstrual Products

Questions to ask in patient assessment and counseling

- What symptoms are you experiencing?
- How severe are they?
- At what time in the menstrual cycle do your symptoms occur?
- Are these symptoms the same as or different from symptoms you have experienced in previous menstrual cycles?
- Are your menses heavier or lighter than usual?
- Have you experienced any unusual bleeding? At midcycle?
- Is your menstrual cycle shorter or longer than usual?
- Have you missed a period?
- Have you experienced an abnormal vaginal discharge? Has it been discolored or accompanied by itching and burning or by an abnormal odor?
- Have you experienced vaginal dryness or difficult or painful sexual intercourse?
- Have you experienced abdominal cramping, lower abdominal pain, or lower back pain?
- Have you experienced one or more of the following symptoms just prior to your period: mood swings, low self-esteem, depression, anger, anxiety, jumpiness, lack of energy, difficulty concentrating, food craving, insomnia, weight gain, fluid retention, breast tenderness, or bloating?
- Are you now experiencing a high fever, dizziness, nausea, vomiting, diarrhea, rash, muscle aches, or mental confusion? Is there a relationship between the onset of these symptoms and your menstrual period?
- Do you use menstrual pads or tampons?
- Do you use contraception? If so, which method?
- What medication(s) are you taking?
- What medication(s) have you taken previously to control your symptoms?
- Are you allergic or hypersensitive to any drugs? If yes, which one(s)?

Vaginal Disorders and Feminine Hygiene

Normal vaginal physiologic mechanisms maintain an environment that discourages the overgrowth of pathogenic organisms. When this environment is altered, the potential for

---

Editor's Note: This chapter is adapted from Leslie A. Shimp and Constance M. Fleming, "Vaginal and Menstrual Products," in Covington, T.R., ed. *Handbook of Nonprescription Drugs,* 11th edition, which is based, in part, on the 10th edition chapter "Menstrual Products," and has been updated and expanded to include discussions of vaginal infections and douching. The core material of these discussions appeared in the 10th edition chapters "Topical Anti-Infective Products," written by Dennis P. West and Susan V. Maddux, and "Personal Care Products," written by Donald R. Miller and Mary Kuzel. For a more extensive discussion of this topic, readers are encouraged to consult Chapter 6 of the *Handbook.*

infection is increased. About 40% of women who experience vaginal symptoms have some type of vaginal infection.

Vaginal Infections

Common symptoms of vaginitis may include vaginal discharge, pruritus, irritation, soreness, dysuria (pain on urination), and dyspareunia (pain during sexual intercourse). Distinguishing one infection from another is often difficult. Symptoms may be similar for different infections, and characteristic symptoms may be absent in some patients. Nevertheless, in view of the large number of women seeking diagnosis and treatment for vaginal infections and the recent Food and Drug Administration (FDA) approval of nonprescription antifungal compounds for vaginal use, it is imperative that the pharmacist be able to help patients decide about the appropriateness of self-treatment and understand the therapeutic management of vaginal infections.

Types of Vaginal Infections

Three types of infections account for most vaginal symptoms: bacterial vaginosis, candidal vulvovaginitis, and trichomoniasis. Infections may also be mixed, with more than one causative organism, and vaginal symptoms may be noninfectious (e.g., atrophic vaginitis, allergic or chemical dermatologic reaction).

Bacterial Vaginosis. Bacterial vaginosis is the most common type of vaginal infection in women of childbearing age. The organisms responsible for this infection are not well defined.

Half of the women with bacterial vaginosis are asymptomatic; the other half report a vaginal discharge with a "fishy" odor that is most prominent following intercourse. Standard diagnostic criteria require that three of four conditions be present: (1) a vaginal pH of greater than 4.5, (2) the presence of clue cells, (3) a positive amine test producing a fishy odor, and (4) a homogeneous vaginal discharge. Predisposing factors are thought to include pregnancy, the use of an intrauterine device, lactation, and sexual activity, particularly the onset of a new sexual relationship or intercourse with multiple partners. In general, bacterial vaginosis is benign. However, it may be associated with pelvic inflammatory disease (PID), preterm labor and premature rupture of the fetal membranes, and urinary tract infections.

Trichomoniasis. Trichomoniasis is caused by the protozoa Trichomonas vaginalis and is classified as a sexually transmitted disease (STD). Repeat occurrences are common. It accounts for 15%–20% of all vaginal infections.

Trichomoniasis is primarily a disease of young women; two thirds of cases occur in women less than 30 years of age. Other predisposing factors are sexual activity, multiple sex partners, pregnancy, and menopause. Between 50% and 75% of women complain of a profuse, frothy, or foamy vaginal discharge. This discharge may be white, yellow, gray, or green and may be malodorous. Less frequently, women report lower abdominal pain, pruritus, or "strawberry" spots. These symptoms most commonly occur during or immediately following menstruation. Between 10% and 50% of women are asymptomatic.

Candidal Vulvovaginitis. About 75% of women experience at least one candidal vaginal infection during their childbearing years, and up to 40% experience a subsequent infection. Less than 5% experience recurrent candidal vulvovaginitis. Candida fungi are the causative organisms of this vaginal infection; about 85% of cases are caused by Candida albicans. The incidence of non-albicans candidal infections has increased in the last two decades, and Candida tropicalis and Candida glabrata now account for a significant minority of candidal vaginal infections. Candidal vulvovaginitis has also been referred to as "yeast infection" and "moniliasis."

The characteristic symptoms are intense pruritus; a thick, whitish vaginal discharge (often referred to as "curdlike" or "cottage cheese–like") with no offensive odor; and vulvar or vaginal erythema. Most symptomatic women experience vaginal or vulvar pruritus or irritation, but fewer than one half report a vaginal discharge and few report an odor to the discharge.

Possible risk factors include pregnancy, the use of estrogen-containing oral contraceptives, diabetes mellitus, treatment with broad-spectrum antibiotics or immunosuppressant drugs, human immunodeficiency virus (HIV) infection, and sexual activity.

Assessment of Vaginal Infections

Candidal vulvovaginitis is the only vaginal infection for which effective nonprescription treatment is available. Many patients prefer to self-treat empirically for presumed vulvovaginal candidiasis. Pharmacists can advise patients when it is appropriate to self-treat for vaginal symptoms and when physician evaluation is indicated.

Self-treatment is most appropriate when the woman (1) has infrequent vaginal symptoms (no more than three vaginal infections per year and no vaginal infection within the last 2 months); (2) has previously had physician-diagnosed candidal vulvovaginitis; and (3) has current symptoms consistent with the characteristic signs and mild to moderate symptoms of candidal vulvovaginitis.

Self-treatment is inappropriate for pregnant women and for girls under 12 years of age. Patients with concurrent symptoms such as fever or pain in the lower abdomen, back, or shoulder should be referred for evaluation by a physician, as should patients who are taking certain medications (e.g., systemic corticosteroids, antineoplastic agents) or who have medical conditions (e.g., diabetes mellitus, HIV infection) that may predispose them to candidal infections.

Self-treatment is not appropriate for recurrent vaginal symptoms (i.e., four or more documented infections within a 12-month period). Recurrent candidal infections often require long-term suppressive prophylactic therapy. Finally, frequent or recurrent episodes of vulvovaginal candidal may be an early sign of HIV infection. The FDA now requires that nonprescription products for the treatment of vulvovaginal candidal infection have a label to that effect.

An algorithm for an appropriate approach to the patient with vaginal symptoms is presented in Figure 1.

Drug Treatment of Vaginal Infections

Vaginal Antibacterial/Antiprotozoal Agents. The treatment of bacterial vaginosis and trichomoniasis usually requires prescription medications. Metronidazole vaginal gel in a 0.75% concentration (MetroGel-Vaginal) and clindamycin vaginal cream in a 2% concentration (Cleocin) are approved for the treatment of bacterial vaginosis. Clindamycin cream is the treatment of choice for women during their first trimester of pregnancy. The standard therapy for trichomoniasis is currently oral metronidazole (Prostat, Flagyl) as a single 2-g dose, as a 1-g dose taken twice a day for 1 day, or as a 250-mg or 500-mg dose taken three times a day for 7 days.

Vaginal Antifungal Agents. Currently, recommended initial therapy for candidal vulvovaginitis is with an imidazole product.

There are currently four topical imidazole derivatives available in the United States for treating candidal vulvovaginitis: butoconazole, clotrimazole, miconazole, and tioconazole. Terconazole is often grouped with the imidazoles but is more appropriately classified as a triazole. At this time, clotrimazole, miconazole, and butoconazole are available as nonprescription medications (Table 1). Studies have shown the imidazoles to be equally effective and without major toxicities; effectiveness rates are approximately 85%–90%. Side effects from topical therapy are minimal, the most common are local burning or itching.

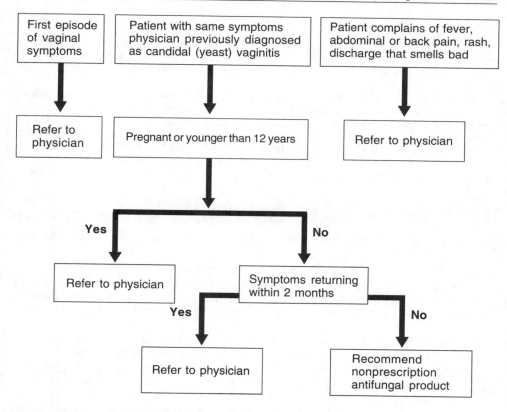

FIGURE 1 Management of patients with symptoms of a vaginal infection.

TABLE 1 Nonprescription vaginal antifungal preparations

Agent (Brand name)	Dosage form
Clotrimazole (Gyne-Lotrimin, Mycelex-7, generic)	1% cream (45 g) 100-mg tablets (7) Combination pack (7 tablets and 7 g of cream)
Miconazole (Monistat-7, generic)	2% cream (45 g) Prefilled applicators 100-mg suppository Combination pack (7 tablets and 7 g of cream)
Butoconazole (Femstat)	2% cream (20 g) Prefilled applicators (35 g)

Reprinted from *Drug Topics Redbook.* Montvale, NJ: Medical Economics; 1995: 526–607.

The success rates of the topical imidazoles and triazoles in the treatment of candidal vulvovaginitis are similar.

Selection of cream, tablet, or suppository formulations can be left to patient preference. If vulvar symptoms are significant, a cream preparation or the combination of a cream and vaginal suppositories/tablets is preferable so that vulvar application can accompany intravaginal administration.

Directions for proper use of these products are listed in Table 2. These directions should be discussed with the patient, preferably in a private counseling area. The pharmacist should also inform the patient of potential local reactions, including temporary burning, itching, and irritation. The patient must be instructed to stop using the antifungal product and call her physician if she develops abdominal cramping, headache, urticaria, hives, or skin rash. Women should be instructed to continue therapy if menses begin during the course of therapy. Some patients object to using the vaginal antifungals during menses;

Table 2 Directions for using vaginal antifungal products

1. Start the treatment at night before going to bed. A supine position will reduce leakage of the product from the vagina.

2. Wash the entire vaginal area with mild soap and water and dry completely before applying the product.

3. Unscrew the cap and place the cap upside down on the end of the tube. Push down firmly until the seal is broken. (For vaginal tablets/suppositories, remove the protective wrapper.)

4. Attach the applicator to the tube by turning the applicator clockwise. (For vaginal tablets/suppositories, place the product into the end of the applicator barrel.)

5. Squeeze the tube from the bottom to force the cream into the applicator. Do this until the inside piece of the applicator is pushed out as far as possible and the applicator is completely filled with cream. Remove the applicator from the tube.

6. Standing with your feet slightly apart and your knees bent or lying on your back with your knees bent, gently insert the applicator into the vagina as far as it will go comfortably. Push the inside piece of the applicator in and place the cream as far back in the vagina as possible. (For vaginal tablets/suppositories, insert the applicator into the vagina and press plunger until it stops to deposit the product.) Remove the applicator from the vagina. You may want to wear a sanitary pad during the time you are using the vaginal product, because some leakage will likely occur. Do not use a tampon to prevent leakage.

7. Recap the tube (if using cream) and clean the applicator by pulling the two pieces apart and washing them with soap and warm water.

8. Continue using the product according to product instructions.

9. Complete the full course of therapy and use on consecutive days, even during menstrual flow.

10. Avoid sexual contact during treatment. If intercourse does occur, do not use condoms, diaphrams, or cervical caps; the antifungal may damage the contraceptive device and increase the risk of pregnancy.

11. If no improvement is noted after 3 days, if symptoms worsen after 3 days, or if symptoms are still present after you have completed the course of therapy, contact your physician.

postponement of treatment may be reasonable. The pharmacist should also emphasize the importance of continuing therapy despite early symptomatic relief.

The patient should also be instructed to obtain a physician evaluation if there has been no improvement or worsening of symptoms after 3 days of therapy, if symptoms are incompletely resolved after the full course of therapy, or if symptoms recur within 2 months of stopping therapy.

Other Drug Treatments for Candidiasis.   Other topical vaginal agents that have been used to treat candidiasis include povidone-iodine, gentian violet, boric acid, and Lactobacillus preparations. Nonspecific nonprescription preparations, including Vagisil and Yeast-Gard (benzocaine and resorcinol) and Vaginex (tripelennamine), are rarely appropriate, given the superior efficacy and other advantages of the imidazole derivatives.

Nondrug Measures

Consumption of yogurt has also been suggested as a measure to decrease candidal vulvovaginitis, particularly for women who experience recurrent infections. Home remedies such as vaginal douches are generally not effective.

Vaginal Douche Products

Douching is a relatively common practice; more than half of all women douche regularly or intermittently. Douche products are available as liquids, liquid concentrates to be diluted with water, powders to be dissolved in water, and powders to be instilled as powders (see product table "Feminine Hygiene Products" in *Nonprescription Products: Formulations & Features*). Premixed douche products in disposable applicators are widely available and convenient to use.

An alternative cleansing method involves gently washing the vagina and vulvar, perineal, and anal regions with the fingers using lukewarm water and mild soap.

Douche Ingredients

Table 3 summarizes the types of ingredients that may be contained in douche products.

Douche Equipment

Two types of syringes are available for douching purposes: the douche bag and the bulb douche syringes. The douche bag (fountain syringe or folding feminine syringe) holds 1–2 quarts of fluid and comes with tubing and a shut-off valve. Two types of tips are supplied, one for enema use (the shorter rectal nozzle) and one for douching. The two tips are not interchangeable.

Bulb douche syringes are available as disposable and nondisposable products. The flow rate is regulated by the amount of hand pressure exerted when the bulb is squeezed. Gentle pressure is recommended because excess pressure may force fluid through the cervix and cause inflammation.

Potential Adverse Effects of Douches

Frequent douching may lead to an increased risk for PID, sterility, and/or ectopic pregnancy. Additional problems include irritation or sensitization from douche ingredients and disruption of normal vaginal flora and vaginal pH. Douching may alter the vaginal chemical environment, leading to an increased risk for acquiring a sexually transmitted disease or cervical cancer. Manufacturers recommend that women who suspect that they have PID or any sexually transmitted disease stop douching and immediately consult a physician.

Table 3 Douche ingredients

Antimicrobial agents

- Examples: benzethonium, benzalkonium, boric acid, cetylpyridinium
- Therapeutic antimicrobial activity highly questionable in concentrations present in these products
- Local irritation, sensitization, and contact dermatitis possible; if these symptoms develop, instruct patient to discontinue use of product and consult a health care provider

Counterirritants

- Examples: eucalyptol, menthol, phenol
- Efficacy as local anesthetic or antipruritic agents has not been substantiated

Astringents

- Examples: ammonium, potassium alums
- Intended to reduce local edema, inflammation, and exudation
- Act as irritants in moderate or high concentrations but ineffective if too dilute

Proteolytics

- Example: papain
- Helps to remove excess vaginal discharge.
- May elicit inflammatory and allergic reactions

Surfactants

- Examples: docusate sodium, nonoxynol 4
- Intended to facilitate spread of douche over vaginal mucosa and penetration of mucosal folds
- Cosmetic or clinical value not readily apparent

Substances affecting pH

- Examples: Sodium perborate (for alkalinity), lactic acid, acetic acid (for acidity)
- Vinegar-and-water douche: prepare by mixing 1/4–1/3 cup household white vinegar with 2 quarts warm water

Povidone-iodine

- Greater potential than acetic acid douches to reduce total bacteria
- May allow pathogenic species to proliferate, increasing the risk for vaginal infection
- Should not be used by individuals allergic to iodine-containing products
- Absorption poses a particular hazard to pregnant women

Douching Guidelines

To use douches safely, appropriately, and effectively, patients should be instructed as follows:

- Strictly follow the manufacturer's instructions.
- Keep all douche equipment clean.
- Use lukewarm water to dilute products.
- Never instill a douche with forceful pressure.
- Do not use these products for birth control.
- Do not douche until at least 8 hours after intercourse if a diaphragm, cervical cap, or contraceptive jelly, cream, or foam is used.
- Do not douche 24–48 hours before any gynecologic examination.

Menstruation and Menstrual Disorders

During their menstrual periods, some women experience abdominal pain and cramping, headache, and fluid retention. Many women use nonprescription products and seek advice from a pharmacist on how best to manage their symptoms. The pharmacist should be familiar with common menstrual symptoms and disorders, as well as with the risks associated with the misuse of menstrual products (e.g., toxic shock syndrome). See pages 98–100 of the *Handbook* for a discussion of the physiology of the menstrual cycle.

Menstrual Disorders

Dysmenorrhea

Dysmenorrhea (i.e., difficult or painful menstruation) occurs in an estimated 50% of postpubescent women.

Types. Dysmenorrhea is divided into primary and secondary disease. Primary dysmenorrhea is idiopathic and is associated with pain at the time of menstruation with no identifiable organic pelvic disease. It usually develops within 6–12 months of menarche and generally affects women during their teenage years and early twenties. Primary dysmenorrhea pain lasts from a few hours up to 48–72 hours. Although it is experienced as lower midabdominal or suprapubic pain, which is cramping in nature, the pain may radiate to the lower back and upper thighs and may be accompanied by symptoms such as nausea, vomiting, fatigue, nervousness, dizziness, diarrhea, and headache.

Secondary dysmenorrhea is usually associated with pelvic pathology. Possible causes include endometriosis, PID, ovarian cysts, benign uterine tumors, endometrial cancer, adhesions, cervical stenosis, and congenital abnormalities. Secondary dysmenorrhea may also be caused by the presence of intrauterine devices. Because symptoms of dysmenorrhea are similar to those of endometriosis, ectopic pregnancy, and PID, physician evaluation is necessary. Secondary dysmenorrhea is suggested if dysmenorrhea initially appears years after menarche or occurs throughout the duration of menstrual flow; if the patient experiences irregular menstrual cycles or menorrhagia; or if the patient has a history of PID or infertility.

Etiology. A number of other factors have been associated with the occurrence or severity of dysmenorrhea. The decrease in incidence and severity of dysmenorrhea with age may be related to pregnancy, because during late pregnancy, uterine adrenergic nerves virtually disappear and only a portion regenerate after childbirth. Lifestyle alterations may also alleviate symptoms to varying degrees. Smoking tobacco or consuming excessive amounts of ethanol has been associated with more severe dysmenorrhea. Evidence regarding the benefit of exercise is conflicting.

Assessment. Before recommending any product to a patient experiencing symptoms of dysmenorrhea, the pharmacist should establish the onset of pain in relation to the onset of menses. Primary dysmenorrhea produces abdominal and lower back pain that begins within 1–2 days before the onset of menses and ceases during the first several days of menstrual blood flow. Pain that does not follow this pattern and that is severe or different from pain occurring during previous menstrual cycles should be evaluated promptly by a physician. It is important that adolescents who experience symptoms be educated about dysmenorrhea and realize this condition can be treated with products that can provide symptomatic relief. They should also be reassured that dysmenorrhea is relatively common.

Treatment. For mild symptoms, an analgesic agent such as acetaminophen or aspirin and the application of local heat to the abdomen or lower back may be adequate.

Before recommending aspirin, the pharmacist should question the patient about allergy or intolerance to aspirin, disease states that are relative contraindications to aspirin therapy (e.g., peptic ulcer disease, gastritis, bleeding disorders, asthma, or renal insufficiency), and current medication usage. Clinically significant aspirin–drug interactions occur with anticoagulants, probenecid, phenytoin, oral hypoglycemics, and high doses of antacids.

The principal nonprescription agents for the treatment of moderate dysmenorrhea are nonsteroidal anti-inflammatory drugs (NSAIDs), which inhibit the production and action of prostaglandins. Three NSAIDs are available as nonprescription products: ibuprofen 200 mg; naproxen sodium 220 mg; and ketoprofen 12.5 mg. Therapy should begin at the onset of pain after menstrual flow begins and be continued for the first 48–72 hours of menstrual flow, because this is when prostaglandin release is maximal. Optimal pain relief is achieved when these agents are taken on a scheduled rather than an as-needed basis.

Each of these agents has a side effect profile: naproxen sodium is more likely to cause drowsiness, shortness of breath, and tinnitus than is ibuprofen or ketoprofen; ketoprofen and naproxen are associated with a greater incidence of fluid retention, constipation, and headache than is ibuprofen; and ketoprofen is more likely to cause gas/bloating, diarrhea, or nervousness/irritability than is ibuprofen or naproxen. Side effects from a few days of use are limited. Those most commonly associated with short-term NSAID therapy include gastrointestinal (GI) symptoms (e.g., upset stomach, vomiting, heartburn, abdominal pain, diarrhea, constipation, and anorexia) and central nervous system side effects (e.g., headache and dizziness). The GI side effects of these agents may be decreased by taking the drugs with food.

Relative contraindications to the use of these NSAIDs include a history of allergy to aspirin (bronchospastic reaction) or to any other NSAID, active GI disease (e.g., peptic ulcer disease, gastroesophageal reflux disease, or ulcerative colitis), and bleeding disorders.

The patient with more severe dysmenorrhea or with dysmenorrhea that does not respond to nonprescription therapy should be referred to a physician.

Amenorrhea

Amenorrhea is defined as the absence or abnormal cessation of menses.

Types. Primary amenorrhea is the term used for the disorder when a female adolescent does not begin menstruation. Amenorrhea is diagnosed if menses has not occurred by age 14 in a female who has not had any secondary sexual development, or by age 16 in a female whose secondary sexual development has occurred. *Secondary amenorrhea* refers to a cessation of menses for 3 months or longer in a woman who was previously having menses.

Etiology. Possible causes include gonadal failure, reproductive tract anomalies, emotional stress, weight loss or gain, poor nutrition, anorexia nervosa, excessive exercise, hyperthyroidism, hypothyroidism, and previous exposure to radiation or chemotherapy used to treat childhood malignancies. Exercise-induced amenorrhea can be manifested as either primary or secondary amenorrhea, depending on the age at which intense athletic training occurs.

Treatment. Treatment of primary amenorrhea caused by gonadal failure may be managed by hormone replacement therapy. Chromosome disorders and reproductive tract anomalies often require a combination of hormone replacement and surgical therapy.

Normogonadotropic amenorrhea can be caused by malnutrition or excessive exercise. To resume menses, these patients should modify their lifestyle; such modifications may include reduced exercise, reduced stress, and adequate intakes of calcium, caloric fat, and protein. Many athletes are reluctant to gain weight or decrease their intensity of physical training. In this case, treatment with combined oral contraceptives may be instituted to protect against the loss of bone mass caused by the low estrogen levels associated with exercise-associated amenorrhea.

Amenorrhea caused by psychologic trauma or emotional stress often resolves with psychotherapeutic counseling.

Menorrhagia

Menorrhagia is excessive menstrual blood loss occurring with either menses lasting for more than 7 days or a total blood loss of more than 60–80 mL of blood. Menorrhagia is one of the most common causes of iron deficiency in women of reproductive age.

Etiology. Systemic illnesses and endocrine disorders (e.g., renal and hepatic disease, uterine tumors or polyps, thyroid dysfunction, and diabetes mellitus) may cause menorrhagia. A number of medications, including anticoagulants, oral contraceptives, postmenopausal hormone replacement therapy, oral or intramuscular progestins, neuroleptics, and chemotherapy, can cause abnormal vaginal bleeding. Intrauterine devices may also cause excessive menses.

Treatment. Estrogen–progestin combination oral contraceptives are effective in reducing menstrual blood loss. NSAIDs are also effective in decreasing menorrhagia. NSAIDs are most effective when given for several days premenstrually and then regularly during menses.

Dysfunctional Uterine Bleeding

Dysfunctional uterine bleeding (DUB) is a syndrome of irregular menses with periods of prolonged, heavy menstrual flow alternating with amenorrhea for which there is no identifiable etiology. DUB most commonly occurs during the first 2 years following menarche and during the perimenopausal period. It is usually the result of anovulatory cycles.

Treatment. In mild cases, therapy is initiated with just iron supplementation. If the condition is more severe, an estrogen–progestin combination oral contraceptive may be prescribed to regulate the menstrual cycle.

Midcycle Pain and Bleeding

This common type of intermenstrual bleeding, which may be accompanied by short-lived abdominal pain, is typically due to the decrease in ovarian estrogen production, which occurs at midcycle. It is self-limited and does not require therapy. Intermenstrual bleeding, commonly referred to as spotting or breakthrough bleeding, is also associated with use of an oral contraceptive, particularly during the first 3 months of therapy. Forgetting to take the pills or taking them at an inconsistent time every day can cause intermenstrual bleeding, as can drug interactions that may reduce the efficacy of the oral contraceptive. A sudden discontinuation of high-dose vitamin C ($\geq$1000 mg per day) can also cause spotting.

Premenstrual Syndrome

Premenstrual syndrome (PMS) can be defined as a cyclic disorder composed of a combination of physical and emotional (mood) changes that occur during the luteal phase of the menstrual cycle and improve significantly or disappear within the first several days of menstrual flow. Many theories have been developed to explain the etiology of PMS, but it remains unknown (see Table 4 on page 104 of the *Handbook*).

Symptoms. Physical or mood changes prior to the onset of menses are part of the normal menstrual cycle and are referred to medically as molimina. Common symptoms include minor weight gain, abdominal bloating, mild fatigue, and irritability. Only a small percentage of women, probably less than 10%, experience symptoms severe enough to meet the criteria in Table 4.

TABLE 4   Medications prescribed for treatment of PMS symptoms

Symptom	Drug therapy
Anxiety	Alprazolam; buspirone; transdermal estradiol
Depression/ mood swings	Vitamin B_6 (50 mg/day); antidepressants (TCA; SSRI); calcium (1000 mg/day); magnesium (360 mg/day); transdermal estradiol; danazol
Fatigue	Vitamin B_6 (50 mg/day)
Fluid retention	Spironolactone
Bloating	Calcium (1000 mg/day); magnesium (360 mg/day); transdermal estradiol; bromocriptine
Irritability	Vitamin B_6 (50 mg/day); calcium (1000 mg/day); danazol
Mastalgia	Evening primrose oil; danazol; bromocriptine; tamoxifen
Suppression of ovulation	Oral contraceptive (combined/progestin-only); progesterone; leuprolide

Information extracted from Parker PD. Premenstrual syndrome. *Am Fam Physician.* 1994; 50(6): 1309–17.

Treatment. The initial treatment of the symptoms of PMS is generally conservative, consisting of education and nondrug measures. Women should be educated about the syndrome and encouraged to elicit family support and understanding. Other recommendations include avoiding stress, developing mechanisms for managing stress, learning relaxation techniques, exercising, and making appropriate dietary alterations (e.g., lowering sodium intake and avoiding caffeine). For symptoms that are not responsive to nondrug therapy, a number of medications have been prescribed with variable and limited success (Table 4). Because PMS is a multisymptom disorder, a single therapeutic agent is unlikely to address all symptoms. Specific agents should be selected to address the major symptoms that the patient is experiencing.

One of the most common premenstrual complaints is fluid accumulation. Three nonprescription diuretics—ammonium chloride, caffeine, and pamabrom—are contained in commercially available menstrual products (see product table "Menstrual Products" in *Nonprescription Products: Formulations & Features*).

Ammonium chloride

■ Acid-forming salt with short duration of effect

■ Dose: up to 3 g/day (divided into three doses) for no more than 6 consecutive days

■ Larger doses can produce significant GI and central nervous system adverse effects

■ Contraindicated in patients with renal or liver impairment

Caffeine

■ Dose: 100–200 mg every 3 to 4 hours

■ Tolerance may develop to the diuretic effect

■ May cause anxiety, restlessness, insomnia, and GI irritation

■ Additive side effects possible with concomitant consumption of caffeine-containing beverages and foods or other caffeine-containing medications

Pamabrom

■ Dose: up to 200 mg/day

■ Contained in combination products with analgesics and antihistamines for the treatment of PMS

The NSAIDs have shown some evidence of efficacy in managing symptoms of PMS. These agents may be most useful for women who experience both dysmenorrhea and PMS; reducing symptoms associated with dysmenorrhea may help improve a woman's ability to tolerate PMS-related symptoms. Several smooth-muscle relaxants, antihistamines, sympathomimetic amines, and herbal preparations have also been evaluated for the treatment of dysmenorrhea and PMS, but none of these agents is classified as safe and effective.

Atrophic Vaginitis and Vaginal Dryness

Etiology and Symptoms. At menopause, vaginal lubrication declines secondary to the decrease in estrogen levels. Atrophic vaginitis is inflammation of the vagina related to atrophy of the vaginal mucosa secondary to decreased estrogen levels. Symptoms include vaginal irritation, burning, itching, and dyspareunia. The most common cause of secondary superficial dyspareunia is also a lack of adequate vaginal lubrication. This condition is most common in postmenopausal women and breast-feeding women. The pharmacist should inquire about the onset of these symptoms; self-treatment is most appropriate for those women who have previously been able to maintain adequate vaginal lubrication. Severe vaginal dryness or dyspareunia should be evaluated by a physician.

Treatment. Vaginal dryness can often be treated with topical lubricants (see product table "Vaginal Lubricants" in *Nonprescription Products: Formulations & Features*). The pharmacist should question patients about the use of any vaginal or feminine hygiene products because such products may cause or worsen vaginal irritation and dyspareunia.

Water-soluble lubricants (e.g., Gyne-Moistrin, K-Y Jelly, and Replens) and moisturizing skin lotions (e.g., Lubriderm and Keri-lotion) are acceptable vaginal lubricants. Vaseline should not be used. If the patient is using a condom or diaphragm, only water-soluble lubricants should be used because other products may impair the efficacy of these contraceptive methods. Water-soluble lubricant gels can be applied both externally and internally. Initially, the patient should be instructed to use a liberal quantity of lubricant (up to 2 tbsp) and then to tailor the quantity and frequency of use to her specific needs. If the patient is treating dyspareunia, the lubricant should be applied to both the vaginal opening and the penis. If nonprescription lubricants do not produce adequate benefit or are aesthetically unappealing to the patient, oral or topical estrogen replacement therapy may be prescribed.

The Pharmacist's Role in Assessment of Menstrual Disorders

Before recommending any product, the pharmacist should obtain a clear and complete description of the patient's current symptoms, including their severity, onset, similarity to symptoms experienced during other menstrual cycles, relationship to onset of menstrual bleeding, and the patient's explanation for their occurrence. The pharmacist should also gather information on current medication therapy, treatment previously tried, outcome of prior therapy (efficacy, dose, duration, side effects), drug allergies, hypersensitivities, or intolerances, and whether symptoms were evaluated by a physician. All conditions of menstrual dysfunction (i.e., amenorrhea, menorrhagia, DUB, and midcycle pain and bleeding), with the exception of minor midcycle pain and bleeding, should be evaluated by a physician. The pharmacist should instruct the patient to see a physician for any of the following problems:

- Abnormal vaginal bleeding or discharge;
- Atrophic vaginitis or vaginal dryness;
- Dyspareunia;
- Irregular menstrual cycles or amenorrhea or dysmenorrhea;
- Significant alterations in mood; and
- Breast tenderness.

Pharmacists discussing premenstrual symptoms with patients should emphasize that minor symptoms such as bloating and weight gain, fatigue, irritability, mood swings, changes in appetite, and breast tenderness are not uncommon. In addition, pharmacists should inquire about prior self-treatment and discuss any potential dangers inherent in prior therapy (e.g., neuropathy associated with vitamin B_6 therapy). Pharmacists should also dispel myths about the effect of the menstrual cycle on the ability of women to function normally.

Menstrual Products and Toxic Shock Syndrome

Feminine Cleansing Products

The pharmacist should be familiar with feminine hygiene products and should know how to advise a patient regarding their appropriate use and which symptoms related to their use require referral to a physician.

Feminine Pads and Tampons

Feminine pads are used to absorb menstrual and other vaginal discharges. They are available in a wide variety of sizes and absorbencies. Frequent changing of sanitary pads and applying powder to the inner thighs may alleviate chafing. Many women prefer the new, less cumbersome light pads for the first and last days of their cycles. These light pads may also be used to protect undergarments from being stained by vaginal creams, vaginal tablets, suppository leakage, or normal vaginal secretions.

Tampons are intravaginal inserts designed to absorb menstrual and other vaginal discharges. They have the advantage over feminine pads of being worn internally, which lessens chafing, odor, bulkiness, and irritation. Some tampons are scented, and some fragrances may cause local irritation and allergic reactions, such as allergic contact dermatitis.

Toxic Shock Syndrome (TSS)

Toxic shock syndrome is a term used to describe a severe multisystem illness characterized by high fever, profound hypotension, severe diarrhea, mental confusion, renal failure, erythroderma, and skin desquamation.

Incidence. TSS is divided into menstrual and nonmenstrual cases. About one third of TSS cases are of the nonmenstrual type. TSS can occur in both men and women; about one third of the nonmenstrual cases occur in men. Menstrual TSS primarily affects women between the ages of 15–19 years. One reason for the greater incidence in young women is the absence of preexisting antibodies to the TSS toxin. By the age of 20–25, more than 90% of both men and women have detectable antibodies to this toxin.

Etiology/Manifestation. TSS is a life-threatening disease. Known to result from infections (at any site) with toxin-producing strains of *Staphylococcus aureus,* TSS is essentially a consequence of the systemic effects of the toxin. The major cause of TSS is TSST-1, an exotoxin produced by 90%–100% of the strains of S aureus associated with menstrual TSS and by 60%–75% of the strains associated with nonmenstrual TSS.

The clinical manifestations of TSS characteristically evolve quite rapidly. Within 8–12 hours an individual can move from a state of good health to full-blown TSS, which includes high fever, myalgias, vomiting and diarrhea, erythroderma, decreased urine output, severe hypotension, and shock. Dermatologic manifestations are characteristic of TSS; both the early rash and subsequent skin desquamation are required for a definite diagnosis. The early rash, which usually appears on the lower abdomen and thighs, is often described as a sunburnlike, diffuse, macular erythroderma that is not pruritic.

Risk Factors. The strongest predictor of risk for menstrual TSS is the use of tampons. To decrease the likelihood of TSS, tampon manufacturers altered the composition and lowered the absorbency of tampons. In addition, the FDA changed the requirement for the labeling of tampons so that terms such as regular and super, which are used to indicate the absorbency of tampons, have a uniform meaning and indicate a specific range of fluid absorbed per tampon. Higher-absorbency products (>15 g) are not prohibited, but no products are currently marketed with these higher absorbencies. The risk for TSS continues to be greater in tampon users than in other individuals, and the greatest risk is associated with the use of higher-absorbency tampons.

In addition to tampons, the risk for TSS has been associated with the use of all barrier contraceptives, including diaphragms, cervical caps, and cervical sponges.

The Pharmacist's Role in TSS Counseling. A pharmacist should be able to counsel a patient about the prevention of TSS, emphasizing that the risk for this condition is quite small; recent data suggest an incidence of 1–2.5 per 100,000 menstruating women. Avoidance or reduction of risk can be accomplished if patients follow the guidelines listed below:

- To reduce the risk for TSS to almost zero, use sanitary pads instead of tampons.
- To lower the risk for TSS while using tampons, use the lowest-absorbency tampons compatible with your needs and alternate the use of menstrual pads (e.g., at night) with the use of tampons. Changing them at least four to six times per day is suggested.
- Wash hands with soap before inserting anything into the vagina.
- Follow instructions for vaginal contraceptive products carefully. A sponge or diaphragm or cervical cap should not be left in place in the vagina longer than recommended and should not be used during a menstrual period.
- Do not use tampons, contraceptive sponges, or a cervical cap during the first 12 weeks after childbirth. It may be best to avoid using a diaphragm as well.
- Read the insert on TSS enclosed in the tampon package and become familiar with the early symptoms of TSS. These include a high fever, muscle aches, a sunburnlike rash, weakness, fatigue, nausea, vomiting, and diarrhea.
- If the early symptoms of TSS occur, remove the tampon immediately and seek emergency medical treatment.

Women who have had TSS are at higher risk for recurrent episodes, especially during the first year after the illness. Prevention of TSS for these patients includes avoidance of tampons; administration of oral antistaphylococcal antibiotics during menses until there is a rise in the TSST-1 titer; and the use of nonbarrier forms of contraception, at least until the TSST-1 titers rise.

CHAPTER 7

Contraceptive Methods and Products

Questions to ask in patient assessment and counseling

- Are you now using a contraceptive method? What type?
- What contraceptive products have you used before?
- What did you like or dislike about your current or previous contraceptive method?
- Are you in a monogamous relationship now?
- What does your partner like or dislike about your current or previous contraceptive method?
- Have you discussed contraception and sexual health matters with your physician or another health care provider?
- Do you belong to a religious faith that has specific guidelines concerning family planning?
- Do you have children? Do you want additional children?
- Do you know what your risks are for being infected with the virus that causes AIDS or with other sexually transmitted diseases?
- How do you protect yourself from sexually transmitted diseases, including AIDS?

Uses for Contraceptive Products

Prevention of Unwanted Pregnancies

Consistent and proper use of a contraceptive, whether prescription or nonprescription, will significantly reduce the incidence of unwanted pregnancies. Oral contraceptives are the most widely used method of conception control in the United States; 39% of all women aged 15 to 44 use the birth control pill as their primary method of contraception. The next most prevalent method is sterilization of either the male or the female. After that, 25% of the women surveyed relied on condoms, 5% used spermicides, 4% used the diaphragm, and 1% had received a hormonal implant. Some patients reported using multiple methods. Overall, 94% of women aged 15 to 44 years reported using some form of birth control.

Prevention of Sexually Transmitted Diseases

Sexually active persons who do not use condoms place themselves at significant risk for acquiring a sexually transmitted disease (STD). Adolescents and young adults under the age of 25 years account for two thirds of all cases of STDs.

Types of Sexually Transmitted Diseases

There are more than 20 STDs, both bacterial and viral, that may have severe, long-standing consequences on the health and reproductive capabilities of those infected. The presence

---

Editor's Note: This chapter is adapted from Louise Parent-Stevens and David L. Lourwood, "Contraceptive Methods and Products," in Covington, T.R., ed., *Handbook of Nonprescription Drugs*, 11th edition, which is based, in part, on the chapter with the same title that appeared in the 10th edition but was written by Louise Parent-Stevens and Roberta S. Carrier. For a more extensive discussion of this topic, readers are encouraged to consult Chapter 7 of the *Handbook*.

of some STDs may increase a person's susceptibility to and risk of acquiring the human immunodeficiency virus (HIV) infection.

AIDS. The known routes of transmission of acquired immunodeficiency syndrome (AIDS) are (1) blood and blood products (via transfusions, the sharing of contaminated needles and syringes, and accidental contamination from needle sticks); (2) mucous membrane exposures (saliva, seminal fluid, and vaginal fluids, including menstrual blood); and (3) perinatal and peripartum transmission to infants. In the United States, at least 65% of HIV infections are transmitted via heterosexual or homosexual intercourse.

Chlamydia. Chlamydia is an obligate intracellular parasite that often does not present with immediate symptoms for the female but may lead to pelvic inflammatory disease (PID), infertility, and chronic pelvic pain. It is the most common STD in the United States. Women infected with chlamydia most often present with a mucopurulent discharge from the cervix.

Men often present with nongonococcal urethritis (NGU). This infection is caused by chlamydia in up to 50% of cases, yet it may also be caused by other sexually transmittable organisms such as *Ureaplasma urealyticum, Trichomonas vaginalis,* and herpes simplex virus. Symptoms include dysuria, urinary frequency, and mucoid-to-purulent urethral discharge. Many men have asymptomatic infections. Several complications, including urethral strictures and epididymitis, may occur.

NGU may be transmitted to female sexual partners. Chlamydia may be transmitted by a pregnant woman to the fetus and result in neonatal infections such as ophthalmia or pneumonia.

Gonorrhea. Men who are symptomatic present with dysuria, increased urinary frequency, and a purulent urethral discharge. Women may have an abnormal vaginal discharge, abnormal menses, or dysuria. Gonorrhea may also present in the pharynx and anus. Up to one fourth of men infected with gonorrhea and as many as three fourths of women may be asymptomatic.

Up to 40% of untreated women with gonorrhea may develop PID. Men, when untreated, are at increased risk for epididymitis, urethral stricture, and sterility. In both sexes, gonorrhea may also disseminate to involve the skeletal, cardiovascular, and nervous systems. Gonorrhea may be transmitted to newborns.

Herpes Infections. Herpes genitalis is caused by herpes simplex virus types 1 or 2.

Both sexes may present with single or multiple vesicles, which are usually quite pruritic. These vesicles, which may appear anywhere on the genitalia, spontaneously rupture to form a shallow ulcer that may be quite painful. Lesions spontaneously resolve. First, or primary, infections often take longer to heal and are more often symptomatic. Subsequent, or recurrent, infections are usually milder and resolve quicker. Recurrent infections may be asymptomatic. Drug therapy for herpes only ameliorates the symptoms and hastens the healing of the ulcers. Patients with herpetic genital infections remain infectious all their lives. Patients are most infectious at the time of active occurrences.

Genital herpes has been associated with an increased risk for contracting HIV infections.

Syphilis. Primary syphilis presents with a painless, indurated chancre located at the site of exposure. In men, this chancre may appear on the penis; in women, the chancre may be difficult to see because it is found on the internal structures of the genital tract. Chancres may also appear inside the anus, in the pharynx, on the lips, or on the fingers.

The secondary stage of syphilis may present as a highly variable skin rash. Latent syphilis is asymptomatic. Sequelae of late disease include neurosyphilis, cardiovascular disease, and localized gumma formation.

Hepatitis B. Hepatitis B can be passed by sexual activity. Heterosexual intercourse is now the predominant mode of hepatitis B transmission.

Most hepatitis infections are asymptomatic. Symptoms, when noted, may include a serum sickness–like prodrome (skin eruptions, urticaria, arthralgia, and arthritis), lassitude, anorexia, nausea, vomiting, headache, fever, dark urine, jaundice, and moderate liver enlargement with tenderness. Long-term complications can include chronic active hepatitis, cirrhosis, hepatocellular carcinoma, hepatic failure, and death.

Trichomoniasis. Trichomoniasis is predominantly noted as a vaginal infection that presents with a frothy, excessive discharge; other symptoms include erythema, edema, and pruritus of the external genitalia. In some women, trichomoniasis may be asymptomatic. Men rarely present with symptoms but may present with urethritis, balanitis, or cutaneous lesions on the penis. Complications of trichomoniasis include common recurrent infections and infections secondary to excoriations. Increased risk of PID, low birth weight, and premature childbirth may occur.

Bacterial Vaginosis. Bacterial vaginosis is caused by several species of vaginal bacteria. Common symptoms include an excessive or malodorous vaginal discharge; erythema, edema, and pruritus of the external genitalia may also be seen. Recurrent infections may be common in untreated patients, as may be secondary infections due to excoriations. An increased risk of PID and premature childbirth may be common in patients with bacterial vaginosis.

Prevention of STDs

As health care practitioners in a position to offer much-needed health information, pharmacists must keep current in their knowledge of all aspects of the prevention and treatment of STDs, especially AIDS.

The only sure way to guard against infection with the HIV through sexual contact is to abstain from sex or to remain in a mutually monogamous relationship with an uninfected individual. If neither action is feasible, the next option is to use latex (not natural membrane) condoms for any oral, anal, or vaginal intercourse.

Laboratory data suggest that the spermicide nonoxynol-9 in proper concentrations may be somewhat effective in killing the AIDS virus and might offer additional protection when used with condoms. However, recent data have also indicated that spermicide-mediated vulvovaginal microabrasions could increase a woman's susceptibility to HIV.

Timing is important in the proper use of the male condom. Seminal fluid can leak from the erect penis in some men. This pre-ejaculatory fluid can contain HIV, other pathogens, and viable sperm. Thus, for proper use in safer sex, the condom must be placed on the penis well before contact is made with the partner's mouth, vagina, anus, or any broken skin. It is very important to emphasize that condom use does not guarantee safety because condoms can break.

Other contraceptive methods have also been studied for their efficacy in preventing transmission of AIDS. They have thus far shown limited protection against AIDS and other STDs (Table 1). Some STDs, such as syphilis and herpes, may be spread via external skin lesions. Condoms and spermicides may not be effective in preventing these types of infection.

Choice of Contraceptive Method

Pharmacists should be aware of the safety, effectiveness, accessibility, acceptability, and cost of the different contraceptive methods to help their patients make informed decisions. Safety factors to consider include the risk of side effects as well as protection against

TABLE 1   Effectiveness of contraceptives on bacterial and viral STDs

Contraceptive method	Bacterial STD	Viral STD
Latex male condoms	Protective	Protective
Polyurethane male condoms	Probably protective	Probably protective
Natural membrane condoms	Protective	Possibly not protective
Female condom	Possibly protective against recurrent vaginal trichomoniasis	Possibly protective
Spermicides	Protective against cervical gonorrhea and chlamydia	Undetermined in vivo
Diaphragms	Protective against cervical infection; associated with vaginal anaerobic overgrowth	Protective against cervical infection
Hormonal	Associated with increased cervical chlamydia, protective against symptomatic PID[a]	Not protective
Intrauterine device	Associated with PID in first month after insertion	Not protective
Natural family planning	Not protective	Not protective

[a]Pelvic inflammatory disease (PID).

Adapted with permission from Hatcher RA, Trussell J, Stewart G, et al. *Contraceptive Technology.* 16th rev ed. New York: Irvington Publishers; 1994: 81.

infectious STDs, including HIV. It is important that sexually active individuals who are infertile, through either surgical or natural causes, be aware that they are still at risk for contracting and transmitting STDs. Other safety considerations are the potential for method-associated adverse effects on future fertility as well as on the fetus, should unintended conception occur.

The effectiveness of a contraceptive method is reported in two ways: the accidental pregnancy rate in the first year of *perfect* use (method-related failure rate) and the accidental pregnancy rate in the first year of *typical* use (use-related failure rate) (Table 2). Reported use-related failure rates may vary, depending on the population studied. Effectiveness increases with increasing length of use of a particular method.

Important factors in determining a method's acceptability include user's religious beliefs and future reproductive plans, partner's support, complexity of method use, degree of interruption of spontaneity, "messiness," and cost. Advantages and disadvantages of the various contraceptive methods discussed below are summarized in Table 3.

TABLE 2   First-year failure/continuation rates of various contraceptive methods[a,b]

Method (1)	% who experience accidental pregnancy in first year of use	
	Typical use[a] (2)	Perfect use[b] (3)
Chance[c]	85	—
Spermicides[d]	21	6
Withdrawal	19	4
Natural family planning	20	—
Calendar (rhythm) method	—	9
Cervical mucus (ovulation) method	—	3
Symptothermal method[e]	—	2
Basal body temperature (postovulation) method	—	1
Cervical cap[f]		
Parous women	36	26
Nulliparous women	18	9
Diaphragm[f]	18	6
Condom[g]		
Male	12	3
Female	21–25[h]	5
Pill	3	—
Progestin only	—	0.5
Combined (estrogen/progestin)	—	0.1
Intrauterine device		
Progesterone T	2.0	1.5
Cu T 380A	0.8	0.6
Depo-Provera	0.3	0.3
Norplant (6 capsules)	0.09	0.09
Sterilization		
Female	0.4	0.4
Male	0.15	0.10

Note. Emergency contraceptive pills: Treatment initiated within 72 hours after unprotected intercourse reduces the risk of pregnancy by at least 75%. The treatment schedule is one dose as soon as possible (but no more than 72 hours) after unprotected intercourse and a second dose 12 hours after the first. The hormones that have been studied in the clinical trials of postcoital hormonal contraception are found in Nordette, Levlen, Lo/Ovral (one dose is four pills), Triphasil, Tri-Levlen (one dose is four yellow pills), and Ovral (one dose is two pills).

Lactational amenorrhea method: This is a highly effective, temporary method of contraception. However, to maintain effective protection against pregnancy, another method of contraception must be used as soon as menstruation resumes, the frequency or duration of breast-feeding is reduced, bottle feeding is introduced, or the baby reaches 6 months of age.

[a]Among typical couples who initiate use of a method (not necessarily for the first time), the percentage who experience an accidental pregnancy during the first year if they do not stop use for any other reason.

[b]Among couples who initiate use of a method (not necessarily for the first time) and who use it perfectly (both consistently and correctly), the percentage who experience an accidental pregnancy during the first year if they do not stop use for any other reason.

Continued on next page

cThe percentages failing in columns (2) and (3) are based on data from populations in whom contraception is not used and from women who cease using contraception to become pregnant. Among such populations, about 89% become pregnant within 1 year. This estimate was lowered slightly (to 85%) to represent the percentage who would become pregnant within 1 year among women now relying on reversible methods of contraception if they abandoned contraception altogether.

dFoams, creams, gels, vaginal suppositories, and vaginal film.

eCervical mucus (ovulation) method supplemented by calendar in the preovulatory phase and by BBT in the postovulatory phase.

fWith spermicidal cream or jelly.

gWithout spermicides.

hExtrapolated from 6-month failure rates.

Adapted with permission from Hatcher RA, Trussell J, Stewart G, et al. *Contraceptive Technology.* 16th rev ed. New York: Irvington Publishers; 1994:113–4.

Condoms

Male Condoms

Condoms—also known as rubbers, sheaths, prophylactics, safes, skins, or pros—are the most important barrier contraceptive device.

Types. Current-day materials include latex, polyurethane and lamb cecum (natural membrane, or skin). Latex condoms have been shown to protect against various STDs, including HIV (Table 1). The polyurethane condom has been shown in vitro to be impermeable to HIV; studies to confirm this effect in vivo are ongoing. Its use should be restricted to patients with latex allergies. Condoms made from lamb cecum provide less protection from STDs and HIV than do latex condoms because the presence of pores in the membrane may allow the passage of viral organisms. They are also more expensive. Skins should be recommended only for those who have a latex allergy or are not at risk for STDs.

Proper Use/Storage. Guidelines for proper condom use are given in Table 4.
 Proper storage of condoms is very important. Condoms must be protected from light and excessive heat. The shelf life of condoms under optimal conditions, as packaged by the manufacturers, is 3–5 years; the user should always check for discoloration, brittleness, or stickiness, and condoms displaying any of these characteristics should be discarded.

Female Condom

The Reality condom is made of polyurethane. It is thinner than the male condom and is resistant to degradation by oil-based lubricants. It is prelubricated and comes with additional lubricant. The condom is secured by a circular ring that fits like a diaphragm over the cervix. An outer ring, which dangles outside the vagina, is designed to protect the external genitalia. The female condom is designed for one-time use and may be inserted up to 8 hours before intercourse. It should then be removed immediately after intercourse and before the woman stands up.

Vaginal Contraceptives

Vaginal contraceptives (spermicides) use surface-active agents to immobilize (kill) sperm. The effective spermicides include nonoxynol-9, octoxynol-9, and menfegol. Nearly all currently available products use nonoxynol-9. No products containing menfegol are currently marketed in the United States.

TABLE 3 Advantages and disadvantages of nonprescription contraceptive methods

Contraceptive method	Advantages	Disadvantages
Male condom	Effective; acceptable; inexpensive; nontoxic	Possible decreased sexual pleasure for the male[a]; latex sensitivity[b]
Female condom	Reduced chance of breakage vs. male condom; less messy than spermicides; no known adverse effects	Cost; cumbersome, unattractive appearance; vaginal irritation; decreased sensation; increased noise if lubrication is inadequate; difficulty with insertion; questionable protection against STDs
Spermicides	Easy to use; relatively inexpensive; useful backup method to condoms, or if a birth control pill has been missed; possibly protective against STDs	Low effectiveness rate when used alone; product-specific directions for use, dosage, and timing of administration; possible allergy to some components; messiness; possible irritation or damage of vaginal and cervical epithelium with frequent use or use of high-concentration product
Natural family planning	Encourages communication within relationship; minimal cost; no chemical risk to fertility or health of couple (or fetus, should pregnancy occur)	Higher pregnancy rates than most other methods; no protection against STDs

[a]Strategies for countering this problem include use of very thin or ridged condoms, or—in a monogamous relationship with an HIV-negative individual—natural membrane condoms.

[b]Occurs in 1%–2% of population. To determine latex sensitivity, patients should be asked if they can wear rubber gloves or blow up a balloon without developing itching. Male or female partner may develop contact dermatitis from use of latex condoms. Symptoms include immediate localized itching and swelling (urticarial reaction) or a delayed eczematous reaction. The reaction may spread beyond the area of physical contact with latex in patients with severe sensitivity. Changing condom brands may alleviate the problem. If it does not, polyurethane or lamb cecum condoms may be used if their limitations are recognized.

Types of Spermicides

Spermicides come in a variety of dosage forms: jelly, cream, foam, suppository, and film (see product table "Spermicidal Products" in *Nonprescription Products: Formulations & Features*). Table 5 describes the dosage forms and guidelines for use of these products.

Failure Rate

Spermicides used alone have a relatively high failure rate among typical first-year users (Table 2). Of these products, vaginal foam appears to be most effective when it is used consistently. Efficacy improves greatly if spermicides are used in conjunction with barrier methods such as diaphragms, cervical caps, or condoms.

TABLE 4 Guidelines for proper condom use

1. *Always* use latex condoms unless you are in a monogamous relationship with someone you *know* is not infected with HIV.

2. Use only fresh condoms (not previously opened) that have been stored in a dry, cool place (not a wallet or car glove compartment).

3. Do *not* attempt to test the condom for leaks before using; this increases the risk of tearing.

4. Be aware that long fingernails or jewelry may tear condoms.

5. Unroll the condom onto the erect penis before it comes into *any* contact with the vagina. *This is very important for preventing both pregnancy and disease.* If you start to put the condom on backward, discard that condom and use a fresh one.

6. If you are not using a reservoir-tipped condom, leave 1/2 inch of space between the end of the condom and the tip of the penis by pinching the top of the condom as you unroll it. This leaves space for the ejaculate and decreases the risk of breakage.

7. If your partner has vaginal dryness, you may want to use additional lubrication. This will help decrease the risk of tears and breakage. Only *water-based lubricants* such as K-Y Jelly and Lubrin are safe for use with condoms. Oil-based lubricants, such as Vaseline and Crisco, weaken condoms and increase the chance of breakage. Spermicidal agents may be used as lubricants with condoms and may increase the effectiveness of the condom as well.

8. After ejaculation, withdraw the penis immediately. Hold on to the rim of the condom as you withdraw to prevent the condom from slipping off, especially if you have used additional lubrication.

9. Check the condom for tears and then discard.

10. If a tear has occurred, *immediately* insert spermicidal foam, cream, or jelly containing a high concentration of spermicide into the vagina. *Do not* use *suppositories* or a vaginal *film*. The delay time for dissolution may decrease the product's efficacy.

Natural Family Planning

Natural family planning methods, also called periodic abstinence, rhythm, or fertility awareness methods, use various techniques to determine a woman's period of fertility.

Natural family planning can be divided into four methods: calendar, basal body temperature (BBT), cervical mucus, and symptothermal. Each of these methods requires the woman to keep detailed records of her menstrual cycles and other symptoms associated with cyclical hormonal levels. With the information acquired over several months, a woman is usually able to predict her most fertile time. With this information, a couple can choose to abstain from sexual intercourse during this period if they want to avoid pregnancy or engage in intercourse if conception is desired.

All these methods, especially the BBT and cervical mucus methods, require extensive training and support from persons who have experience with them. For a discussion of natural family planning methods and a list of organizations providing information on family planning, see pages 123–7 and page 131, respectively, of the *Handbook*.

TABLE 5 Types of spermicides

Vaginal creams and jellies

Creams have better lubricating and spreading qualities; gels may be less messy.

Allergic reactions may be experienced by either partner; however, they are very rare.

For use without a diaphragm or cervical cap

Choose a product with a high concentration of spermicide.

Deposit a full applicator of spermicide high in the vagina.

May insert product up to 30–60 minutes in advance of intercourse; it is effective immediately.

Reapply product if intercourse is repeated or occurs more than 60 minutes after initial application.

Do not douche until at least 8 hours after the last act of intercourse.

For use with a diaphragm or cervical cap

Fill barrier one-third full with spermicide and position over cervix (up to 1 hour before intercourse).

Leave diaphragm in place for at least 6 hours after intercourse. Insert additional spermicide without removing diaphragm if coitus is repeated within 6 hours.

If 6 hours have elapsed since intercourse, remove and wash diaphragm and apply new spermicide before reuse.

The cervical cap may be left in place up to 48 hours.

Vaginal foams

May be used in combination with condoms, oral contraceptives, and newly inserted intrauterine devices (IUDs).

When used alone, may have higher efficacy rates than other vaginal contraceptives.

May provide less lubrication than creams and jellies and therefore be less suitable for women experiencing vaginal dryness.

Insert up to 1 hour before coitus; effective immediately upon insertion.

Apply as close to the cervix as possible.

Delay douching for at least 8 hours after the last act of intercourse.

Vaginal suppositories

Pharmacist should make certain the user understands the directions (e.g., unwrap product, insert in vaginal orifice)

Product must be inserted high in the vagina.

Efficacy of vaginal suppositories is low; they are generally not recommended.

Contraceptive film

Insert on tip of finger and place at the cervix at least 5 minutes before intercourse; product is activated by vaginal secretions.

Product is effective for 2 hours.

Do not place the film over the penis for insertion.

Comparative effectiveness of film vs. other vaginal contraceptive products is unknown.

Adjunctive Contraceptive Methods

Lactational Infertility. When the infant receives only breast milk and the mother has not menstruated, protection against conception may persist for up to 6 months. However, if breast feedings are supplemented with bottle feedings, lactational amenorrhea may not be a reliable form of contraception. In general, if a breast-feeding woman is sexually active, other contraceptive measures should be used no later than 5 weeks postpartum.

In-Home Ovulation Prediction Tests. Ovulation prediction test kits, which are designed to aid couples in conceiving, detect the surge in urinary secretion of LH that occurs shortly before ovulation. Because the life expectancy of sperm may be longer than 72 hours, these ovulation predictors do not give warning of impending ovulation with enough accuracy to be effective contraceptive agents when used alone.

Home urine assays for estrogen and pregnanediol have been developed to detect the beginning and end, respectively, of the fertile phase. These tests can warn of impending ovulation at least 3 days before its occurrence and can also detect the rise in progesterone that signals the end of the fertile period. Urine assays are not yet commercially available.

Ineffective/Unrecommended Methods of Contraception

Withdrawal

Coitus interruptus (withdrawal), involves coital activity until ejaculation is imminent, followed by withdrawal of the penis and ejaculation away from the vagina or vulva. Accidental pregnancy rates with this method are in the range of 19 pregnancies per 100 couples in the first year of use.

Douching

Postcoital douching has no effect in removing sperm from the upper reproductive tract and could, in fact, force or propel sperm higher up in the tract.

Pharmacoeconomics of Contraceptive Products

A recent study has demonstrated that all forms of contraception are cost-effective when viewed against the costs of an undesired pregnancy.

Differences among methods depend on the willingness of both members of a couple to use a product properly. Significant cost savings for barrier methods can be achieved by minimizing imperfect use.

The Pharmacist's Role in Contraceptive Selection

Pharmacists can be invaluable in contributing to the reproductive health and knowledge of people in their communities. Toward this end, they should:

■ Familiarize themselves with the proper use of nonprescription contraceptive products;

■ Provide opportunities for consultation with patients and a private area for education and counseling;

■ Make special efforts to offer contraceptive information and services to adolescents, who are especially likely to be uninformed or misinformed about reproductive matters;

■ Provide verbal instruction, since printed instructions are often written above the reading level of most adolescents and many adults;

■ Stress condom use as a method of disease prevention for everyone who is sexually active, including persons already using prescription methods of birth control;

- Suggest the diaphragm, cervical cap, or natural family planing methods as possible acceptable contraceptive methods for persons who are in a stable relationship, keeping in mind that the first two methods require special fitting and that the latter requires referral to those with experience in training; and
- Remind couples of medications that may interfere with physical signs and symptoms monitored in natural family-planning techniques (e.g., phenothiazines, aspirin, and other medications may alter body temperature; vaginal foams, gels, creams, and douches interfere with cervical mucus).

CHAPTER 8

Cold, Cough, and Allergy Products

Questions to ask in patient assessment and counseling

Allergic Rhinitis

- What symptoms do you have?
- Are the symptoms present year-round or only during selected times of the year?
- What factors aggravate the symptoms?
- Are the symptoms better or worse at home? At work? At school?
- Does anyone in your family have a history of allergies?
- Do you have a fever, sore throat, cough, vomiting, or diarrhea?
- What prescription and nonprescription medications are you taking?
- What prescription and nonprescription medications have you taken in the past to treat your symptoms? Did any of them relieve your symptoms?
- Are you allergic to any medications?
- Do you have any dietary restrictions?

Congestion

- What are your symptoms?
- Is your nasal discharge thick or discolored?
- What medications have you used to treat your symptoms?
- Are you taking any other medications?
- Are you allergic to any medication?
- Have you ever experienced an adverse reaction to any medication?
- Have you ever had more congestion after using a spray decongestant?
- Do you have hypertension or other cardiovascular diseases? Angle-closure or open-angle glaucoma? Diabetes? Thyroid disease? Benign prostatic hypertrophy? A seizure disorder?
- Are you being treated for depression? If so, are you taking isocarboxazid (Marplan), phenelzine (Nardil), or tranylcypromine (Parnate)?
- Are you pregnant or breast-feeding?
- If the medication is for a child, how old is the child?
- Do you participate in sporting events?

Editor's Note: This chapter is adapted from Karen J. Tietze, "Cold, Cough, and Allergy Products," in Covington, T.R., ed., *Handbook of Nonprescription Drugs,* 11th edition, which is based, in part, on a chapter with the same title that appeared in the 10th edition but was written by Bobby G. Bryant and Thomas P. Lombardi. For a more extensive discussion of this topic, readers are encouraged to consult Chapter 8 of the *Handbook.*

Allergic Rhinitis

The hallmark of allergic rhinitis is a temporal relationship between exposure to allergens and the development of nasal symptoms. Although approximately two thirds of individuals with allergic rhinitis develop symptoms of the disease before age 30, symptoms may develop at any time except during the first year of life. Approximately 2 years of allergen exposure are needed before allergic rhinitis occurs.

Etiology

There are no universally accepted diagnostic criteria for allergic rhinitis. The condition may, however, be classified according to whether symptoms occur throughout the year (perennial allergic rhinitis) or during specific seasons (seasonal allergic rhinitis).

Perennial Allergic Rhinitis

Perennial allergic rhinitis is caused by continual exposure to many types of allergens. Allergens commonly associated with perennial allergic rhinitis include those from house dust mites, molds, cockroaches, and house pets.

Seasonal Allergic Rhinitis

Seasonal allergic rhinitis is caused by windborne plant (e.g., tree, grass, and ragweed) pollens. Although the duration of the pollinating season varies geographically, the onset is about the same in all regions. Ragweed begins to pollinate in mid-August and persists until the first frost. Other weed pollens appear in late summer and early fall and also last until the first frost. Other common pollens include tree pollens, which appear in late March and last through May, and grass pollens, which appear in May and last through June or early July.

Pathophysiology

Immunologic Response

A complete discussion of the immunologic response appears on page 138 of the *Handbook*.

Patient Assessment

The pharmacist should ask the patient the questions listed at the beginning of the chapter to determine the specific symptoms experienced, the severity and pattern, if any, of those symptoms, predisposing factors, and current and past treatment regimens.

Symptoms

Major ocular symptoms include itching, lacrimation, mild soreness, puffiness, chemosis, and conjunctival hyperemia. Major nasal symptoms include nasal congestion, watery rhinorrhea, itching, sneezing paroxysms, and postnasal drip. Major head and neck symptoms include loss of taste and smell, mild sore throat secondary to postnasal drip, earache, sinus headache, itching of the palate and throat, and repeated clearing of the throat. Major systemic symptoms include malaise and fatigue.

The symptoms associated with perennial allergic rhinitis are similar to but less severe than those associated with seasonal allergic rhinitis. Symptoms may be associated with specific activities such as mowing the lawn or exacerbated by nonspecific irritants such as cigarette smoke. Patients may be symptom-free at work or school but extremely symptomatic in other environments. Patients should be asked what factors they associate with their symptoms and what patterns their symptoms seem to show. Aggravating factors should be identified.

Uncomplicated allergic rhinitis does not cause fever, significant sore throat, vomiting, or diarrhea. Table 1 compares symptoms of allergic rhinitis with those of other rhinitis syndromes. Patients with the latter should be referred to their physicians for evaluation and treatment.

Complications

Chronic obstruction around the sinus ostia and eustachian tubes increases the risk of sinusitis, recurrent otitis media, and eustachian tube dysfunction. Poor tympanic membrane compliance and significant hearing loss may result from fluid collections in the middle ear. Patients who develop fever, purulent nasal discharge, frequent headaches, or earache should be referred to their physicians.

TABLE 1 Features of common rhinitis syndromes

	Allergic rhinitis	Infectious rhinitis	Vasomotor rhinitis	Rhinitis medicamentosa
Etiology	Allergens	Viral or bacterial	Unknown	Tachyphylaxis to topical decongestants
Symptoms	Rhinorrhea, congestion, sneezing, pruritus (nose or roof of mouth), allergic shiners, allergic salute, cough with postnasal drip, ocular itching and lacrimation	Fever[a], constitutional symptoms, mucopurulent rhinorrhea, scratchy throat, congestion, cough	Rhinorrhea, congestion	Congestion
Pattern	Perennial or seasonal	Any time	Any time	Temporal relationship with use of topical decongestants
Associated factors	Concurrent atopic disease, family history	None	Affects primarily women; precipitated by strong odors, alcohol, stress, and changes in temperature, humidity, and barometric pressure	Overuse of topical decongestants, concurrent antihypertensive therapy

[a]Rare; more common in children.

Adapted from Fireman P. Pathophysiology and pharmacotherapy of common upper respiratory diseases. *Pharmacotherapy*. 1993 Nov-Dec; 13 (16 pt 2): 101S–9S.

Physical Assessment

Patients may have "allergic shiners," which are dark circles beneath the eyes secondary to venous and lymphatic congestion. A horizontal crease across the lower third of the nose may be visible in patients who repeatedly rub their noses upward. Severe nasal obstruction may result in chronic mouth breathing. The nasal mucosa appear pale and swollen; the nasal secretions are clear and watery. The eyes may be watery and there may be periorbital edema.

Diagnostic Testing

A discussion of diagnostic testing appears on page 139 of the *Handbook*.

Disease Management

The first step in managing allergic rhinitis is avoidance of the offending allergens. Pharmacotherapy is used if avoidance measures are not feasible or do not adequately relieve the symptoms. Treatment should be targeted at specific symptoms (Table 2). Immunotherapy is indicated for patients whose symptoms cannot be adequately controlled with medications or whose symptoms occur most days of the year.

Preventive Measures

Patients allergic to outdoor allergens should follow pollen count reports, keep house and car windows closed, and use air conditioners.

Patients with grass allergies should not work or play in grassy areas, especially during early summer. Patients with outdoor mold allergies should avoid mowing the lawn and raking leaves and should not disturb leaf or compost piles. Indoor mold exposure can be reduced by venting bathrooms and kitchens, using dehumidification, and eliminating moldy areas of the indoor environment (e.g., wet basements).

House dust mite exposure can be minimized by controlling the indoor environment. Indoor humidity should be reduced to less than 50%. Pillows, mattresses, and box springs should be encased in plastic airtight covers that are cleaned weekly with a damp cloth. Items that collect dust, such as rugs, stuffed furniture, stuffed toys, and open bookshelves and television or stereo cabinets, should be removed from sleeping areas. All bedding, including mattress pads, should be washed weekly in hot water. Vacuum cleaners should be equipped with high-efficiency particulate air cleaner (HEPA) filters to avoid aerosolizing the house dust mite feces when vacuuming. HEPA filters can also be installed in the central

TABLE 2 Symptomatic nonprescription drug treatment of allergic rhinitis

Symptoms	Treatment
Ocular itching, lacrimation, puffiness	Ophthalmic antihistamines, systemic antihistamines
Chemosis, conjunctival redness	Ophthalmic decongestants
Rhinorrhea, nasal itching, postnasal drip	Systemic antihistamines
Nasal congestion	Systemic decongestants (topical is an option but overuse potential is high)
Headache, earache, sinus pain	Systemic analgesics (decongestants may relieve sinus pain due to sinus congestion)

ductwork of homes with forced air or can be freestanding units. Because they are expensive, however, patients should be encouraged to rent HEPA filters before purchasing them. Acaricides such as tannic acid and benzyl benzoate can be used to treat furniture and carpeting, but treatment needs to be repeated frequently.

Animal allergen exposures can be limited by removing pets from the household or at least by totally excluding the pet from the patient's bedroom.

Antihistamines

Antihistamines are first-line agents for the prophylaxis and treatment of allergic rhinitis. Antihistamines are effective for reducing sneezing and itching and somewhat less effective for reducing rhinorrhea. They have no effect on nasal congestion.

Classification. Antihistamines may be classified by chemical structure, relative sedative properties, or generation. The second-generation, nonsedating antihistamines (astemizole [Hismanal], cetirizine [Zyrtec], fexofenadine [Allegra], loratadine [Claritin], and terfenadine [Seldane]) differ from the first-generation antihistamines in that they are highly specific for histamine-1 receptors and do not have any anticholinergic, antiemetic, or local anesthetic activity.

Side Effects. Side effects associated with the cholinergic blockage achieved with first-generation antihistamines include dryness of the eyes, mouth, and nose; blurred vision; urinary retention; and tachycardia. These agents cross the blood-brain barrier and are associated with significant sedation and impaired mental performance. Second generation antihistamines do not cross the blood-brain barrier and are less sedating. Torsade de pointes, a cardiac arrhythmia reported with terfenadine and astemizole, has rarely been observed with the older antihistamines.

Product Selection Guidelines. Of the first-generation antihistamines, the alkylamines (chlorpheniramine, brompheniramine, and pheniramine) are the least sedating and the ethanolamines (diphenhydramine, doxylamine, and phenyltoloxamine) are the most sedating. The second-generation agents astemizole, cetirizine, fexofenadine, loratidine, and terfenadine are available by prescription only.

Decongestants

Decongestants, which are sympathomimetics, reduce nasal congestion. They have no effect on histamine or any other mediator involved in the allergic reaction. Therefore, decongestants are commonly administered in combination with antihistamines.

Side Effects. Rebound congestion (rhinitis medicamentosa), or rebound nasal mucosal edema, is a common problem when decongestants are administered topically for more than 3–5 days. Treatment consists of slow withdrawal of the topical decongestant (one nostril at a time); replacement of the decongestant with topical normal saline, which is believed to soothe and moisten the nasal mucosa; and, if needed, topical corticosteroids and systemic decongestants. The mucous membrane returns to normal in 1–2 weeks.

Systemic decongestants constrict all vascular beds and stimulate the central nervous system. Diseases potentially aggravated by sympathomimetics include high blood pressure, heart disease, diabetes mellitus, and hyperthyroidism. Monoamine oxidase inhibition intensifies sympathomimetic activity; oral sympathomimetics are contraindicated in patients who are taking monoamine oxidase inhibitors for the treatment of depression, other psychiatric or emotional conditions, or Parkinson's disease except under the advice and supervision of a physician.

Headache has been reported with systemic decongestants, especially when they are used with other sympathomimetic medications.

Product Selection Guidelines. Product selection depends on the expected duration of treatment and the presence of concomitant disease. Patients with seasonal or allergic rhinitis generally require decongestants throughout the entire period of exposure to allergens.

Topical dosage forms include sprays, drops, and inhalers. Nasal sprays are the preferred dosage form for older children and adults. Topical decongestants are effective; however, the risk of rebound congestion greatly limits their usefulness. Topical drug administration may be used, however, to control acute symptoms on a short-term (3–5 day) basis. Nasal obstruction greatly reduces the effectiveness of topical agents. Physical abnormalities such as severe septal deviation may interfere with drug administration.

Patients with hypertension and other cardiovascular diseases, diabetes mellitus, benign prostatic hypertrophy, or hyperthyroidism should use oral sympathomimetics only under the supervision of a physician. Pseudoephedrine has less effect on blood pressure than does phenylpropanolamine. Short-acting products may be safer for patients with cardiovascular disease. Persons with diabetes may confuse hypoglycemia or hyperglycemia with the side effects of decongestants (e.g., nervousness, tremor, anxiety, dizziness).

Decongestants are considered stimulants; patients who participate in official athletic events should avoid phenylephrine (Neo-Synephrine), ephedrine (various), pseudoephedrine, and propylhexedrine (Benzedrex). Physical performance may be impaired by first-generation antihistamines (owing to their sedating and anticholinergic effects) and by immunotherapy (owing to discomfort at site of injection).

Decongestants should be used during pregnancy only if the potential benefit justifies the potential risk to the fetus. It is not known how much decongestant is excreted into breast milk following topical or systemic administration. Women who breast-feed should use decongestants with caution.

Topical Anti-Inflammatory Drugs

Corticosteroids and cromolyn sodium are topical agents used for allergic rhinitis. Both are available only by prescription. Nasal corticosteroids do not usually have the systemic side effects associated with oral corticosteroids. Local irritation or epistaxis may be a problem.

Expectorants and Mucolytics

Mucolytics thin mucus, making it easier to expel secretions. Water cannot be incorporated into mucus after the mucus has been formed, but hydration will aid in the formation of a less viscid mucus. Hydration can be accomplished by maintaining an adequate fluid intake; steam inhalation may soothe irritated membranes. The efficacy of the expectorant guaifenesin in allergic rhinitis has not been proved.

Immunotherapy

Immunotherapy is indicated for patients whose symptoms are not controlled by drugs, who have severe conditions or perennial symptoms, or who are allergic to allergens that are difficult to avoid. Patients may improve as early as 3 months after initiation of immunotherapy. About 80% of patients have significant relief while receiving immunotherapy; approximately 60% will remain symptom free after the immunotherapy is discontinued.

Patient Counseling

Patients with allergic rhinitis generally prefer to use sustained-release products. Saline sprays may provide some relief from drying and crusting. All products should be kept out of the reach of children.

Antihistamines

The pharmacist should emphasize the following points to patients taking antihistamines:

- Antihistamines provide symptomatic relief only. They will not cure or prevent the disease.
- Compliance with long-term therapy is essential. Patients with seasonal allergic rhinitis should start taking antihistamines before their specific allergy season begins; patients with perennial allergic rhinitis may need to take antihistamines year-round.
- Sedation associated with some agents can be minimized by (1) administering a full dose at bedtime and using minimally recommended doses combined with a decongestant during the day; or (2) starting with low doses and gradually increasing the dose as tolerated over a several-day period.
- Patients taking first-generation antihistamines should be advised against driving, performing tasks that require alertness, and consuming alcohol or other sedative drugs. Although less likely, sedation and/or decreased mental alertness may also occur with the second-generation antihistamines; thus, the same cautions are needed.
- The very young and the elderly may be particularly sensitive to antihistamines. First-generation antihistamines may cause paradoxical reactions such as nervousness, irritability, and restlessness in these patients.
- Antihistamines should be used during pregnancy only if the potential benefit outweighs the possible risks.
- Antihistamine use by breast-feeding patients is generally not recommended.
- Antihistamines with anticholinergic properties may cause excessive drying or crusting of secretions, making it more difficult for patients with chronic bronchitis or emphysema to clear secretions.
- First-generation antihistamines may exacerbate symptoms of benign prostatic hypertrophy.
- Antihistamines may alter the results of skin and serologic testing. Therefore, patients should inform their physicians that they are taking antihistamines before they undergo any of these diagnostic tests.

Decongestants

The following points should be emphasized when counseling patients on use of decongestants:

- Patients using topical decongestants should be advised to limit use to no more than 3–5 days.
- If patients experience rebound congestion, they need to be counseled on how to withdraw from the medication.
- Patients who have problems sleeping should limit the use of decongestants to the daytime hours and take an antihistamine alone before bedtime.
- Women who are pregnant or breast-feeding should not take these medications without the supervision of a physician.

Patients should also be given the following general guidelines on administering topical decongestants, as well as specific instructions for administering the dosage form chosen.

General Administration Guidelines
- Check the expiration date before using the product.
- Discard the product if it is discolored or if deterioration is suspected.
- Do not share the product with another person.
- Blow the nose before using the product.
- Wait at least a few minutes after administering a dose before blowing the nose.

Sprays
- Do not shake the bottle.
- Remove the cap before using the spray.
- Gently insert the tip of the bottle into one nostril.
- Keep the head upright.
- Inhale deeply while squeezing the bottle.
- Repeat with the other nostril if necessary.
- Rinse the bottle tip with hot water but do not let water enter the bottle.
- Replace the cap.

Metered Dose Pumps
- Do not shake the bottle.
- Remove the cap, then prime the pump (depress it several times with the nozzle pointed away from the face) before using it for the first time.
- Hold the bottle with the nozzle between the first two fingers and the thumb on the bottom of the bottle.
- Gently insert the tip of the pump into the nose.
- Keep the head upright.
- Inhale deeply while depressing the pump once.
- Repeat with the other nostril if necessary.
- Rinse the spray tip with hot water but do not let water enter the bottle.
- Replace the cap.

Drops
- Squeeze the rubber bulb on the dropper to withdraw medication from the bottle.
- Tilt head back while standing or sitting, or lie on the bed with the head tilted back over the side.
- Place the drops into each nostril.
- Gently tilt the head from side to side.
- Rinse the dropper with hot water and let it air dry.

Inhalers
- Warm the inhaler in the hand.
- Remove the cap before using the inhaler.
- Inhale the vapor up one nostril at a time while occluding the other nostril.
- Inhale deeply.

■ Wipe the inhaler clean after each use.
■ Replace the cap.
■ Discard the inhaler after 2–3 months.

Corticosteroids

Topical corticosteroids should be used regularly. Maximal benefit may not occur until after 2–6 weeks of regular treatment.

Pediatric Considerations

The FDA recommends that children age 6 to under 12 years receive one half the adult dose, and those children age 2 to under 6 years receive one fourth the adult dose. Because the potential consequences of airway obstruction are so severe in young children, all children under the age of 2 should be referred to a physician. These dosage recommendations do not take the weight of the child into consideration. Doses may need to be modified for children who are small or large for their age.

Topical and systemic decongestants should not be used in young children without the advice of a physician; topical decongestants should be used for no longer than 3 days. Isotonic saline drops and the gentle aspiration of secretions with a nasal syringe can temporarily relieve nasal obstruction in infants and young children; nasal drainage may be enhanced by letting infants and young children sleep upright in car seats.

The Common Cold

Etiology

The five viruses that commonly infect the upper respiratory tract include the rhinovirus types 2, 9, and 14; the coronavirus type 229E; and the respiratory syncytial virus. There is no single mode of transmission. Factors associated with an increased susceptibility to viral upper respiratory infections include smoking and psychologic stress.

Patient Assessment

The first symptom of a cold is sore throat, followed by nasal symptoms (stuffiness, rhinorrhea, postnasal drip), watering eyes, sneezing, and cough. The sequence of symptoms is the same, regardless of the infecting virus; however, the timing, frequency, and severity vary with the infecting virus. The majority of patients will experience nasal symptoms, regardless of the infecting virus. Patients will be symptomatic for approximately 1–2 weeks.

Table 3 contrasts the symptoms of bacterial and viral sore throats. Table 4 contrasts the symptoms of cold and influenza.

Disease Management

Cold symptoms are usually self-limiting and resolve in 1–2 weeks whether treated or not. General therapeutic measures such as rest and an adequate fluid intake are the mainstays of therapy. Treatment should be symptom specific (Table 5).

Decongestants

Decongestants. (See the discussion of decongestants in the section Allergic Rhinitis.)

TABLE 3 Bacterial versus viral sore throats

Characteristic	Bacterial sore throat	Viral sore throat
Onset	Rapid	Slower
Soreness	Marked	Usually less severe
Constitutional symptoms	Marked	Mild
Upper and lower respiratory symptoms	Not always present	Usually present
Lymph nodes	Large, tender	Slight enlargement, not tender

Adapted from Bulteau V. Sore throat. *Med J Aust.* 1966 Nov; 2:1053–5.

Analgesics and Antipyretics

Patients may complain of feeling feverish, but the common cold is rarely associated with a temperature greater than 100°F (37.8°C). Analgesics/antipyretics are effective treatments. Children and teenagers should avoid aspirin and aspirin-containing products.

Expectorants and Mucolytics

Increasing fluid intake (six to eight 8-oz glasses of fluid per day) and maintaining adequate humidification are important for the production and expectoration of respiratory secretions. Unless directed by a physician, one should not give expectorants to children under 12 if there is a persistent or chronic cough such as occurs with asthma or if the cough is accompanied by excessive mucus.

Antitussives

Antitussives are indicated for the suppression of nonproductive coughs.

Antitussives are sometimes used to suppress productive coughs that prevent sleep or are especially bothersome. However, antitussives may be counterproductive when used to treat a productive cough because cough suppression may impair the expectoration of secretions. Active ingredients in antitussives are as follows:

Codeine. Codeine is the standard antitussive against which all other antitussives are compared. The dose required for cough suppression (10–20 mg) is less than the analgesic dose. Codeine, under usual conditions of use as a cough suppressant, has low-dependency potential. The most common side effects include nausea, drowsiness, lightheadedness, and constipation.

Dextromethorphan. Dextromethorphan has no significant analgesic properties and does not depress respiration; the addiction potential is low. Dextromethorphan is generally well tolerated; drowsiness and gastrointestinal upset are the most common complaints. Patients taking monoamine oxidase inhibitors should not use products containing dextromethorphan without the supervision of a physician.

TABLE 4 Comparative symptoms of the common cold and influenza

Symptom	Common cold	Influenza
Fever	Rare	Sudden onset; temperature >102–104°F (38.8–40°C)
Headache	Mild or absent	Prominent
Myalgia or arthralgia	Mild or absent	Prominent
Fatigue, weakness, and exhaustion	Mild or absent	Extreme
Rhinorrhea	Common	Less common
Nasal congestion	Common	Less common
Sneezing	Common	Less common
Sore throat	Common	Common
Cough	Less common; usually nonproductive	Common; persistent nonproductive
Ocular	Watery eyes	Pain on motion of eyes; photophobia; burning
Duration	5–10 days	1 wk
Complications	Sinus congestion; earache	Bronchitis; pneumonia

Reprinted from Dolan R. In: Isselbacher KJ et al, eds. *Harrison's Principles of Internal Medicine.* 13th ed. New York: McGraw-Hill, Inc; 1994: 803–7, 814–9.

Diphenhydramine. The most common side effects of diphenhydramine hydrochloride are sedation and anticholinergic effects. Diphenhydramine hydrochloride should not be taken by individuals in whom the use of anticholinergics are contraindicated (e.g., those with narrow-angle glaucoma or benign prostatic hypertrophy) or in situations in which mental alertness or physical coordination and dexterity are required.

Topical Antitussives. Camphor and menthol are the only two monograph topical antitussives. Camphor and menthol are also approved for steam inhalation, and menthol is also approved in a lozenge or compressed tablet formulation.

Anesthetics and Antiseptics

Antiseptics are ineffective against viral infections. Products containing local anesthetics may be used every 3 or 4 hours for temporary symptomatic relief. Alternatives include hard candy, which stimulates salivary flow and acts as a soothing demulcent, warm saline gargles (1–3 tsp of salt per 8–12 oz of warm water), and fruit juice.

Humidifiers

Inhalation of heated or unheated humidified air may soothe airways and improve airway hydration. Application of hot humidified air directly to the nasal passages is of no benefit.

TABLE 5 Symptomatic nonprescription drug treatment of the common cold

Symptom	Treatment
Nasal congestion and discharge	Decongestants
Cough	Hydration, demulcents, antitussives, expectorants, cool mist/steam vapors
Sore throat	Demulcents, saline gargles, local anesthetics, systemic analgesics
Laryngitis	Cool mist/steam vapors
Feverishness and headache	Systemic analgesics

Patient Counseling

Patients using topical decongestants should be counseled on the appropriate administration technique and advised to limit use of these products to 3–5 days. Patients should be referred to a physician if they have symptoms such as sore throat that persists for longer than 1 week, high fever, rash, or persistent headache, which reflect the possibility of a more serious condition.

The first step in controlling cough associated with the common cold is to maintain an adequate fluid intake. The tickling sensation in the pharynx may be controlled with a demulcent such as hard candy or cough drops. A cough suppressant may be indicated if the cough is dry and nonproductive, and if it interferes with work or sleep. Sore throats may be treated with demulcents, saline gargles, or local anesthetic lozenges or solutions.

Headache and fever may be treated with usual doses of aspirin, acetaminophen, ibuprofen, or naproxen. Patients should be referred to their physician if the fever persists for more than 24 hours or if the cold symptoms do not improve in about a week.

Patients with complicating diseases and women who are pregnant or breast-feeding should not take these medications without the supervision of a physician.

Pediatric Considerations

The risk of toxicity from cough and cold medications is higher in infants and young children than in adults. Acetaminophen is the analgesic and antipyretic of choice for children. Children with a history of febrile seizures should be given an antipyretic. Children and teenagers less than 15 years of age should not be given aspirin because of the potential association with Reye's syndrome.

The American Academy of Pediatrics Committee on Drugs has advised against the use of combination cough and cold medications. Simple, soothing, inexpensive, and safe remedies such as tea with lemon and honey, chicken soup, and hot broths should be used. Supportive measures for infants include clearing the nose with a bulb syringe, positioning the infant so that the secretions drain from the nose, maintaining adequate fluid intake, increasing the humidity of inspired air, and using saline nose drops.

CHAPTER 9

Asthma Products

Questions to ask in patient assessment and counseling

- *Has a physician diagnosed your condition as asthma? (If patient answers "no," proceed with questions for undiagnosed asthma. If "yes," proceed with questions for diagnosed asthma.)*

Undiagnosed Asthma

- *Have you had an attack or recurrent attacks of wheezing?*
- *Do you have a troublesome cough at night?*
- *Do you cough or wheeze after exercise?*
- *Do you cough, wheeze, or have chest tightness after exposure to airborne allergens or pollutants?*
- *Do your colds "go to the chest" or take more than 10 days to clear up?*

Diagnosed Asthma

- *Are you under the care of a physician?*
- *Do you have a written asthma care plan?*
- *Do you have other medical problems, such as heart disease, seizures, high blood pressure, hyperthyroidism, or diabetes?*
- *What prescription or nonprescription medications are you taking?*
- *During the past year, how many days have you missed from school or work because of asthma?*
- *How many nights per week do you awake with asthma?*
- *In the last year, have you been to the emergency room or hospital because of asthma?*
- *Does asthma affect your ability to exercise (even brisk walking)?*
- *Have you used any asthma products in the past? If so, which ones? Were they effective? Did they cause any side effects? If so, what were they?*
- *How often each day or week do you use a bronchodilator inhaler for symptoms of asthma? Would you demonstrate how you use your inhaler? How do you clean it?*
- *Do you use a spacer device? If so, would you demonstrate how you use it?*
- *Do you have a peak flow meter? If so, is it a manual or electronic meter? How do you use it?*

Editor's Note: This chapter is adapted from Dennis M. Williams and Timothy H. Self, "Asthma Products," in Covington, T.R., ed., *Handbook of Nonprescription Drugs*, 11th edition, which is based, in part, on the chapter with the same title that appeared in the 10th edition but was written by H. William Kelly and Mary Beth O'Connell. For a more extensive discussion of the etiology and pathophysiology of asthma, and the nonprescription products used to treat it, readers are encouraged to consult Chapter 9 of the *Handbook*.

An estimated 10 million persons in the United States, including 3 million children, have asthma. The annual age-adjusted death rate from asthma increased 40% in the United States between 1982 and 1991. An increase in morbidity and mortality from asthma in the United States and worldwide has been a major concern and was the impetus for the National Heart, Lung, and Blood Institute (NHLBI) to establish the National Asthma Education Program, now known as the National Asthma Education and Prevention Program (NAEPP). NAEPP has developed guidelines for the diagnosis and management of asthma.

Epidemiology, Pathophysiology, and Etiology

The NAEPP report defines asthma as a lung disease with the following characteristics:

■ Airway obstruction that is reversible (but not completely so in some patients) either spontaneously or with treatment;

■ Airway inflammation; and

■ Increased airway responsiveness to a variety of stimuli.

Symptomatic asthma is more common in children than in adults, with the age of onset being under 10 years of age for 50% of all subjects. The prevalence rate is slightly higher in males until puberty, at which time the gender ratio is approximately equal. Symptoms often significantly decrease in severity as patients age; 50%–70% of children with asthma have a permanent or temporary symptom-free remission by adulthood. Evidence increasingly suggests that chronic asthma may result in irreversible chronic obstruction.

Asthma is a chronic inflammatory disease that involves the airways and is further characterized by recurrent exacerbations. Although the cellular defect in asthma is still unknown, unchecked inflammation of the airways is known to be the principal cause of their excessive reactivity to various triggering events.

The etiology of asthma is not known; however, epidemiologic studies suggest a genetic component. Atopy is the strongest identified predisposing factor in the development of asthma.

Factors that sensitize the airways and lead to the onset of asthma include indoor allergens, including house dust mites, furred animals, and fungi. Outdoor allergens, including dust, pollens, and fungi, are also sensitizers. Other important sensitizers are occupational agents and drug or food additives. Once patients have been sensitized, they are susceptible to asthma triggers. Asthma is generally exacerbated by respiratory tract infections (primarily viral), inhaled allergens, inhaled air pollutants, smoking (active and passive), exercise, or occupational and industrial irritants, sulfites, or drugs.

Symptoms

Asthma is episodic in nature. Periods of airway obstruction may last from a few minutes to several days. The severity of obstruction is highly variable (Figure 1). Cough, wheezing (a fine, whistling sound), dyspnea (difficulty breathing), and chest tightness are common symptoms of asthma. An increased bronchomotor tone, which is usually reversible with a bronchodilator, is often present. During acute asthma attacks, patients demonstrate a marked decrease in all measures of expiratory flow rate and may complain of a tightness in their chest as well as dyspnea. Approximately 30%–50% of patients with asthma complain of excessive sputum production. Some patients develop irreversible airflow limitation over a period of several years.

Clinical features before treatment[a]	Daily medication(s) required to maintain control	Step 4: Severe persistent asthma
Continuous symptoms Frequent exacerbations Frequent nocturnal asthma symptoms Physical activities limited by asthma symptoms PEF or FEV_1: ≤60% predicted; variability >30%	Multiple daily controller medications: high doses of inhaled corticosteroid, long-acting bronchodilator, and long-term use of oral corticosteroid	

Clinical features before treatment[a]	Daily medication(s) required to maintain control	Step 3: Moderate persistent asthma
Daily symptoms Exacerbations affect activity and sleep Nocturnal asthma symptoms occur >1 time a week Daily use of inhaled short-acting beta$_2$-agonists PEF or FEV_1: >60%–<80% predicted; variability >30%	Daily controller medications: inhaled corticosteroid and long-acting bronchodilator (especially for nocturnal symptoms)	

Clinical features before treatment[a]	Daily medication(s) required to maintain control	Step 2: Mild persistent asthma
Symptoms occur ≥1 time a week but <1 time a day Exacerbations may affect activity and sleep Nocturnal symptoms occur >2 times a month PEF or FEV_1: ≥80% predicted; variability 20%–30%	One daily controller medication; a long-acting bronchodilator could be added to anti-inflammatory medication (especially for nocturnal symptoms)	

Clinical features before treatment[a]	Daily medication(s) required to maintain control	Step 1: Intermittent asthma
Intermittent symptoms occur <1 time a week Brief exacerbations lasting from a few hours to a few days Nocturnal symptoms occur <2 times a month Lung function between exacerbations is asymptomatic and normal PEF or FEV_1: ≥80% predicted; variability <20%	Intermittent reliever medication taken only as needed: inhaled short-acting beta$_2$-agonists Intensity of treatment depends on severity of exacerbation; oral corticosteroids may be required	

[a]The presence of one of the clinical features of a category is sufficient to place a patient in that category.

FIGURE 1 Classification of asthma severity. Reprinted from National Heart, Lung, and Blood Institute. Global Initiative for Asthma. Pub No 95–3659. Bethesda, Md: US Department of Health and Human Services; 1995.

Patient Assessment

Medical diagnosis of asthma is essential to rule out other causes of pulmonary symptoms such as physical obstruction from a tumor, congestive heart failure, and chronic bronchitis. Patients presenting with new symptoms of asthma should be referred to their physician or other health care provider. The following scenarios demonstrate the importance of a medical diagnosis of asthma prior to initiation of nonprescription drug therapy:

- Patients with a history of hypertension or heart disease and new pulmonary symptoms should be referred to a physician immediately.
- Patients who awaken in the middle of the night with dyspnea and cough resulting from pulmonary edema may have congestive heart failure.
- Shortness of breath and chest pain in women taking oral contraceptives may be signs of pulmonary emboli.
- Patients with chronic bronchitis and emphysema experience symptoms similar to those of asthma. These symptoms, however, are usually continuous instead of episodic.

The first set of questions at the beginning of this chapter should be helpful in differentiating asthma from other pulmonary conditions.

Asthma is frequently unrecognized, especially in children. Pharmacists can play a major role in identifying potential patients with asthma and referring them for appropriate care. Symptoms such as recurrent wheezing, periods of dyspnea, coughing, chest tightness, and repeated respiratory tract infections warrant additional assessments. Many patients have mild asthma that does not progress; in others, the condition may worsen and be accompanied by dyspnea and wheezing, cough, apprehension, chest distention, tenacious sputum, flaring nostrils, and sinus tachycardia.

If a diagnosis of asthma has been previously established, it is important to determine the frequency and severity of symptoms and which self-treatment approaches have already been attempted. Patients with any of the following symptoms need immediate medical attention:

- Shortness of breath that makes it impossible to complete a full sentence without stopping;
- Discomfort that persists while they are at rest after using a bronchodilator;
- Symptoms that worsen despite the use of a bronchodilator; or
- Progressive dyspnea and wheezing with dependence on nonprescription bronchodilators.

Treatment

The use of nonprescription medications for the management of asthma symptoms is controversial. If indicated, nonprescription medications are reserved only for patients with mild, intermittent symptoms. Even in this situation, many clinicians prefer to recommend a prescription, short-acting, inhaled, selective beta$_2$-agonist (e.g., albuterol) based on its greater potency, longer duration of effect, and fewer adverse effects.

The Pharmacist's Role in Managing Asthma

A report by the NHLBI states that areas of involvement for pharmacists in the management of asthma include:

- Educating patients about asthma medications;
- Instructing patients in proper inhalation techniques;
- Monitoring medication use and refill intervals to identify patients with poorly controlled asthma;

- Referring patients for appropriate care;
- Assisting patients in using peak flow meters properly;
- Assisting patients in incorporating the meters in a self-management plan designed by a physician;
- Helping patients discharged from hospitals understand their asthma management plan; and
- Serving as a resource for physicians by sharing current expert guidelines about asthma management.

These areas should be the primary focus of pharmaceutical care for the asthma patient.

To assist with the appropriate treatment plan for a specific asthma patient, the pharmacist must consider the goals of treatment, the severity of the disease, specific patient characteristics, past medical history, and the benefits and risks of the various drug classes for asthma treatment.

It is extremely important for the pharmacist to determine the pattern of use for patients using nonprescription bronchodilator inhalers. Self-treatment may delay the patient's seeking necessary medical care and result in resistant, acute, severe asthma attacks. Patients with symptoms that occur more often than one to two times weekly and those with nocturnal asthma should be *strongly encouraged* to seek medical advice. If the symptoms are new and the patient has not been diagnosed by a physician as having asthma, medical referral for evaluation is essential.

Stepped-Care Treatment

A stepped-care approach to asthma treatment, as outlined by the NAEPP, may be instituted. Guidelines are also available from NHBLI's *International Consensus Report on Diagnosis and Treatment of Asthma* and its *Global Initiative for Asthma.* The latter two publications are more recent. The steps in this approach are as follows:

Prevention of Inflammatory Response

The primary focus of asthma therapy is prevention of the inflammatory response. Patients should be instructed on the home use of a peak flow meter so that therapy can be initiated as soon as significant obstruction develops. If as-needed or chronic medications do not abate the asthma attack, the patient should be instructed to seek medical attention early. Caregivers and significant others of patients with asthma should also be educated on how to assess the severity of and treat asthma attacks. Patients should learn what triggers their asthma attacks so that they can either avoid these triggers or premedicate appropriately prior to exposure. Patients with asthma should receive annual immunizations against influenza virus, preferably each fall, unless they have a history of adverse reactions to the vaccine.

As-Needed Drug Therapy

Mild asthma can be treated using a short-acting beta$_2$-agonist inhaler when needed. The patient can use the inhaler either to prevent attacks when exposure to known triggers associated with difficulty in breathing are anticipated or to abate dyspnea. The patient should maintain a record of inhaler usage and peak flow measurements.

Chronic Drug Therapy

If a patient with moderate asthma has at least two episodes of asthma symptoms a week, chronic therapy with an anti-inflammatory should be initiated. The anti-inflammatory should be combined with an as-needed or a regularly scheduled inhaled bronchodilator.

For moderate to severe asthma, combinations of drugs that work on the different phases of asthma (i.e., inflammation and bronchoconstriction) are essential. These patients require a fast-acting agent for relief of acute symptoms (short-acting, inhaled $beta_2$-agonist) for as-needed use and an inhaled anti-inflammatory agent as a controller.

For patients with severe asthma, chronic multiple drug use is required. Chronic use of both a long-acting, inhaled $beta_2$-agonist and a high-dose inhaled corticosteroid, supplemented as needed with an additional inhaled short-acting $beta_2$-agonist, is often required. Theophylline, salmeterol, an oral $beta_2$-agonist, and oral steroids may also be needed.

Rescue Therapy

Rescue therapy refers to the management of asthma exacerbations characterized by progressively worsening shortness of breath, cough, wheezing, or chest tightness. The most commonly used agents are short-acting inhaled $beta_2$-agonists and systemic corticosteroids (e.g., prednisone).

Step-Down Therapy

Asthma may improve spontaneously or as a result of therapy. When asthma control is achieved and maintained for at least 3 months, it is reasonable to attempt to identify the minimum therapy required to maintain control by gradually reducing doses or discontinuing medication. Integral components of this approach are patient education and evaluation of patient compliance and response.

Use of Peak Flow Meters in Asthma Management

Delay in seeking medical care is a major contributor to asthma mortality. Subjective symptoms of wheezing and dyspnea are poor measures of lung function and contribute to such delay. Thus, the NAEPP panel has recommended home monitoring of peak expiratory flow rate (PEFR) with portable peak flow meters in all patients with chronic, moderate to severe asthma.

The PEFR correlates well with a patient's forced expiratory volume exhaled in one second (FEV_1) and provides an objective at-home measurement of airway obstruction. Proper use of these devices is important, and pharmacists should ensure proper technique (Table 1). The pharmacist should evaluate individual products before recommending their use.

The patient and physician should determine the patient's best peak flow value. Once it has been determined, the "three-zone" system may be used to relate peak flow readings to

TABLE 1 Correct use of peak flow meters

1. Set the meter indicator on the bottom of the scale before each forced expiration.
2. Take all measurements while standing, if possible.
3. Make sure that the hole in the back of the meter is not covered.
4. Take a deep breath.
5. Seal your lips tightly around the mouthpiece (do not let any air leak out).
6. Rest the mouthpiece on the tongue but do not obstruct the opening of the mouthpiece with the tongue.
7. Expire hard and fast (forcefully).
8. Record the best of three efforts as the peak flow value.

asthma management (Table 2). However, this color-coded scheme, which uses a traffic light analogy, should serve only as a guideline: the patient and his or her physician should individualize the system by defining the peak flow values for each zone. A key point in peak flow monitoring is the establishment of the patient's baseline, because this represents a more practical parameter than a population value. Until the patient's best peak flow value is determined, the use of population averages (based on age, height, and gender) is helpful.

Pharmacologic Agents

General Pharmacology

Asthma medications can be categorized by their ability to inhibit the early asthmatic response (EAR) and/or late asthmatic response (LAR). Medications that prevent the EAR are bronchodilators or inhibitors of mast cell mediator release. Medications that modify the LAR inhibit the inflammatory response that is characteristic of asthma. Table 3 lists the various prescription and nonprescription asthma medications according to which phase they prevent or reverse. Only those drugs that inhibit the LAR can reduce bronchial hyperreactivity (BHR). A comparison of the dosage forms, receptor activity, and duration of action of the nonprescription versus prescription bronchodilators is presented in Table 4.

Beta$_2$-agonists relieve spasms of bronchial smooth muscle caused by the EAR. The nonprescription, and some prescription, beta-agonists also influence other adrenergic receptors (Table 4). The alpha-adrenergic stimulation produces bronchoconstriction, vasoconstriction, urinary retention, and mydriasis, which are not beneficial in asthma. Long-term use of beta$_2$-agonists may produce minor degrees of tolerance or tachyphylaxis.

Asthma medications classified as mast cell stabilizers, anti-inflammatories, and bronchodilators other than epinephrine and ephedrine are available only by prescription. Because asthma is predominantly an inflammatory disease, inhaled corticosteroids have become the mainstay of chronic asthma therapy.

Ingredients in Nonprescription Products

Based on lack of data concerning the efficacy of theophylline at doses available in nonprescription products, the FDA has recently ruled that all nonprescription products containing theophylline be withdrawn.

TABLE 2 Three-zone system of asthma management

Zone	Peak flow values	Patient guideline
Green	≥80–100% of the patient's personal best, or the predicted flow value indicated by a standard chart	*Go!* Continue regular activity and regular asthma maintenance therapy
Yellow	50–80% of the patient's personal best, or the predicted flow value indicated by a standard chart	*Caution!* You may require additional medication or increase in regular maintenance therapy
Red	<50% of the patient's personal best, or the predicted flow value indicated by a standard chart	*Stop!* Seek medical advice or medication immediately

TABLE 3 Phase activity of asthma medications

Medication	EAR	LAR
Beta$_2$-agonist	+	-[a]
Theophylline	+	-
Steroids	-	+
Cromolyn	+	+
Nedocromil	+	+
Anticholinergics	+	-
H$_1$-antihistamines	-	-

Key:

Early asthmatic response (EAR)

Late asthmatic response (LAR)

+ means medication inhibits this response

- means medication does not inhibit this response

[a]Long-acting beta$_2$-agonists may inhibit the LAR

Information extracted from:

Lipworth BJ, McDevitt DG. *Br J Clin Pharmacol.* 1992; 33: 129–38.

Twentyman OP, Finnerty JP, Harris, A, et al. *Lancet.* 1990 Dec 1; 336: 1328–42.

Remaining nonprescription oral products will contain only ephedrine. The worldwide phase out of chlorofluorocarbon (CFC) use, however, will affect current epinephrine-containing metered-dose inhalers (MDIs). Therefore, all current nonprescription products for asthma could be unavailable in the near future.

Because current asthma management emphasizes anti-inflammatory medications for moderate and severe chronic asthma and, perhaps, in mild asthma as well, the utility of currently available nonprescription therapies has been appropriately questioned. The only apparent clinically relevant effect of epinephrine and ephedrine is bronchodilation.

Epinephrine

The FDA has classified the following agents as Category I: epinephrine, epinephrine bitartrate, and epinephrine hydrochloride (racemic) in pressurized, metered-dose aerosol dosage forms and aqueous solutions equivalent to 1% epinephrine for use with hand-held rubber-bulb nebulizers.

Mechanism of Action. Epinephrine has equipotent alpha-, beta$_1$-, and beta$_2$-agonist effects, all of which are dose-dependent. The peak effect of epinephrine aerosol for inhalation occurs within 5 to 10 minutes after use; the duration of action is less than 30 minutes.

Indications. No significant difference exists between prescription and nonprescription epinephrine inhalation products. Acute, severe asthma attacks can be treated by subcutaneous injection or by inhalation. However, inhalation of beta$_2$-agonists is currently the therapy of first choice for both indications.

TABLE 4 Selected characteristics of bronchodilator drugs

Drug	Route of administration	Availability	Sympathomimetic Alpha	Sympathomimetic Beta$_1$	Sympathomimetic Beta$_2$	Anticholinergic	Duration of action (h)
Albuterol[a]	Inhalation	Rx	—	+	+++		3–6
	Oral: tablets	Rx		+	+++		5–8
Atropine	Inhalation	Rx	—	—	—	+++	4
Bitolterol[a]	Inhalation	Rx	—	+	+++		4–6
Epinephrine[a]	Inhalation	OTC	+++	+++	+++		1–3
	Subcutaneous	Rx	+++	+++	+++		1–4
Ephedrine	Oral: syrup, capsules, tablets	OTC	+++	++	++		3–5
	Intramuscular, subcutaneous	Rx	+++	++	++		<1
Ipratropium	Inhalation	Rx	—	—	—	+++	4–6
Isoproterenol[a]	Inhalation	Rx		+++	+++		0.5–2
	Sublingual	Rx		+++	+++		1–2
Isoetharine[a]	Inhalation	Rx		++	+++		1–3
Metaproterenol[a]	Inhalation	Rx		+++	+++		2–4
	Oral: tablets, syrup	Rx		+++	+++		4
Pirbuterol[a]	Inhalation	Rx		+	+++		4–6
Salmeterol	Inhalation	Rx		+	+++	—	12
Terbutaline[a]	Inhalation	Rx		+	+++		3–6
	Oral: tablet	Rx		+	+++		4–8
	Subcutaneous	Rx		+	+++		1.5–4
Theophylline[b] (various salts) (sustained release)	Oral: liquid, tablets	Rx	+	++	++		8–24

+ indicates relative intensity of effect.

[a]Inhalation confers more bronchial activity than systemic administration.

[b]Although theophylline is not a sympathomimetic drug, it causes the release of endogenous catecholamines.

Contraindications. Epinephrine products should not to be used unless a physician has made a diagnosis of asthma, the patient has never been hospitalized for asthma, and no other medications are being taken for asthma unless directed by a physician. Patients with preexisting disease or conditions such as heart disease, high blood pressure, thyroid disease, diabetes, or difficulty in urinating due to enlargement of the prostate should avoid self-treatment with these products, as should patients taking a prescription anti-hypertensive or antidepressant drug.

Dosage.

- For adults and children 4 years of age and older, the dosage recommendation adopted for metered-dose delivery systems is one inhalation followed by a second inhalation if symptoms have not been relieved after at least 1 minute; usage should not then be repeated for at least 3 hours.

- When an aqueous solution at a concentration equivalent to 1% epinephrine base is used with a hand-held rubber-bulb nebulizer, the inhalation dosage for adults and children 4 years of age or older is one to three inhalations no more often than every 3 hours.

- For children under 4 years of age, no dosage recommendations exist.

- The solution should not be used if it is brown or cloudy.

Adverse Effects. Adverse effects are rare when epinephrine is administered by inhalation at recommended levels. Adverse effects observed in patients experiencing a drug overdose may include tachycardia, cardiac arrhythmias, hypertension, tremor, or anxiety.

Precautions. Epinephrine products require statements that warn against exceeding the recommended dosages unless directed by a physician. Many clinicians consider the nonselective adrenergic properties and short duration of action of epinephrine to be adequate reasons not to recommend these products.

Antihistamines

The role of antihistamines in asthma management has also changed substantially in recent years. The prevailing opinion is that antihistamines may offer modest benefit for the patient with asthma and associated allergies. Although the labeling of most prescription and nonprescription antihistamine products still contain warnings about their use in patients with asthma, these products are generally considered safe.

Good control of concurrent allergic rhinitis helps control asthma, whereas poorly controlled allergic rhinitis may worsen asthma. The second-generation prescription anti-histamines cetirizine and azelastine also have anti-inflammatory activity. These agents produce less sedation than the first-generation antihistamines.

Expectorants

Many asthma products contain expectorants, especially guaifenesin and potassium iodide. Guaifenesin, at proper doses, is considered to be safe and effective. Other nonprescription expectorants, however, are probably no more effective than is adequate hydration. A change in mucus production may be a sign of worsening asthma or infection and requires medical evaluation. An FDA advisory panel has recommended that iodide-containing expectorants be restricted to prescription status. The FDA also states that, unless ordered by a physician, guaifenesin should not be taken for a persistent or chronic cough that occurs with asthma.

Antitussives

Antitussives should generally not be used for asthma because a productive cough has a highly useful effect. The reflex cough induced by bronchospasm is often relieved by bronchodilators, not antitussives. According to the FDA, codeine should not be taken by patients with a chronic pulmonary disease or shortness of breath unless directed by a physician. Similarly, dextromethorphan should not be used without a physician's prescription if a cough persists for longer than 1 week; tends to recur; or is accompanied by fever, rash, or persistent headache.

Delivery Systems

Traditional Inhalers

MDIs deliver approximately 10%–15% of the dose to the lower airway. Thus, it is essential that proper technique be used.

The open-mouth technique is advocated to decrease the amount of drug making contact with and adhering to the back of the throat; the risk with this technique is that patients may miss their mouth when they spray. Inhaling more slowly, holding the breath longer, and exhaling slowly increase the amount of drug retained in the airways. Waiting between inhalations allows the bronchodilator to work and may increase delivery of the drug to the airways with subsequent inhalations. When using multiple inhalers, a practical rule is to use the fastest-acting bronchodilator first, followed by the second bronchodilator (if applicable), followed by the nonbronchodilator medications.

A means of determining the need for a refill is to calculate the number of days that the medication should last or estimate the number of as-needed doses that an inhaler usually contains.

Nontraditional Inhalers, Spacers, and Other Devices

Because of the prevalence of suboptimal MDI technique by patients, the use of assist devices or alternative delivery systems may be considered. The most commonly used add-on spacer devices (Aerochamber, InspirEase, and Inhal-Aid) are available only by prescription. The distance between the inhaler mouthpiece and the mouth allows the CFC to evaporate, resulting in smaller droplet sizes and greater lung deposition. Use of a spacer lessens impaction of the drug on the oropharynx and thereby decreases the incidence of oral candidiasis that can occur with regular use of a steroid.

Spacers or extender devices used with MDIs can improve delivery of the drug to the airways.

For best results, patients should be instructed to actuate the MDI once and inhale the drug immediately after actuating the aerosol into the device. The inhalation technique for dry powder inhalers such as Rotahaler is significantly different from that for MDIs. After inserting the device in the mouth the patient should breathe in deeply and rapidly.

Specific Patient or Disease Considerations

Geriatric Patients

Elderly patients may have decreased beta-agonist activity. Lower doses of theophylline should be initiated and the therapy should be monitored by determining serum theophylline concentrations. An elderly patient's medication profile should be closely scrutinized for potential drug interactions with theophylline.

Specialized inhaler instruction should be repeatedly given. Spacers or nebulizers should be used with elderly patients who are unable to use inhalers correctly.

Pediatric Patients

Many children under the age of 5 will not be able to use an MDI correctly; they may need nebulizers. An MDI attached to a spacer device can be mastered by some preschool age asthma patients. Children over 8 years of age can generally use an inhaler without a spacer. The child's technique should be assessed often and the need for a spacer ascertained.

Pregnant/Lactating Patients

The use of asthma medications in a pregnant or lactating patient with asthma is based on the balance between adverse drug reactions and the sequelae of an asthma attack on the developing fetus or nursing infant. The pharmacist should determine the FDA risk category of a product before recommending it to a pregnant woman.

Certain asthma medications can be delivered to a nursing infant via mother's milk. The American Academy of Pediatrics Committee on Drugs lists the following medications as potentially problematic: atropine, dexbrompheniramine maleate with d-isoephedrine, iodinated glycerol, pseudoephedrine, prednisone, prednisolone, terbutaline, theophylline, and triprolidine.

Exercise-Induced Asthma

Exercise-induced asthma may be treated by modifying the exercise regimen or using inhaled beta$_2$-agonists or cromolyn sodium. Patients with exercise-induced asthma may minimize the adverse impact of exercise by choosing exercises that are conducted in warm, humid areas (e.g., swimming); extending their warm-up period; increasing their fitness level; refraining from food ingestion 2 hours before exercise; or wearing a face mask.

Nocturnal Asthma

In some patients, additional pharmacologic therapy may be required to provide treatment throughout the sleeping period. Long-acting inhaled beta-agonists (e.g., salmeterol), sustained-release beta-agonists and sustained-release theophylline can be used. Most patients' nocturnal asthma will improve by increasing their daytime anti-inflammatory therapy with cromolyn or inhaled steroids.

Product Selection Guidelines

Once the assessment of asthma has been confirmed, the pharmacist should ask the patient a series of questions to gather the necessary information for product choice and to determine whether the patient needs medical attention. The pharmacist may consider using a nonprescription asthma drug if the patient has never been to an emergency room or hospitalized for asthma treatment, is not receiving prescription asthma medications, and does not have any of the following conditions:

■ Hypertension;

■ Diabetes;

■ Uncontrolled thyroid disease;

■ Heart disease; or

■ Difficulty in urinating due to an enlarged prostate.

The pharmacist must also determine that the patient has symptoms no more than once a week and has very infrequent nocturnal symptoms. The patient's pharmacy profile and use of other nonprescription medications must then be reviewed for drugs that interact with any of the products available in the nonprescription drugs and any allergies or hyper-sensitivities to the nonprescription products, including aspirin or other nonsteroidal anti-inflammatory drugs (NSAIDs). Specific patient factors such as age, pregnancy, lactation, and finances also need to be considered.

Using nonprescription drugs to treat bronchospasm from asthma presents a dilemma, because nonprescription bronchodilators are usually effective only in mild disease; however, mild disease can progress to more moderate to severe disease if not appropriately treated with anti-inflammatories. In addition, nonprescription bronchodilators may mask worsening asthma. To tread this fine line can be dangerous, and the patient and the patient's family should know when to abandon self-treatment and immediately seek medical care. Patients should be encouraged to rely heavily on peak flow measurements, rather than subjective judgments, in making treatment decisions.

In some patients with bronchospasm and rhinorrhea, decongestant effects of ephedrine or epinephrine may be desirable; however, these patients may be treated more effectively with an alpha-adrenergic nasal spray for the short term and with intranasal cromolyn or corticosteroids for chronic allergic rhinitis.

Patient Counseling

The pharmacist should provide general information about the use and storage of medications, instructions on the use and care of inhalers, and pertinent pharmacologic information.

Patients should be told the following about the use of medications:

■ Do not exceed dosages stated on the labeling.

■ Store asthma medications away from a child's access.

■ Do not store medications in damp or hot places or in direct sunlight.

■ Discard outdated medications away from a child's access.

■ Contact a health care practitioner if you experience decreased responsiveness to a drug.

To educate patients adequately on inhaler use, pharmacists should provide demonstrations of correct technique along with both written (Table 5) and verbal

---

TABLE 5 Correct inhaler technique

1. Remove dust cap.
2. Shake canister.
3. Position inhaler with mouthpiece at the bottom.
4. Tilt head back slightly.
5. Breathe out slowly.
6. Close lips on inhaler or hold inhaler 1 to 2 inches from open mouth.
7. Actuate while inhaling slowly and deeply.
8. Hold breath as long as possible, up to 10 seconds.
9. Breathe out slowly.
10. Wait 30 seconds to 1 minute before administering second inhalation.
11. If steroid inhaler is being used, rinse mouth after use.

instructions. Patients should then demonstrate their inhaler technique to the pharmacist. Resources such as videotaped demonstrations are available from several pharmaceutical manufacturers.

If a patient's technique is not adequate after repeated inhaler instruction, the pharmacist should suggest the use of a spacer. If epinephrine aerosols are being used, the patient should be advised to wait at least 1 minute between inhalations. Patients should also be told that rinsing the mouth after using an inhaler (with or without a spacer) may prevent dryness as well as oral candidal infections.

Care and disposal of the canister are also important. Because of several reports of patients aspirating small objects, including coins, lodged in the mouthpiece, the dust cap should be kept over the mouth piece of the inhaler. Table 6 lists guidelines for canister care.

An important element in educating patients about their asthma therapy is telling them which precautions to take with their medications, what side effects might occur, and what foods, beverages, and medications might contain sulfites. For example, precaution should be taken with the use of antihistamines, which may be associated with increased CNS side effects if taken with other CNS medications (e.g., phenobarbital, pain medications, alcohol).

Some asthma patients develop bronchospasm induced by aspirin. A cross-sensitivity may exist with other NSAIDs (e.g., ibuprofen, ketoprofen, naproxen). Patients should be cautioned that some nonprescription allergy, cough/cold, and analgesic preparations contain aspirin. Aspirin-sensitive patients can usually take acetaminophen as an analgesic.

Asthma patients also need to be educated about the potential of sulfites and sulfur dioxide to elicit bronchospasm. Sulfites are used as preservatives in the pharmaceutical, food, and fermentation industries. Certain medications also contain sulfites; however, by FDA regulations, such medications must list sulfites as an ingredient in the package insert.

Finally, patients should be advised to seek immediate medical intervention if they experience any of the following:

- Inability to complete a full sentence without stopping;
- Persistent discomfort after using a bronchodilator, even while at rest;
- Incomplete relief of symptoms after using a bronchodilator;
- Worsening of dyspnea after using a bronchodilator.

Various pharmaceutical companies, agencies, and foundations offer patient education materials and services. A complete list of educational material can be obtained from the National Asthma Education and Prevention Program, Office of Prevention, Education, and Control, National Heart, Lung, and Blood Institute, National Institutes of Health, Bethesda, MD 20892.

TABLE 6   Care of canister

Wash the inhaler mouthpiece daily with warm water to prevent clogging. Keep the mouthpiece free of particles.

Routinely clean and air-dry inhaler devices.

Do not puncture the unit; the contents are under pressure.

Do not store the canister near heat (≥120°F [≥48.9°C]) or open flames.

Do not discard canisters into fires or incinerators.

Be aware that canisters left in freezing temperatures will release large aerosol particles after actuation. Allow the canister to come to room temperature (59–86°F [15–30°C]) before use.

Chapter 10

Sleep Aid and Stimulant Products

Questions to ask in patient assessment and counseling

Sleep Aid Products

- How long have you had trouble sleeping?
- How severe is your sleep disturbance?
- Do you generally have trouble falling asleep? Do you wake up frequently or too early?
- Do you feel rested when you awake in the morning?
- Do you have trouble staying alert during the day?
- Do you take naps? How often?
- What do you think is causing your sleep problem?
- Has there been increased stress in your life lately?
- Do you have any health problems?
- Do you take any prescription and nonprescription medications? If so, what are they?
- Do you drink coffee or other caffeinated beverages? How often and at what times?
- Do you drink alcoholic beverages? If so, how much and how often?
- Do you smoke?
- Have you ever been treated for psychiatric illness?
- Would you describe yourself as a nervous or anxious person?
- Have you recently felt depressed or disinterested in your usual activities?
- Have you ever been told you snore loudly or are a restless sleeper?
- What methods or medications have you used to treat your sleep disturbance? How long did you use them? Were they effective?

Stimulant Products

- Why do you want to use this product?
- How long do you intend to use this product?
- Have you ever used a stimulant product? Did you experience any adverse effects?
- Do you regularly drink coffee, tea, cola, or other caffeinated beverages? Have you experienced adverse effects from drinking them?
- Do you take any prescription and nonprescription medications? If so, what are they?
- Are you under a physician's care? What medical problems do you have?
- Do you have anxiety, irritability, or any other nervous condition?
- Do you have problems sleeping? (If patient has problems sleeping, see Sleep Aid Products questions.)

Editor's Note: This chapter is adapted from M. Lynn Crismon and Donna M. Jermain, "Sleep Aid and Stimulant Products," in Covington, T.R., ed., *Handbook of Nonprescription Drugs,* 11th edition. For a more extensive discussion of sleep physiology, sleep disorders, and sleep aid and stimulant products, readers are encouraged to consult Chapter 10 of the *Handbook.*

- *Are you pregnant or breast-feeding?*
- *Do you smoke cigarettes or chew tobacco?*
- *Do you drink alcohol? If so, how much and how often?*

Sleep Disorders

Although insomnia is the most common cause of difficulty in sleeping, patients with other sleep disorders may also seek a nonprescription sleep aid from the pharmacist. Among these disorders are sleep apnea, narcolepsy, nocturnal myoclonus, and restless legs syndrome.

Insomnia

Insomnia is not a disease. It is a symptom or patient complaint for which there are no precise criteria or definitions. Patients may complain of difficulty falling asleep, frequent nocturnal awakening, early morning awakening, or poor quality of sleep. There is no ideal duration of sleep, and patients complaining of a sleep disturbance may actually sleep for the same length of time as other individuals who feel they sleep well. However, these patients usually report that it takes them more than 30 minutes to fall asleep, and their sleep duration is less than 6–7 hours nightly. Moreover, their perceived sleep pattern and quality of daytime functioning may be more important than their duration of sleep. Thus, patients with insomnia are those who feel they sleep poorly at night and function poorly during the day.

Insomnia can be classified as transient, short-term, or chronic. It is extremely important that the pharmacist ask the patient questions to determine the etiology and duration of the insomnia. Although nonprescription sleep products have not been extensively evaluated, it is assumed they work best in transient and short-term insomnia.

Transient insomnia is commonly caused by environmental changes or life stresses. Transient insomnia is often self-limiting, lasting less than 1 week. If more severe stresses are present, transient insomnia may become short-term insomnia, which usually lasts 1–3 weeks.

Chronic or long-term insomnia lasts from more than 3 weeks to years and is often the result of medical problems, psychologic dysfunction, or substance abuse. Faulty sleep habits may also be a cause. For example, the elderly often take daytime naps, which may contribute to nocturnal sleep disturbance.

Sleep Apnea

Sleep apnea is characterized by poor sleep quality, gasping, snoring, and daytime fatigue and sedation. This disorder, which occurs more often among the elderly, appears to be more common in men. Significant morbidity is associated with obstructive sleep apnea.

Narcolepsy, Nocturnal Myoclonus, and Restless Legs Syndrome

Narcolepsy is characterized by daytime sleep attacks, cataplexy (sudden loss of muscle tone), hypnagogic hallucinations, and sleep paralysis. The patient with nocturnal myoclonus experiences jerky leg movements throughout the night. Restless legs syndrome is manifested by an uncomfortable feeling in the calves and thighs and irresistible leg movements in the evening hours. Nocturnal myoclonus and restless legs syndrome may occur concomitantly. Patients who complain of any of these types of symptoms should be referred to a physician. Formal assessment by a sleep laboratory can be extremely useful.

Patient Assessment

The pharmacist should evaluate the patient carefully before deciding whether to recommend a nonprescription product. Questions such as those at the beginning of this chapter should be asked. Medical and psychiatric problems are often associated with long-term insomnia (Table 1); this is particularly relevant for elderly patients. Numerous medications and recreational drugs may induce sleep disturbance (Table 2); for this reason, the pharmacist should perform a careful history to rule out the possibility of drug-induced sleep dysfunction. If, during questioning of a patient, the pharmacist discovers a medical, psychiatric, or drug-induced reason for the insomnia, or if the patient has long-term insomnia, the pharmacist should encourage the patient to see a physician for a complete evaluation. Whether a sleep product is recommended or not, the pharmacist should counsel the patient regarding sleep hygiene (Table 3).

TABLE 1   Etiology of chronic (long-term) insomnia

Medical problems

Pain

Angina pectoris

Arthritis

Cancer

Chronic pain syndromes

Cluster headaches

Migraine

Peptic ulcer/gastrointestinal reflux

Postoperative pain

Respiratory difficulty

Asthma

Bronchitis

Chronic obstructive pulmonary disease

Congestive heart failure

Other medical problems

Constipation

Epilepsy

Hyperthyroidism

Nocturia

Parkinson's disease

Peptic ulcer disease

Renal insufficiency

Tachyarrhythmias

Psychiatric problems (30%–70% of cases)

Anxiety disorder

Bipolar disorder

Dementia

Depression

Posttraumatic stress disorder

Schizophrenia

Substance abuse

Sleep disorders

Sleep apnea

Nocturnal myoclonus

Delayed sleep phase syndrome (night-shift workers)

Drug-related insomnia

Psychophysiologic insomnia (idiopathic insomnia)

Restless legs syndrome

TABLE 2   Drugs that may exacerbate insomnia

Drugs that may cause insomnia	Drugs that may produce withdrawal insomnia
Alcohol	**Alcohol**
Antidepressants	**Antihistamines**
Buproprion	**Barbiturates**
Monoamine oxidase	**Benzodiazepines**
Serotonin-specific reuptake inhibitors	
Tricyclic antidepressants	**Hypnotics (miscellaneous)**
Venlafaxine	Bromides
Antihypertensives	Chloral hydrate
Beta blockers (especially propanolol)	Ethchlorvynol
Clonidine	Glutethimide
Diuretics (at bedtime)	
Methyldopa	**Monoamine oxidase inhibitors**
Reserpine	
Hypnotic use (chronic)	**Tricyclic antidepressants**
Nicotine	**Miscellaneous**
Sympathomimetic amines	Amphetamines
Amphetamines	Cocaine
Appetite suppressants	Marijuana
Beta-adrenergic agonists	Opiates
Caffeine	Phencyclidine
Decongestants (e.g., phenylpropanolamine, phenylephrine)	
Miscellaneous	
Anabolic steroids	
Antineoplastics	
Corticosteroids	
Histamine$_2$-receptor antagonists	
Levodopa	
Methysergide	
Oral contraceptives	
Phenytoin	
Quinidine	
Theophylline	
Thyroid preparations	

Sleep Aid Products

The primary indication for nonprescription sleep aids is the symptomatic management of transient and short-term insomnia. Antihistamines are the most common nonprescription treatment for insomnia; however, a phytomedicinal product, valerian, and the hormone melatonin are also marketed as sleep aids.

TABLE 3 Principles of good sleep hygiene

1. Follow a regular sleep pattern: go to bed and arise at about the same time daily.
2. Make the bedroom comfortable for sleeping. Avoid temperature extremes, noise, and lights.
3. Make sure the bed is comfortable.
4. Engage in relaxing activities prior to bedtime.
5. Exercise regularly but not late in the evening.
6. Use the bedroom only for sleep and sexual activities, and not as an office or game room.
7. If tense, practice relaxation exercises.
8. Avoid eating meals or large snacks immediately prior to bedtime.
9. Eliminate daytime naps.
10. Avoid caffeine after noon.
11. Avoid alcohol or nicotine use late in the evening.
12. If unable to fall asleep, leave the bedroom and participate in relaxing activities until tired.

Antihistamines

Diphenhydramine (hydrochloride or citrate) is the only agent that the Food and Drug Administration (FDA) deems safe and effective for nonprescription use. Although the safety of doxylamine has not been fully established and no published studies supporting the efficacy of doxylamine as a sleep aid are currently available, the FDA has allowed it to remain on the market.

Pharmacokinetics

Both diphenhydramine and doxylamine are well absorbed from the gastrointestinal (GI) tract and have short to intermediate half-lives. Significant drowsiness has been shown to last from 3 to 6 hours after a single 50-mg dose of diphenhydramine whereas impairment in performance on psychomotor tests lasts only 2 to 4 hours. This may indicate that patients can be assured that their ability to perform tasks requiring mental alertness and cognitive ability will not be impaired for any longer than they feel drowsy.

Efficacy

Of the published clinical trials with diphenhydramine, most indicate efficacy. Because no published efficacy and safety studies are available documenting the value of doxylamine as a sleep aid, only diphenhydramine should be recommended to patients for such use at the present time.

Although poorly studied, tolerance to the hypnotic effects of diphenhydramine appears to result with repeated use. Most adult patients should be advised not to exceed 50 mg nightly, and all patients should limit their use of diphenhydramine to no more than 7–10 consecutive nights. Patients complaining of continuing insomnia after 10 days of non-prescription sleep aid use and good sleep hygiene measures should be referred to a physician for a more thorough evaluation.

Adverse Effects/Toxicity

The primary side effects of diphenhydramine and doxylamine are anticholinergic. Common adverse effects include dry mouth and throat, constipation, blurred vision, and tinnitus. Older male patients should be asked about prostatic hypertrophy and difficulty urinating. Narrow- (closed-) angle glaucoma is also a contraindication. Patients with cardiovascular disease may be particularly susceptible to the anticholinergic adverse effects of ethanolamine sleep aids such as diphenhydramine and doxylamine. A patient's concomitant medication regimen should be reviewed before a pharmacist recommends diphenhydramine. A patient who is taking other anticholinergics should be alerted to the potential for additive side effects.

Patients should be cautioned not to drive an automobile or operate machinery until their response to the drug is known. They should also be warned of the additive central nervous system (CNS) depressant effects of alcohol and encouraged not to drink alcoholic beverages while taking these drugs. Some patients may develop excitation from diphenhydramine and other highly anticholinergic antihistamines.

Antihistamine dosage excess can result in potentially lethal anticholinergic toxicity. This may occur as a result of drug interactions, the purposeful ingestion of a large amount of the medication, or individual sensitivity. Anticholinergic toxicity is particularly common in children, in whom the symptoms are usually more severe. CNS anticholinergic toxicity is one of the primary presenting features of antihistamine excess. Physical signs may include dilated pupils, flushed skin, hot and dry mucous membranes, and elevated body temperature. Tachycardia is common. In more severe cases, delirium, coma, or seizures may occur.

Use during Pregnancy/Lactation

The safety of antihistamines during pregnancy has not been clearly established. Pharmacists should advise pregnant women to consult their physician regarding any sleep disturbance.

There appears to be an increased risk of CNS side effects from antihistamine use in neonates. For this reason, and because such drugs may inhibit lactation, pharmacists should recommend that nursing mothers not use antihistamines for sleep.

Miscellaneous Products

L-Tryptophan

In 1990, the FDA recalled all products containing L-tryptophan except protein supplements, infant formulas, and parenteral and enteral nutritional products. L-tryptophan has been associated with eosinophilia-myalgia syndrome (EMS) and serotonin storm. The symptoms of EMS include myalgia, fatigue, shortness of breath, cough, skin rash, arthralgias, peripheral edema, and eosinophilia. The concomitant use of L-tryptophan and serotonin reuptake inhibitors or monoamine oxidase inhibitors has resulted in a serotonin storm. Symptoms of this drug interaction include agitation, restlessness, tremor, hyperthermia, diarrhea, and cramping. Given its questionable efficacy and known adverse effects, pharmacists should be reluctant to recommend L-tryptophan as a sleep aid.

Valerian

Valerian is an herbal remedy that has been used for some time in several European countries as a sleep aid. Valerian is not included in the 1989 FDA-approved monograph on nonprescription sleep aids. Pharmacists should not recommend valerian as a sleep aid or sedative until there is more information available.

Melatonin

Melatonin, an endogenous hormone produced by the pineal gland, shifts circadian rhythm by a mechanism that is nearly opposite to that of light exposure. Melatonin also decreases body temperature and mental alertness. These findings have aroused interest in examining the effects of this hormone in sleep disorders, especially sleep phase shifts, jet lag, and mood disorders. There is some evidence to support a hypothesis that physiologic doses of melatonin are associated with sleep induction.

If recommending melatonin for use in a patient with insomnia, the pharmacist should stipulate that doses no greater than 0.1–1 mg be taken. Patients should also be cautioned not to drive or operate machinery after taking the sleep aid. Pharmacists should be aware that these recommendations are made without benefit of FDA review.

Alcohol

Ethanol is a CNS depressant. After occasional evening consumption of one or two drinks, alcohol is effective in decreasing sleep latency; however, with heavy or continuous consumption, alcohol disrupts the sleep cycle.

Alcohol is present in some nonprescription combination cold products. Products of this type are marketed and sometimes recommended by physicians and pharmacists to induce sleep. Data are limited regarding their efficacy and safety as sleep aids.

Approximately 10%–15% of chronic insomniacs have problems with substance abuse, especially alcohol abuse. Patients who abuse alcohol are also frequent abusers of other CNS depressants. The pharmacist must acquire the patient's medication history to evaluate the possibilities of additive CNS depression between alcohol and other medications and of substance abuse. Patients who drink regularly should be referred to a physician. Most clinicians advise that alcohol never be used as a sleep aid or an adjunct to a sleep aid program.

Stimulant Products (Caffeine)

Caffeine is a common ingredient in coffee, tea, soft drinks, and chocolate products. It is also present in many prescription and nonprescription drugs, including headache and cold remedies, menstrual pain relief products, diet aids, and stimulant preparations. Caffeine is the only FDA-approved stimulant for nonprescription use.

Physiologic Effects

Central Nervous System Effects

Caffeine doses of 50–200 mg can increase alertness and decrease fatigue and drowsiness. At higher doses, caffeine may produce tremulousness, nervousness, headache, irritability, and insomnia.

Caffeine's effect on sleep varies greatly among individuals. Caffeine also has varying effects on mood. Aggressive behavior has been reported to decrease with caffeine reduction. Caffeine may exacerbate anxiety, thus potentially worsening symptoms in patients with anxiety or panic disorder.

Cardiovascular Effects

Caffeine stimulates heart muscle; however, this action is often opposed by simultaneous medullary vagal stimulation. As the caffeine dose is increased, the myocardium stimulation overcomes the vagal effect.

Pharmacokinetics

Caffeine is rapidly and completely absorbed from the GI tract, and peak plasma concentrations occur 30–60 minutes after ingestion. Caffeine crosses the blood–brain barrier rapidly. It is extensively metabolized in the liver. In adults, the average half-life of caffeine is 4–6 hours. In infants under 3 months of age, the half-life may be as long as 100 hours.

Indications

Caffeine is commercially available as the sole ingredient in most CNS stimulant products as well as one of the ingredients in many combination products such as headache remedies. As a CNS stimulant, caffeine is marketed to help patients stay awake and to restore mental alertness. Oral doses of 100–200 mg are needed to achieve mild CNS stimulation in adults. The recommended adult dose of timed-release products is 200–250 mg. Before recommending caffeine as a CNS stimulant, the pharmacist should ask the patient the questions outlined at the beginning of this chapter. Given the paucity of data supporting the efficacy of caffeine and the well-known effects of caffeine excess, pharmacists should carefully consider whether caffeine products should be recommended.

Adverse Effects

The primary adverse events associated with caffeine are CNS stimulant effects and GI irritation. Adverse CNS effects include insomnia, nervousness, restlessness, excitement, tinnitus, muscular tremor, headache, lightheadedness, and mild delirium. These effects are more pronounced in children. Adverse GI effects include nausea, vomiting, diarrhea, and stomach pain. Other adverse effects include diuresis, extrasystoles, palpitations, and tachycardia.

Dependence/Withdrawal

Physical dependence may result from prolonged caffeine consumption; withdrawal symptoms can occur following abrupt cessation. The most common withdrawal symptoms are fatigue and headache. Anxiety, nausea, vomiting, impaired psychomotor function, and irritability are also noted. Withdrawal symptoms generally occur 12–24 hours after cessation of caffeine ingestion, peak in 20–48 hours, and may persist for a week.

Toxicity

Serious symptomatology can occur after caffeine overdose. Symptoms include nervousness, restlessness, insomnia, excitement, diuresis, facial flushing, muscle twitching, GI disturbance, tachycardia or cardiac arrhythmia, "rambling" flow of thought and speech, psychomotor agitation, or periods of inexhaustibility. The lethal dose in adults is 150–200 mg/kg of body weight.

Drug Interactions

Patients should be informed that caffeine's metabolism is inhibited by alcohol, disulfiram, mexiletine, cimetidine, norfloxacin, enoxacin, ciprofloxacin, and oral contraceptives containing estrogen.

GI distress is increased when nonsteroidal anti-inflammatory drugs, aspirin, corticosteroids, or alcohol is administered along with caffeine. Blood pressure may be increased when caffeine and phenylpropanolamine are coadministered. Monoamine oxidase inhibitors in combination with caffeine are of concern because patients may develop life-threatening cardiac complications. Caffeine does not typically affect the efficacy of medications used to treat hypertension but may interfere with the benefit of antiarrhythmic agents. Caffeine and diazepam coadministered have antagonizing effects.

Therapeutic Concerns

Pediatric Considerations

Although there appear to be no behavioral problems reported in normal children consuming caffeine, there is no indication that children have been intentionally given caffeine as a stimulant.

Geriatric Considerations

In the elderly, caffeine consumption may be a factor in subjective insomnia. If calcium intake and balance are maintained, caffeine does not pose a risk for osteoporosis.

Use during Pregnancy/Lactation

Teratogenic Effects. The FDA issued a warning in 1980 advising pregnant women to limit or avoid caffeine consumption. However, no consistent teratogenic effects have been reported in animal studies that used massive caffeine doses.

Overall, information is incomplete and the data are conflicting, but no direct correlations can be made between caffeine consumption and birth defects. However, it is prudent to recommend limiting caffeine intake to 300 mg per day or less, because decreases in birth weight are reported to occur when intake exceeds this amount.

Concentration in Breast Milk. Caffeine passes into breast milk; however, the caffeine concentration in breast milk is only 1% of the mother's plasma concentration. No adverse effects have been reported in infants of nursing mothers consuming 200–336 mg per day of caffeine. Caffeine, whether from medicinal or food sources, should be ingested immediately after nursing, and consumption should be moderate.

Benign Breast Disease

Fibrocystic breast disease may be associated with caffeine consumption.

Guidelines for Patient Education and Counseling

Pharmacists should be aware of the various prescription and nonprescription products containing caffeine and should advise patients of the additive effects of dietary and medicinal caffeine. Elderly patients who are receiving other CNS stimulants should ingest caffeine with caution.

Patients need to be advised of the possible drug interactions, as outlined above, that may occur with caffeine. The combination of caffeine and alcohol ingestion needs to be addressed. Contrary to folklore, caffeine will not "sober up" a person intoxicated on alcohol.

Caffeine is contraindicated in patients with known hypersensitivity to the drug. It should be used cautiously in patients who have or have had peptic ulcer disease and in individuals with symptomatic cardiac arrhythmias and palpitations. High-dose caffeine intake may result in a hyperglycemic event because it may increase blood glucose concentrations. Lower doses should be used in patients with renal dysfunction. Caffeine has been shown to worsen mental status in some patients with psychiatric disorders.

Caffeine should never be recommended as a substitute for adequate sleep and rest.

CHAPTER 11

Acid-Peptic Products

Questions to ask in patient assessment and counseling

- Can you describe the pain? How severe is it?
- How long have you had this pain?
- Is the pain constant, or does it come and go?
- When does the pain occur? Do you experience it immediately after meals or several hours later? Does the pain wake you up at night? Is it worse when you lie down? When you bend over?
- Is the pain relieved by food? Do certain foods, coffee, or carbonated beverages make it worse?
- Do you have any other signs and symptoms?
- Do you drink alcohol? How much? Is the pain worse after drinking alcohol?
- Have you lost any weight recently?
- Have you vomited blood or black material that looks like coffee grounds?
- Have you noticed red blood in the stool, or have the stools been black or tarry?
- Have you had any difficulty or pain when swallowing?
- Have you seen a health care provider about these symptoms? If so, what did your health care provider tell you to do?
- Have you ever used an antacid or histamine$_2$-receptor antagonist (for example, Zantac) to treat this pain? Which one? How were you taking the product? Did it relieve the pain?
- What prescription and nonprescription drugs do you take? Have you recently taken aspirin, naproxen sodium, or ibuprofen products?
- Do you smoke? How much?
- Have you or has anyone in your family ever had an ulcer?
- Do you have any medical problems such as diabetes or kidney or heart disease? Are you currently under a health care provider's care for any medical conditions?
- Are you on a special diet?

Self-care is an important part of the management of upper abdominal pain and discomfort. Antacids are useful for the short-term relief of indigestion, heartburn, and excessive eating and drinking, as well as for the relief of symptoms associated with gastroesophageal reflux disease (GERD) and peptic ulcer disease (PUD). The pharmacist should be able to distinguish between those patients who are appropriate for self-treatment and those who need medical attention and select appropriate antacids, histamine$_2$-receptor antagonists (H$_2$RAs), and/or antiflatulent products.

Editor's Note: This chapter is adapted from Julianne B. Pinson and C. Wayne Weart, "Acid-Peptic Products," in Covington, T.R., ed., *Handbook of Nonprescription Drugs,* 11th edition. For a more extensive discussion of the physiology of the gastrointestinal tract, acid-peptic disorders, and acid-peptic products, readers are encouraged to consult Chapter 11 of the *Handbook.*

Acid-Peptic Disorders

The maintenance of normal, healthy gastroduodenal mucosa is often described as a balance between the aggressive forces of acid and pepsin and the defensive forces of the gastric mucosal barrier. Virtually all factors implicated in the etiology of gastric diseases affect this critical balance in some way.

Peptic Ulcer Disease

PUD is a group of chronic disorders characterized by ulcerating mucosal lesions in the upper GI tract. The most common sites of PUD are the duodenum and the stomach. Duodenal ulcers (DUs) typically affect persons 25–55 years of age, while the peak incidence of gastric ulcers (GUs) occurs around 55–65 years of age.

Pathogenesis

Acid was previously thought to be the most important factor in the development of peptic ulcers. Today, it is recognized that although acid must be present for ulcers to develop, it does not usually cause ulcers in the absence of factors that disrupt the gastric mucosal barrier. The two most important factors that disturb this barrier and thus promote ulcer development are *Helicobacter pylori* (*H pylori*) and nonsteroidal anti-inflammatory drugs (NSAIDs).

Helicobacter pylori. Virtually all patients (95%–100%) with DUs and more than 95% of patients with GUs that are not caused by NSAIDs harbor the organism.

PUD has historically been viewed as a chronic disease. However, mounting evidence demonstrates dramatic reductions in recurrence rates in patients in whom *H pylori* has been eradicated.

NSAIDs. NSAIDs are the most common cause of ulcers in patients who are not infected with *H pylori*. Most NSAID-induced ulcers occur in the stomach. The risk of developing NSAID-induced ulcers or complications increases with age, previous history of peptic ulcer or GI bleeding, higher doses of NSAIDs, concomitant cardiovascular disease, and concomitant use of corticosteroids.

Other Factors.

■ Smoking doubles the incidence of PUD, increases ulcer recurrence, and reduces ulcer healing with H₂RAs.

■ Alcohol is not a proven risk factor for PUD except in patients with cirrhosis.

■ The role of stress and psychologic factors in PUD remains controversial.

Signs and Symptoms

■ Upper abdominal pain is the most frequent symptom of PUD.

■ Pain is usually relieved within 5–10 minutes of eating or taking antacids.

■ Fifty–eighty percent of ulcer patients report being awakened with pain at night.

■ Nausea and vomiting, diarrhea, a sense of fullness, and abdominal distention are fairly common with GUs but less so with DUs.

■ Symptoms do not correlate well with ulceration.

■ Asymptomatic disease is particularly likely in elderly patients.

The most common complication of PUD is bleeding. Other major complications include perforation, penetration, and gastric outlet obstruction.

Treatment

Patients who describe a history and symptoms consistent with PUD or NSAID-induced gastropathy should be referred to a health care provider. This is especially important for elderly patients and those with symptoms suggestive of ulcer complications. Patients who have experienced significant weight loss should also be advised to consult a health care provider.

Use of Prescription Drugs. The goals of therapy for PUD have been to promote ulcer healing, relieve pain, prevent complications, and prevent recurrences. Since 1977, H_2RAs have been the preferred agents to achieve these goals. When used as maintenance therapy, these agents are effective at reducing recurrence rates. Sucralfate is as effective as the H_2RAs in healing and reducing recurrence rates of DUs but is not approved for healing or maintenance of GUs. Ulcer healing may also be accomplished with proton pump inhibitors, which tend to achieve faster symptomatic relief and healing rates than H_2RAs.

Eradication of Helicobacter pylori. Increasingly, the goals for PUD are being met by eradication of *H pylori*. The NIH Consensus Panel recommended that ulcer patients with *H pylori* infection be treated with antibiotics in addition to antisecretory agents, regardless of whether they are suffering from the initial presentation of the disease or a recurrence. Eradication of *H pylori* modestly reduces time to ulcer healing, enhances healing of refractory ulcers, and substantially reduces the rate of ulcer recurrence.

Antacids. Antacids were the mainstay of therapy for PUD until the late 1970s, when H_2RAs became available. It was not until 1977, however, that high doses of antacids were actually proven effective in healing DUs and GUs. Antacids also heal most small NSAID-induced ulcers within 12 weeks, whether or not NSAIDs are continued.

Despite an equal ability to heal ulcers, antacids are not favored as first-line therapy over prescription agents for PUD.

When antacids are recommended for supplemental pain relief, patients should be advised to take doses providing 40–80 mEq neutralizing capacity. These doses may be taken on an as-needed basis and may be titrated upward. Because antacids can reduce the bioavailability of H_2RAs, doses should be separated by 1–2 hours. Most patients will need supplemental antacids for pain relief only for the first 7–14 days of treatment; however, healing cannot be expected before 4–6 weeks. Pharmacists should educate patients regarding the poor correlation between pain relief and ulcer healing. Patients who are taking antacids or other medications and whose pain has not yet resolved should contact their health care providers, but should not discontinue their medication.

Nonprescription H_2-Receptor Antagonists. Nonprescription H_2RAs are not approved for the healing or maintenance of PUD, nor are they indicated for symptomatic relief of pain associated with ulcers. Patients wishing to self-medicate with these agents should be questioned about their symptoms, history of GI disorders, and use of prescription medications. Some patients may not understand that nonprescription H_2RAs are simply lower doses of the prescription agents they are already taking.

It is unlikely that nonprescription H_2RAs will prevent NSAID-induced ulcers. It is possible, however, that H_2RAs would relieve dyspeptic symptoms associated with NSAID use. It is prudent for the pharmacist to refer patients with NSAID-associated dyspeptic symptoms for medical evaluation if they are at high risk for, or would not tolerate, complications of an NSAID-induced ulcer. Such patients include the elderly, smokers, those using corticosteroids concomitantly, those with a history of PUD or GI bleeding, those using high doses of NSAIDS, and those with concomitant cardiovascular disease.

Nondrug Measures. Bland diets and small meals eaten at frequent intervals appear to have no benefit. Patients should be encouraged to eat three meals a day of their own choosing and should avoid eating snacks at night. Caffeine-containing beverages, alcohol, and smoking should be discouraged. The frequent use of milk as a buffer to acid has been suggested in patients with PUD. However, milk is a very poor buffering agent, and the calcium and protein in milk actually stimulate acid secretion.

Gastroesophageal Reflux Disease

The reflux of gastric contents into the esophagus, or gastroesophageal reflux, is generally a benign physiologic process. Patients who suffer symptoms or tissue damage as a result of gastroesophageal reflux are said to suffer from GERD. What distinguishes patients with GERD from those with normal physiologic reflux is the frequency and duration of reflux episodes, resulting in related signs and symptoms and/or esophageal tissue damage. The typical complaint of patients with reflux esophagitis is heartburn; however, all patients with heartburn do not necessarily have reflux esophagitis.

Pathogenesis

Many factors may promote reflux by reducing lower esophageal sphincter (LES) tone, delaying gastric emptying, increasing acid secretion, or impairing the gastroesophageal pressure gradient (Table 1).

Signs and Symptoms

- Heartburn, the classic symptom of PUD, is usually described as a burning sensation or pain in the lower chest.
- Pain may radiate up into the chest, the back, and less often, the throat.
- Pain may occur soon after meals, upon lying down or stooping, and after some forms of exercise. Many patients state that the pain wakes them from sleep.
- Chest pain, not typical of heartburn, may resemble anginal pain.
- Regurgitation is an extension of the reflux process. Patients may complain of an acid, bitter taste or a "sour stomach."
- Delayed gastric emptying is evidenced by bloating, early satiety, belching, and nausea.
- Dysphagia (a sensation of slowed or blocked passage between the mouth and esophagus) may indicate an esophageal stricture, cancer, or motility disorder.
- Odynophagia (pain on swallowing) may occur and usually suggests severe mucosal damage in the esophagus.

Complications of GERD include acute and chronic bleeding from esophageal ulcers, esophageal strictures, and pulmonary complications (e.g., cough, bronchitis, pneumonia).

Treatment

Any patient who describes difficulty or pain when swallowing may have developed complications from GERD and should be referred to a health care provider. Gastric cancer might be suspected in patients who report significant, unintentional weight loss or in patients older than 45 years who report a new onset of symptoms. Patients whose symptoms are suggestive of anginal pain also warrant referral.

TABLE 1 Factors that promote gastroesophageal reflux disease

Reduced lower esophageal sphincter tone

Smoking

Beverages and foods
  Alcohol
  Caffeine
  Chocolates
  Fatty, greasy foods
  Spearmint
  Peppermint

Medications
  Anticholinergic agents
  Beta$_2$-agonists
  Calcium channel antagonists
  Diazepam
  Dopamine
  Estrogen
  Meperidine
  Morphine
  Nitrates
  Progesterone
  Prostaglandins
  Tricyclic antidepressants

Delayed gastric emptying

Anticholinergic medications
Overeating
Motility disorder

Increased acid secretion

Smoking

Beverages and foods
  Alcohol
  Citrus fruits
  Coffee
  Garlic
  Milk
  Onions
  Soda
  Spicy foods
  Tomatoes, tomato-based foods

Hypersecretory conditions
  Duodenal ulcers
  Endocrine adenomas
  Zollinger-Ellison syndrome

Impaired gastroesophageal pressure gradient

Supine body position
Obesity
Tight-fitting clothing

Adapted from *Pepcid AC New Product Bulletin*. Washington, DC: American Pharmaceutical Association; August 1995.

The management of GERD may be viewed as a stepped-care approach, with antacids, nonprescription H$_2$RAs, and nondrug measures forming the basis for the first step (Figure 1).

Antacids. Antacids have long been the mainstay for patients needing symptomatic relief for mild to moderate GERD.

Treatment ranging from high doses of liquid aluminum-magnesium antacids (80–160 mEq acid-neutralizing capacity [ANC] given seven times daily) to low doses of antacid tablets (14–30 mEq ANC/tablet) taken as needed have been reported to provide symptomatic relief. It is reasonable to advise patients to begin with 40–80 mEq as needed for symptoms. If necessary, these doses may be titrated to a scheduled regimen, such as 40–80 mEq after meals and at bedtime.

Some antacid products contain alginic acid. They are not as effective when patients are supine; therefore, patients receiving such products should be instructed not to lie down immediately after taking them. Products containing alginic acid are best suited for use throughout the day, whereas antacids may be taken throughout the day and/or at bedtime.

Antireflux surgery			**Phase 3:** Refractory disease

| Lansoprazole 30 mg/day _or_ Omeprazole 20–40 mg/day | Cimetidine 800 mg bid or 400 mg qid _and/or_ Ranitidine 150 mg qid Famotidine 40 mg bid Nizatidine 150 mg bid | Cisapride 10–20 mg ac & hs _or_ Metoclopramide 10–20 mg ac & hs | **Phase 2B:** Severe mucosal damage |

| Cimetidine 400 mg bid or 300 mg qid _and/or_ Ranitidine 150 mg qid Famotidine 20 mg bid Nizatidine 150 mg bid | Metoclopramide 10–20 mg ac & hs _or_ Cisapride 10–20 mg ac & hs | **Phase 2A:** Persistent symptoms Mucosal damage |

| Diet modification Weight loss Elevate head of bed Avoid drugs that decrease _and_ LES tone Restrict smoking & alcohol Avoid lying down after eating Avoid tight-fitting clothes | Antacids ± alginic acid 40–80 mEq pc & hs _or_ Cimetidine 200 mg bid Famotidine 10 mg bid Ranitidine 75 mg bid Nizatidine 75 mg bid | **Phase 1:** Mild/ occasional symptoms Do not seek medical help |

Lower esophageal sphincter (LES); acid neutralizing capacity (ANC).
Before meals (ac); after meals (pc); bedtime (hs); twice daily (bid); four times daily (qid).

FIGURE 1   Stepped-care approach to managing gastroesophageal reflux disease.

Nonprescription H_2-Receptor Antagonists.   The nonprescription H_2RAs ranitidine, cimetidine, and famotidine are approved for the relief of heartburn, acid indigestion, and sour stomach. Famotidine and cimetidine are also approved for prevention of these symptoms associated with food and beverages. The nonprescription form of nizatidine is approved only for the prevention of these symptoms.

Medical Referral.   When patients have pain that does not respond to conservative treatment with lifestyle modifications, antacids, and/or nonprescription H_2RAs, they should be referred for medical evaluation. Moderate-to-severe GERD requires very high doses of prescription H_2RAs or proton pump inhibitors because damaged mucosa in the esophagus is more difficult to heal than that in the duodenum. Patients with recurring disease require maintenance therapy with full doses of H_2RAs, proton pump inhibitors, or antireflux surgery.

Nondrug Measures. Some patients with mild GERD can be managed with nondrug measures alone. Those who respond to antacids or nonprescription H$_2$RAs should also be educated about lifestyle modifications which may significantly reduce or eliminate symptoms.

Nonpharmacologic interventions for patients with GERD attempt to reduce or eliminate factors that promote reflux. Patients should be instructed to elevate the head of the bed 6 in. either with blocks or by placing a foam wedge under the head. Sleeping on extra pillows is not recommended because this will cause the patient to bend at the waist and actually increase intragastric pressure. Eating the evening meal at least 3 hours before going to bed reduces reflux during sleep. Dietary suggestions for GERD are to (1) avoid foods that reduce LES tone (e.g., chocolate, mints, fats), (2) avoid foods that are direct irritants (e.g., citrus juice, tomato products, coffee), (3) reduce the size of meals, and (4) avoid lying down after meals. Patients should be encouraged to stop smoking and limit their alcohol intake. It may be helpful to avoid chewing gum, sucking on hard candy, and drinking carbonated beverages. Finally, patients with GERD should be questioned about the use of drugs that decrease LES pressure. When a drug is implicated in causing reflux, switching to a drug with similar therapeutic benefit but without an effect on the LES should be considered.

Gastritis

Gastritis may be classified as either acute erosive gastritis or chronic nonerosive gastritis. Acute erosive gastritis is a short-lived inflammatory process characterized by superficial erosions or ulcerations of the stomach. Chronic nonerosive gastritis is classified into two types based on the anatomical location in the stomach. Type A gastritis is an autoimmune disease characterized by chronic inflammation of the acid-secreting mucosa of the fundus and body of the stomach. Type B gastritis affects the mucus-secreting epithelial cells that line the antrum of the stomach.

Pathogenesis

The agents most often responsible for acute gastritis erosions are alcohol and aspirin and other NSAIDs.

Type B gastritis is generally believed to be caused by *H pylori*. *H pylori*–associated gastritis is also present in more than 99% of patients with DUs.

Signs and Symptoms

Most patients with acute erosive gastritis are asymptomatic. A few complain of epigastric pain. The most common complication of acute erosive gastritis is upper GI bleeding.

Most patients with chronic non-erosive gastritis do not have symptoms. Gastritis is slow in progression, may last for years or decades, and rarely heals spontaneously.

Treatment

Acute erosive gastritis usually heals spontaneously within a few days when the offending agent or condition is removed. Removing the cause of the condition, therefore, is the most important step in managing acute erosive gastritis; pharmacologic agents are rarely needed.

Nonulcer Dyspepsia

Clinicians and patients use the word "dyspepsia" to describe any abdominal discomfort, including epigastric pain, heartburn, nausea, bloating, belching, and indigestion.

Pathogenesis

Nonulcer dyspepsia is a disease in search of a cause. Studies have not found a clear relationship between nonulcer dyspepsia and *H pylori*, stress, emotions, personality, food, environmental factors (e.g., smoking, alcohol, caffeine), genetic factors, or other diseases.

Signs and Symptoms

The typical patient with nonulcer dyspepsia presents with a chronic history (>3 months) of widespread abdominal symptoms, usually in relation to meals. Nonulcer dyspepsia may persist for years. There is no evidence that it leads to PUD or any other disorder.

Treatment

Despite the widespread use of antacids for dyspeptic symptoms, there is little objective proof of their benefit. Trials with prescription H_2RAs have yielded inconsistent results, and there are no published trials with nonprescription H_2RAs.

Intestinal Gas

Intestinal gas, which may present as excessive belching, abdominal discomfort, bloating, and/or flatulence, is a common complaint. The pathogenesis is poorly understood and treatment is far from satisfactory.

Patient Assessment

Patients presenting with dyspeptic symptoms should be questioned to rule out pain related to ischemic heart disease, complications of GERD or PUD, or other serious conditions that warrant medical attention. Factors to consider include:

- The type, severity, and location of the pain;
- Whether the pain radiates;
- The presence of other symptoms, such as nausea, vomiting, bloody stools, weight loss, or pain or difficulty on swallowing;
- Whether symptoms are exacerbated by certain foods, lying down, or exercise;
- Whether the symptoms are relieved by food, antacids, or H_2RAs;
- Medication history; and
- Personal and family history of acid-peptic disorders.

The pharmacist should ask specific questions to determine whether the classic features of ischemic pain are present. For example, severe, crushing chest pain, especially if accompanied by sweating, strongly suggests ischemic pain and possibly myocardial infarction. Other complaints or symptoms for which patients should be referred to a physician are as follows:

- Known allergy to H_2RAs;
- Possibility of being pregnant;
- Severe abdominal or back pain;
- Unexplained weight loss;
- Abdominal pain or heartburn that is unresponsive to antacid or nonprescription H_2RAs within 2 weeks or that recurs soon after stopping;
- Chest pain that is indistinguishable from heartburn;
- Difficulty or pain on swallowing;

- Presence or history of vomiting blood;
- Black, tarry stools (if not taking iron or bismuth subsalicylate);
- Temperature >100°F (37.8°C); and
- Blood in urine.

Referrals should be suggested for elderly patients taking NSAIDs with the following risk factors for NSAID-induced ulceration and complications: concomitant use of corticosteroids, history of PUD, history of GI bleeding, concomitant cardiovascular disease, high doses of NSAIDs, smoking. Finally, children under 12 years of age should be referred to a physician.

It is important to question the patient about the use of both prescription and nonprescription drugs, paying special attention to NSAID use. If the patient is taking a nonprescription drug, the brand name should be specified.

Once serious disorders have been ruled out, the pharmacist should assess whether the patient's symptoms are related to minor acid-peptic disorders. The patient should be questioned about the relationship of the pain to eating. The pain may also be worsened by lying down or bending over, and it may waken patients at night. Patients who describe this type of pain are appropriate candidates for self-treatment with nonprescription acid-peptic products.

If antacids or H_2RAs are recommended and the patient does not experience prompt relief, the pharmacist should refer the patient to a physician. Symptoms that are relieved by these products but return often probably warrant medical attention.

Pharmacologic Agents

The primary aim of nonprescription medications in the treatment of acid-peptic disorders is to provide symptomatic relief, either alone or in conjunction with prescription medications.

Antacids

Antacids only neutralize existing acid; they do not affect the amount or rate of gastric acid secreted. Antacids may also have healing and protective actions beyond and independent of their neutralizing capacities.

Potency

The neutralizing capacities of antacid products vary considerably (Table 2). Antacids should be dosed according to the mEq ANC rather than by the volume or number of tablets. Aluminum-magnesium combination products offer adequate neutralizing capacity with the least potential for side effects.

Onset and Duration of Action

An antacid's onset of neutralizing action depends on how fast it dissolves in gastric acid. Sodium bicarbonate and magnesium hydroxide dissolve quickly. Aluminum hydroxide and calcium carbonate dissolve slowly. Suspensions generally dissolve more easily than do tablets or powders.

If taken on an empty stomach, antacids have a duration of action of only 20–40 minutes. Gastric emptying is greatly slowed by the presence of food. When taken 1 hour after meals, antacids may neutralize acid for up to 3 hours. Sodium bicarbonate and magnesium hydroxide have the shortest duration of neutralizing action, while aluminum hydroxide and calcium carbonate have the longest.

TABLE 2 Potency of antacid products

Antacid suspensions	mEq ANC per ml[a]	Equiv- alent volume[b]	Antacid tablets	mEq ANC per tablet[a]	Equivalent number of tablets[b]
Riopan Extra Strength	6	13.3	Maalox TC	28	3
Extra Strength Maalox			Riopan Plus 2	30	3
Plus	5.8	13.8	Extra Strength		
Maalox-TC	5.44	14.7	Maalox	23.4	4
Mylanta II	58	15.7	Mylanta II	23	4
Gelusil-II	4.8	16.7	Gelusil-II	21	4
Camalox	3.7	21.6	Camalox	18	5
ALternaGEL	3.2	25	Amphojel (600 mg)	16	5
Riopan Plus	3	26.7	Riopan Plus	13.5	6
Milk of Magnesia	2.8	28.6	Temp	14.4	6
Maalox	2.66	30	Tums E-X	15	6
Mylanta	2.54	31.5	Basaljel	13	7
Di-Gel	2.45	32.7	Mylanta	11.5	7
Gelusil	2.4	33.3	Maalox Plus	11.4	7
Basaljel	2.4	33.3	Tums	10	8
Titralac Plus	2.2	36.4	Gelusil	11	8
Kolantyl Gel	2.1	38.1	Maalox	9.7	9
Amphojel	2	40	Rolaids Sodium-Free	8.5	10
Gaviscon	0.8	100	Titralac	7.5	11
			Gaviscon	0.5	160

[a]Acid-neutralizing capacity (ANC), as stated by the product's manufacturer.
[b]Equivalent volumes (mL) or number of tablets calculated to provide 80 mEq ANC.

Formulation

Antacid formulations, liquids (suspensions) and tablets, differ significantly with regard to neutralizing capacity and patient acceptance.

Dissolution rate or ease of solubility is an important determinant of ultimate neutralizing capacity. Suspensions provide a larger surface area and are more rapidly and effectively dissolved in gastric acid. These are more potent than tablets of the same antacid on a milligram-for-milligram basis.

Despite the higher potency, many patients prefer tablets. Patients should be instructed to chew antacid tablets thoroughly and follow with a full glass of water to ensure maximum therapeutic benefit.

Other formulations do not offer any advantages over liquids and tablets.

Palatability

Because antacids often must be taken frequently, their taste is a critical factor in improving compliance. Recommendations for improving taste include refrigerating the product and using high-potency liquid antacids, which can be taken in smaller quantities.

Primary Ingredients

Four primary neutralizing compounds are found in antacid products: sodium bicarbonate, calcium carbonate, aluminum salts (hydroxide, phosphate), and magnesium salts (hydroxide, chloride).

Sodium Bicarbonate. Sodium bicarbonate should be used only for short-term relief of symptoms of overeating or indigestion. It differs from other antacids in that it is completely absorbed into the systemic circulation and can alter systemic pH. In patients with poor renal function, sodium bicarbonate can accumulate and cause a clinically significant metabolic alkalosis or offset the metabolic acidosis of renal failure.

A particular form of the systemic alkalosis caused by high doses of sodium bicarbonate is the milk-alkali syndrome. It can occur whenever a high intake of calcium is combined with any factor producing alkalosis. Many reports involve calcium carbonate as the sole source of both calcium and alkali. Sodium bicarbonate can cause alkalosis (and the milk-alkali syndrome) when ingested with calcium but not when ingested alone.

Symptoms of the milk-alkali syndrome include hypercalcemia, alkalosis, irritability, headache, vertigo, nausea, vomiting, weakness, and myalgia. If calcium and alkali ingestion continues, neurologic symptoms (e.g., memory loss, personality changes, lethargy, stupor, coma) may develop. Renal dysfunction occurs early in the course of the disorder and is present in all stages of it. Most of the symptoms are reversed rapidly after calcium and alkali ingestion is discontinued; however, renal damage may be irreversible.

Another problem occurring as a result of systemic absorption of sodium bicarbonate is sodium overload. Accordingly, sodium bicarbonate is contraindicated in patients with edema, congestive heart failure, renal failure, and cirrhosis and in those on low-salt diets. Hypertensive patients should also avoid the therapeutic use of sodium bicarbonate.

Calcium Carbonate. Calcium carbonate dissolves more slowly in the stomach than sodium bicarbonate does, but it produces a potent and more prolonged neutralization of gastric acid.

Clinically significant alkalosis from calcium carbonate ingestion does not usually develop. However, as previously discussed, calcium carbonate may contribute to the milk-alkali syndrome.

Although the amount of calcium that does not react with intestinal bicarbonate and is absorbed systemically is minimal (10%), enough may be absorbed after several days of high-dose antacid ingestion to cause hypercalcemia. Patients with impaired renal function may develop hypercalcemia from as little as 4 g per day.

Calcium carbonate has not been shown to cause constipation, as commonly believed.

Aluminum. Aluminum hydroxide is slowly dissolved in the stomach. Systemic alkalosis is a minimal risk. Patients with impaired renal function who take aluminum antacids chronically may fail to clear the aluminum, resulting in hyperaluminemia. In patients with normal renal function, the reduction in phosphate absorption caused by aluminum antacids may lead to clinically significant phosphate depletion.

The most frequent side effect of aluminum-containing antacids is constipation. It can be managed with stool softeners or laxatives, or with combination aluminum-magnesium antacids.

Magnesium. Magnesium antacids should not be used in patients with marked renal failure. The most frequent and limiting side effect of magnesium-containing antacids is dose-related diarrhea, which may be severe enough to cause fluid and electrolyte imbalances. Efforts to minimize this diarrhea include using combination aluminum-magnesium antacid products or alternating aluminum-magnesium therapy with an aluminum-only antacid.

Aluminum-Magnesium Combinations. Many antacid products contain a mixture of aluminum and magnesium. Because constipation from aluminum and diarrhea from magnesium are both dose related, combining these two agents allows for potent ANC while using lower doses of each agent. The optimal ratio between magnesium and aluminum to achieve this balance has not been found. The risk of side effects other than those affecting the GI system are not reduced with combination products.

Additional Ingredients

Sugars. Some antacids contain sugars or saccharin. When taken in large amounts over long periods, enough sugar is ingested to alter glucose control in patients with labile diabetes. When recommending an antacid for diabetic patients, the pharmacist should consider the sugar content.

Sodium. Most antacids contain sodium, but the amount differs considerably among products. Many products have been developed that contain less than 0.04 mEq (1 mg) sodium per 5 mL or no sodium at all. These should be used in patients with hypertension, congestive heart failure, renal failure, edema, or cirrhosis, and in those on salt-restricted diets.

Simethicone. See the section on Antiflatulents below.

Alginic Acid. The addition of alginic acid to antacids appears to be effective in relieving symptoms of GERD. When using antacid-alginic acid combination tablets, patients should chew the tablets, follow with a glass of water, and remain upright.

Antacid-Drug Interactions

Antacids interact with drugs by a variety of mechanisms. Factors that influence whether an antacid interacts with another drug include the valence of the cation in the antacid, the dose used, the chronicity of dosing, and, most important, the timing of the administration or consumption of the antacid in relation to the other drug. Several drug interactions and clinical implications are summarized in Table 3.

Miscellaneous Uses of Antacids

Overindulgence/Hangover. The FDA has reviewed nonprescription oral antacids and antacid-acetaminophen combination products for the relief of symptoms associated with overindulgence in food and drink and has endorsed the use of these products for such purposes. It has reversed a previous recommendation and placed in Category II all combination products for hangover that contain both an antacid and caffeine.

H$_2$-Receptor Antagonists

Four H$_2$RAs are available for prescription and nonprescription use in the United States: cimetidine, ranitidine, famotidine, and nizatidine. The oral doses approved for non-prescription use—famotidine 10 mg (up to 20 mg per day), cimetidine 100 mg (up to 400 mg per day), ranitidine 75 mg (up to 150 mg per day), and nizatidine 75 mg (up to 150 mg per day)—are substantially lower than those indicated in the management of PUD and GERD.

Antisecretory activity of the H$_2$RAs usually begins within 1 hour of administration and persists for 6–12 hours. Both the degree and the duration of acid suppression achieved with H$_2$RAs depend upon the dose and drug used.

The pharmacokinetic profiles of the H$_2$RAs are all very similar in healthy, normal volunteers. These drugs are all rapidly absorbed from the small intestine, with peak concentrations occurring from 1 to 3 hours after oral administration. Elimination occurs by

TABLE 3 Antacid-drug interactions

Drug	Antacids					Effect	Clinical implication
	Al	Mg	Al-Mg	CaCO₃	NaHCO₃		
Allopurinol	✓					↓ absorption in 3 patients on chronic hemodialysis with failure to reduce uric acid	Monitor patient for ↓ allopurinol response. Separate doses by ≥2 h
Amphetamine					✓	↓ urinary excretion, allowing potential for retention & intoxication	Avoid concurrent use
Antibiotics							
Nitrofurantoin	✓		✓			↓ rate & extent of absorption	Separate doses by ≥2 h
Tetracycline and quinolones	✓	✓	✓	✓		↓ absorption (up to 90%), resulting in ↓ serum and urine concentrations	May result in treatment failures. Separate doses by ≥2 h, preferably 4–6 h
Anticoagulants		✓				↑ absorption of dicumarol by 50%; no effect on warfarin absorption	Patients needing antacids & anticoagulants should receive warfarin
Anticonvulsants							
Phenytoin	✓		✓			↓ rate & extent of absorption with large doses of antacid; no effect with small doses	Monitor phenytoin effects/levels
Valproic acid	✓	✓	✓			↑ absorption by 12%	Potential for valproic acid toxicity
Beta-blockers							
Propranolol	✓					↓ bioavailability by 50% in 4 of 5 subjects; no effect in another study	Clinical significance of long-term therapy not assessed
Metoprolol			✓			↑ bioavailability by 25% after single dose in 6 healthy volunteers	Probably not significant
Atenolol	✓		✓	✓		↓ bioavailability from 37–51%	May be clinically significant; separate doses by at least 1 h
Benzodiazepines							
Diazepam	✓		✓			↑ absorption & ↑ sedative effects; ↓ rate, but not extent, of absorption	May result in delay in sedative effect. Important only in acute anxiety with single doses, not in chronic dosing
Chlordiazepoxide			✓			↓ rate, but not extent, of absorption	
Clorazepate			✓			↓ rate & extent of absorption	
Captopril			✓			↓ absorption by 42% in 10 healthy volunteers	No evidence of compromised efficacy
Chlorpromazine			✓			↓ absorption & serum concentration; ↓ therapeutic response reported	Monitor for ↓ therapeutic response. Separate doses by ≥2 h
Corticosteroids							
Dexamethasone		✓				↓ absorption	Evidence conflicting & clinical significance questionable
Prednisone	✓		✓			↓ absorption in one study, but not confirmed	

Drug	Antacids					Effect	Clinical implication
	Al	Mg	Al-Mg	CaCO$_3$	NaHCO$_3$		
Digoxin	✓	✓	✓			↓ absorption of digoxin up to 30% in some reports, but no effect in others. May be more likely to occur with tablets than capsules	Clinical significance uncertain. Monitor patients for ↓ digoxin effect when antacids are given concurrently. Space doses to avoid possible interaction
H$_2$RAs Cimetidine Ranitidine Famotidine Nizatidine	✓ ✓		 ✓ ✓ ✓			↓ absorption & peak concentration by 10–40%; clinical failures not reported	Separate doses by at least 1–2 h
Iron	✓	✓		✓	✓	↓ absorption by 50–60%	May interfere with patient's response to iron replacement therapy. Separate doses by ≥2 h
Isoniazid	✓	✓				↓ absorption, particularly with aluminum antacids	Separate doses by ≥1 h
Ketoconazole	✓		✓		✓	↓ ketoconazole absorption	Separate doses by ≥2 h
Levodopa			✓			↑ absorption in some patients, but effect is variable	May be clinically useful in certain patients with delayed gastric emptying. Monitor patient response when adding or stopping antacid
NSAIDs Aspirin			✓	✓		↓ serum concentrations by 30–70%	Monitor serum salicylate levels & observe symptoms when sustained levels are important (e.g., rheumatoid arthritis, systemic lupus erythematosus)
Enteric-coated aspirin			✓			Premature rupture of enteric coating & dissolution in the stomach	Separate doses in patients at risk for NSAID gastropathy
Indomethacin Naproxen Diflunisal	 ✓ ✓	✓	✓ ✓			Delayed absorption & possible ↓ peak concentrations	Not clinically important
Pseudoephedrine						↑ rate, but not extent, of absorption in 6 healthy volunteers	Clinical significance unknown
Quinidine		✓		✓	✓	↑ serum concentrations; toxicity has been reported	Use with caution. Monitor levels & patient response
Sodium polystyrene sulfonate		✓		✓	✓	Metabolic alkalosis	Concurrent use may be dangerous. Separate doses by ≥2h
Sucralfate						↓ dissolution & possible loss of efficacy	Separate doses by ≥30 min
Theophylline						↑ & ↓ in rate, but not extent, of absorption observed, depending on the theophylline preparation	Not important in chronic dosing

Key:
✓ indicates interactions reported in humans. However, interactions may be likely with other antacids in which interactions are not yet reported.

↑ = increased; ↓ = decreased.

Information extracted from:
Gugler R, Allgayer H. Clin Pharmacokin. 1990; 18 (3): 210–9. Gibaldi M et al. Clin Pharmacol Ther. 1974; 16: 520–5. Tatro DS, ed, Drug Interaction Facts. St. Louis: Facts and Comparisons Division, J B Lippincott; 1990. Hansten PD, Horn JR. Drug Interactions. 6th ed. Philadelphia: Lea & Febiger; 1989.

a combination of renal and hepatic metabolism. Dosage adjustment is not necessary in patients with liver disease who have normal renal function.

Adverse Effects

H_2RAs are among the most studied and hence the safest agents ever marketed. The most common adverse effects reported with standard doses of H_2RAs are headache, drowsiness, constipation, diarrhea, nausea, vomiting, and abdominal pain/discomfort. Serious CNS reactions are extremely rare in ambulatory patients.

Drug Interactions

Of the H_2RAs, cimetidine has the greatest potential to interact with other drugs. Because cimetidine binds to several isoenzymes of the cytochrome P-450 enzyme system, it impairs the hepatic metabolism of drugs that are normally cleared by this system. The magnitude of inhibition depends on the dose, the age of the patient, and the patient's hepatic enzyme status. Concomitant administration of cimetidine is of particular concern with theophylline, phenytoin, and warfarin.

The magnitude of changes occurring in drug metabolism with nonprescription doses of cimetidine is likely to be small. However, the potential for adverse clinical consequences exists, particularly in elderly patients. The potential for drug interactions is magnified if patients exceed the recommended dosage. Accordingly, the product label for nonprescription cimetidine includes a warning for patients who take theophylline, phenytoin, or warfarin to consult a physician before taking the product.

When patients who are taking theophylline, cimetidine, or warfarin wish to self-medicate with an H_2RA, it may be simpler and more cost-effective to recommend one other than cimetidine.

All the H_2RAs can affect the bioavailability of certain drugs by raising gastric pH. Concomitant administration of H_2RAs has been reported to reduce the bioavailability of enoxacin, cefpodoxime proxetil, itraconazole, and ketoconazole. There are no data to determine whether these interactions occur with nonprescription H_2RAs, or to what extent. In the absence of such data, it is wise to avoid concomitant administration of H_2RAs with these agents.

Nonprescription H_2RAs offers the convenient option of self-care for patients with dyspeptic symptoms, and may especially benefit patients in underserved areas where there is a shortage of health care providers. There may be significant cost savings as well. Clearly, the consequences of the shift of H_2RAs to nonprescription status in the United States are uncertain, and there is some risk involved. Pharmacists can minimize this risk by recognizing and triaging patients who are at risk for serious GI disease, by guiding patients at risk for cimetidine-drug interactions to other agents, and by counseling and educating patients about the appropriate use of these agents.

Bismuth

Bismuth compounds have recently attracted attention because of their ability to suppress *H pylori* infection and their potential for cytoprotection. Bismuth subsalicylate (BSS) (Pepto-Bismol) is the only nonprescription bismuth compound available in the United States. It is indicated for common diarrhea, traveler's diarrhea, and occasional relief of upset stomach or upper GI symptoms.

Bismuth compounds react with hydrogen sulfide to produce bismuth sulfide, a highly insoluble black salt responsible for the darkening of the tongue or grayish black stools.

Antiflatulents

Use of antiflatulents is largely empiric and evidence supporting their benefit is limited.

Simethicone

The ability of simethicone to reduce intestinal gas is equivocal. Nonetheless, the use of simethicone may be encouraged on a trial basis as some patients subjectively report benefit from it.

Many antacid products contain a combination of simethicone and antacids, but use of both agents is often unnecessary and the efficacy of such combination products has not been well studied. The FDA considers simethicone safe and effective as an antiflatulent, but simethicone has no activity as an antacid.

alpha-Galactosidase

Beano is a solution of the enzyme alpha-galactosidase. It is recommended as a prophylactic treatment of intestinal gas symptoms produced by high-fiber diets (e.g., whole grains, lentils, broccoli, peas, cabbage). Evidence for this product's efficacy is far from conclusive, and the safety of alpha-galactosidase remains to be determined.

Other Drugs

Sucralfate is the only agent approved for the treatment of PUD that does not reduce or neutralize gastric acid. It may be approved for nonprescription use in the future.

Numerous other agents that are useful for the management of acid-peptic disorders are available only by prescription. These agents include prescription-dose H_2RAs, proton pump inhibitors (omeprazole, lansoprazole), misoprostol, cisapride, and various antibiotics in combination with antisecretory drugs.

Product Selection Guidelines

Since there is no evidence that either antacids or nonprescription H_2RAs are more effective, the choice should be based on patient factors and individual preferences.

The patient's medication history is important in selecting an acid-peptic product. Antacids and cimetidine have the greatest potential to cause drug interactions, and patients taking numerous medications may best be treated with one of the other H_2RAs. Financial restraints may dictate the choice of agents as antacids are substantially less expensive.

Currently, only antacids are indicated for supplemental pain relief in patients taking prescription agents for healing or maintenance of PUD. Because most patients with PUD are already taking antisecretory agents, the addition of nonprescription H_2RAs is unlikely to provide a significant benefit. In patients with severe GERD and/or reflux esophagitis, neither antacids nor nonprescription doses of H_2RAs are likely to provide additional benefit to prescription antisecretory medications.

Antacids

Selection of an antacid should be guided by consideration of the chemical properties of the ingredients, the GI and systemic side effects of the ingredients, potency, formulation, taste, drug interactions, and cost. High-potency antacids are generally preferred. Care should be taken to select a formulation that is palatable to the patient.

Contents to consider before selecting an antacid for a patient include sodium, lactose, potassium, magnesium, and sugar. All antacids pose a risk of systemic side effects or electrolyte imbalances in patients with chronic renal failure. Products containing large amounts of sodium (i.e., sodium bicarbonate) or more than 50 mEq per day of magnesium are to be avoided in such patients. Similarly, sodium bicarbonate antacids should be avoided in patients with congestive heart failure, hypertension, or edema and in patients on low-salt diets. Lactose content should be evaluated when choosing an antacid for patients with lactose intolerance, whereas sugar content is important to evaluate for diabetic patients.

Patients complaining of constipation or hemorrhoids should be given antacids containing magnesium or magnesium-aluminum combinations. Patients with a history of diarrhea (e.g., Crohn's disease, irritable bowel syndrome) should avoid magnesium-containing antacids.

H$_2$-Receptor Antagonists

There are no data to support either superior efficacy or the side-effects profile of one H$_2$RA over another when used for heartburn, acid indigestion, and sour stomach. Although significant drug-drug interactions at low doses of cimetidine are unlikely, patients receiving medications that have known interactions with cimetidine may be better managed with famotidine, ranitidine, or nizatidine.

Although a specific H$_2$RA may be labeled for *treatment only, prevention only,* or *treatment and prevention* of heartburn, sour stomach, or indigestion, it is likely that all the nonprescription H$_2$RAs are effective in both preventing and treating these conditions.

Antiflatulents

The selection of an antiflatulent product should be guided by the pattern of symptoms, cost, and concurrent disease states. Since alpha-galactosidase is intended for use as a preventive measure, patients experiencing symptoms of gas who need immediate relief will be better managed with simethicone. Because alpha-galactosidase produces carbohydrates, patients with galactosemia or diabetes should avoid this product and use simethicone instead.

Therapeutic Considerations in Special Populations

Geriatric Patients

Frequent use of acid-peptic products by elderly patients is to be expected because many GI disorders occur more often in this age group. In addition, constipation is common in the elderly.

Symptoms of PUD in elderly patients are different from those in younger patients and can be quite misleading. Many elderly patients with ulcers, and most patients with NSAID-induced ulcers, have no symptoms. If symptoms are present, they are more likely to be vague abdominal discomfort, weakness, dizziness, anorexia, and severe weight loss. It is common for bleeding to be the first sign of an ulcer. The elderly patient should be questioned about signs or symptoms of these complications. An adequate drug history, especially with regard to NSAID use, should be obtained. The pharmacist should have an increased awareness of the risk factors for GI diseases in this population and should evaluate even vague or minor complaints. If the pharmacist cannot determine that the symptoms are related to overeating, eating spicy foods, or occasional reflux, it is wise to refer the patient to a physician.

Elderly patients are less likely to tolerate a large sodium load, more likely to experience side effects from antacids, and more likely to be taking a drug that can interact with antacids. If constipation is frequent, magnesium-containing antacids should be recommended, provided the patient does not have severe renal impairment. Patients should be aware that diarrhea and constipation are possibilities from antacid use and should be encouraged to switch antacids if these side effects occur. Because many elderly patients are on low-salt diets, they should avoid sodium bicarbonate, even for short-term use. Doses of antacids do not need to be altered in elderly patients because of age-related changes in drug elimination, but may need to be reduced because of side effects.

Elderly patients with acid-peptic complaints may be safely treated with nonprescription H_2RAs. The nonprescription doses of H_2RAs are low enough that dosage reductions are not necessary to compensate for age-related reductions in elimination and metabolism. The most important concern is that elderly patients are more likely to be taking medications that interact with cimetidine and possibly ranitidine.

Pregnant/Lactating Patients

Many pregnant women have symptomatic gastroesophageal reflux. Antacids have not produced teratogenic effects and are generally considered safe in pregnancy as long as chronic high doses are avoided.

Controlled data regarding the safety of H_2RA use in pregnancy are limited. Cimetidine, ranitidine, and famotidine have received FDA pregnancy risk category B ratings; nizatidine has a pregnancy risk category of C. Pregnant women seeking a nonprescription product for an acid-peptic disorder should be directed to use antacids rather than H_2RAs unless a health care provider has instructed otherwise.

Simethicone has been assigned a pregnancy risk category of C. Data regarding the safety of alginic acid or alpha-galactosidase in pregnancy are not available. Neither aluminum nor magnesium hydroxide enters breast milk significantly, and no problems have been reported in lactating women. The American Academy of Pediatrics considers cimetidine compatible with breast-feeding.

Pediatric Patients

Gastroesophageal reflux is common in infants and children. Antacids, with or without alginic acid, have been widely used in pediatric patients for this disorder as well as for esophagitis and PUD; however, their safety in pediatric patients has not been clearly established.

Although many cases of reflux in infants are benign, important complications can occur. Any parents or caregivers who are seeking to use antacids for infants or children should be referred to their physicians or pediatricians.

Because the nonprescription H_2RAs are not available in liquid formulations, they are not useful for pediatric patients. These products are not to be used in children younger than 12 years unless directed by a physician.

Although its efficacy is questionable, simethicone is not absorbed from the GI tract and is considered safe for use in infants and children.

The safety and efficacy of alpha-galactosidase have not been evaluated in infants and children.

Patient Counseling

Antacid/Antacid-Alginic Acid Combinations

The patient who purchases an antacid product should be given the following specific advice:

■ Patients using antacids for relief of indigestion, upset stomach, or heartburn should take 40–80 mEq as needed. Some patients may experience relief from a scheduled dose, such as 40–80 mEq immediately after meals and at bedtime.

■ Patients should not eat within 3 hours of going to bed; further, they should elevate the head of the bed 6–8 in. with blocks.

■ Patients should not lie down for approximately 3 hours after eating.

■ Patients should avoid smoking, caffeine, alcohol, fatty foods, tomato-based foods, chocolate, and peppermint/spearmint.

■ Patients should avoid wearing tight-fitting clothing.

■ If obese, patients should lose weight.

■ Patients with PUD who are using antacids for supplemental ulcer pain relief should take 40–80 mEq ANC as needed for symptoms. If an H_2RA is being taken concomitantly, it should be given 1–2 hours before the antacid to avoid a possible reduction in H_2RA bioavailability.

■ In general, patients should be advised not to take more than 500–600 mEq ANC of antacid per day.

■ Antacids should not be taken for longer than 2 weeks. If they do not relieve symptoms promptly or if symptoms return often, a health care provider should be contacted.

■ If a product with alginic acid is recommended, the patient should drink a glass of water after taking it and wait 1–2 hours before lying down or going to bed. Alginic acid products are best suited for daytime use.

■ Because antacids may cause constipation or diarrhea, the patient should seek advice on switching antacids if one of these side effects develops.

■ Patients on low-salt diets should know the amount of sodium in an antacid product and take only those products with a low sodium content. Patients with renal or cardiac disease should also be wary of potassium and magnesium content.

■ Antacid tablets are not as potent as liquids. Patients who find liquids difficult to carry may take antacid tablets during the day at work and more potent liquids at night.

■ Chewable antacid or antacid-alginic acid tablets should be chewed thoroughly and followed with a full glass of water. Effervescent tablets should be dissolved completely in water and the bubbles should subside before the patient drinks the liquid.

■ Patients should space doses of antacids at least 2 hours apart from interacting drugs, such as tetracyclines, iron, and digoxin. When possible, antacids should be spaced at least 4–6 hours apart from quinolone antibiotics; if spaced only 2 hours apart, the quinolone should be given first.

H_2-Receptor Antagonists

The patient who purchases an H_2RA should be given the following specific advice:

■ H_2RAs are not antacids, and they work differently to relieve acid-related symptoms. Nonprescription H_2RAs are the same medications as prescription H_2RAs; they are simply lower doses.

- In patients who anticipate heartburn or indigestion, one dose of any of the H$_2$RAs can be taken 1 hour before eating.

- H$_2$RAs should not be taken for more than 2 weeks continuously except under the advice and supervision of a health care provider. Patients whose symptoms do not resolve with H$_2$RAs or who experience difficulty swallowing or persistent abdominal pain should consult a health care provider.

- H$_2$RAs should not be given to children younger than 12 years of age, pregnant women, or lactating women without the advice of a health care provider.

- The most common side effects reported with nonprescription doses of H$_2$RAs are headache, dizziness, nausea, and diarrhea.

- Patients who are taking phenytoin, theophylline, or warfarin and who wish to take cimetidine 200 mg should consult their health care providers before taking the product. Alternatively, patients should be advised to take famotidine, ranitidine, or nizatidine.

Antiflatulents

The patient who purchases an antiflatulent product should be given the following specific advice:

- Patients using simethicone should take one tablet after meals and at bedtime. Patients should not take more than 500 mg simethicone per 24 hours.

- Dosage recommendations for simethicone drops for infants younger than 2 years of age are 0.3 mL four times daily after meals and at bedtime. To facilitate administration, the suspension may be mixed with 1 oz of cool water, infant formula, or other liquid. Children older than 2 years of age should be given 0.6 mL four times daily after meals and at bedtime.

- Patients using alpha-galactosidase solution should add three to eight drops to the first bite of the offending food. Because temperatures >130°F may inactivate the enzyme, the solution should be added after the food has cooled, and patients should be advised not to cook with the product.

- Patients using alpha-galactosidase tablets may be instructed to swallow, chew, or crumble two to three tablets with the first bite of problem foods. One tablet is equivalent to five drops of alpha-galactosidase solution (≥175 units galactose). For larger meals, more tablets may be used.

CHAPTER 12

Laxative Products

Questions to ask in patient assessment and counseling

- *Why do you feel you need a laxative?*
- *How long has constipation been a problem?*
- *Have you experienced abdominal discomfort or pain, bloating, weight loss, nausea, or vomiting?*
- *Do you have any other symptoms?*
- *Are you being treated by a health care provider for any illness?*
- *Have you recently had abdominal surgery?*
- *Are you pregnant?*
- *How often do you normally have a bowel movement? Have you noticed a change in frequency?*
- *How would you describe your bowel movements? Have they recently changed in any way?*
- *Has the appearance of your stools changed? In what way?*
- *Have you attempted to relieve the constipation by eating more cereals, bread with a high fiber content, fruits, or vegetables?*
- *How much physical exercise do you get?*
- *How many glasses of water or other fluids do you drink each day?*
- *Have you previously used laxatives to relieve constipation?*
- *Are you using a laxative now? How often and how long have you used a laxative?*
- *Have you had any unwanted effects from laxatives, such as diarrhea or stomach pain?*
- *Are you taking any prescription or nonprescription medications? If so, what are they?*
- *Are you allergic to any medication?*

Laxatives facilitate the passage and elimination of feces from the colon and rectum. Many people use laxatives inappropriately to alleviate what they consider to be constipation. Because laxative products are both widely used and abused, the pharmacist can also provide a valuable service by educating patients about their appropriate use.

Constipation

Constipation is defined as a decrease in the frequency of fecal elimination and is characterized by the difficult passage of hard, dry stools. It usually results from the abnormally slow movement of feces through the colon with a resultant accumulation in the descending colon. Typical symptoms of constipation include anorexia, dull headache,

---

Editor's Note: This chapter is adapted from Clarence E. Curry, Jr., and Demetris Tatum-Butler, "Laxative Products," in Covington, T.R., ed., *Handbook of Nonprescription Drugs,* 11th edition. For a more extensive discussion of the etiology of constipation and the pathophysiology of the lower gastrointestinal tract, as well as recommended adult and pediatric dosages of laxative products, readers are encouraged to consult Chapter 12 of the *Handbook.*

lassitude, low back pain, abdominal distention, and lower abdominal distress. Abdominal discomfort and an inadequate response to an increasing variety and dosage of laxatives are common complaints.

The frequency of bowel movements in humans generally ranges from three times a day to three times a week. Therefore, constipation cannot be defined solely in terms of the number of bowel movements in any given period. Regularity is what is typical for the individual who experiences none of the classic symptoms of constipation.

Etiology

Causes of constipation are numerous. Idiopathic constipation often begins in childhood or adolescence. Elderly persons often suffer constipation owing to inappropriate diet, lack of exercise, or lack of muscle tone in the colon. Dietary issues related to the development of constipation include insufficient fluid intake, low fiber content of the diet, and excessive ingestion of foods (e.g., processed cheese) that harden stools.

Constipation of recent onset suggests a possible organic or drug-induced cause. Table 1 lists a number of drugs that may induce constipation. Constipation is often a problem in patients with ulcerative colitis that is limited to the rectum. The use of antidiarrheal agents in these patients may result in colonic dilation and the accumulation of hard stool in an area of the bowel not affected by disease. Constipation may be caused by numerous pathologic conditions, including hypothyroidism, megacolon, stricture, or benign or malignant lesions. Laxatives are contraindicated in such cases; proper diagnosis and medical treatment should be obtained.

Patient Assessment

Before making any recommendations, the pharmacist should ask the patient the questions in the front of this chapter.

The pharmacist should exercise caution when recommending a laxative for a patient receiving prescription drug products because of the possibility of drug interactions (e.g., decreased absorption of other drugs, counteraction of the therapeutic effect of the laxative [Table 1], laxative effect of certain drugs [e.g., magnesium-containing antacids, misoprostol, antiadrenergic drugs]).

Patients should be referred to a physician when

■ Symptoms persist more than 2 weeks;

■ Symptoms recur after dietary or lifestyle changes or after laxative use;

■ The patient reports blood in the stool; or

■ There is doubt or insufficient information about the patient's disease status (e.g., the patient has recently undergone surgery involving the gastrointestinal [GI] tract).

Treatment

Nondrug Measures

Constipation that does not have an organic etiology can often be alleviated with lifestyle modifications such as increased fiber in the diet, adequate fluid intake (i.e., 32–128 oz daily), and exercise (preferably aerobic). Both insoluble fiber (such as whole-grain breads, prunes, raisins, and corn) and soluble fiber (such as beans, oat bran, barley, peas, carrots, citrus fruits, and apples) have been thought to be helpful. The pharmacist should advise patients that increasing bran in the diet may lead to erratic bowel habits, flatulence, and abdominal discomfort during the first few weeks. Some people, moreover, do not respond to the addition of fiber.

TABLE 1 Drugs that may induce constipation

Analgesics (including NSAIDs)

Anesthetics

Antacids (calcium and aluminum compounds)

Anticholinergics (including felbamate and gabapentin)

Anticonvulsants

Antidepressants

Barium sulfate

Benzodiazepines (especially alprazolam and estazolam)

Bismuth

Diuretics

Ganglionic blockers

Hematinics (especially iron)

Hyperlidemia agents (e.g., cholestyramine, pravastatin, and simvastatin)

Hypotensives (e.g., agiotensin-converting enzyme inhibitors, beta-blockers, and calcium channel blockers)

Laxative excess

Monoamine oxidase inhibitors

Metallic intoxication (arsenic, lead, mercury, phosphorus)

Muscle paralyzers

Opiates

Parasympatholytics

Parkinsonism agents (e.g., bromocriptine and selegiline)

Psychotherapeutic drugs (e.g., phenothiazines, butyrophenones)

Adapted with permission from Fordtran JS, Sleisenger M, eds. *Gastrointestinal Disease.* Philadelphia: WB Saunders; 1993: 844.

For those persons who achieve a beneficial effect from one of these measures, heeding the urge to pass the stool is paramount. When these measures prove ineffective, a laxative may be indicated.

Pharmacologic Agents

The most meaningful classification of laxative drugs is the mechanism of action, whereby laxatives are classified as bulk forming, emollient, lubricant, saline, hyperosmotic, and stimulant.

Bulk-Forming Laxatives

Because they most closely approximate the physiologic mechanism in promoting evacuation, bulk-forming products are the recommended choice as initial therapy for most forms of constipation. These laxatives are usually effective in 12–24 hours, but they may require as long as 3 days in some individuals.

Polysaccharides and Cellulose Derivatives. Bulk-forming laxatives are derived from agar, plantago (psyllium) seed, kelp (alginates), and plant gums. Synthetic cellulose derivatives (methyl cellulose and carboxymethyl cellulose sodium) are being used more often, and many preparations that contain these drugs also contain stimulant and/or fecal-softening laxative drugs (e.g., docusate).

Calcium Polycarbophil. Calcium polycarbophil is often used to treat constipation associated with irritable bowel syndrome and diverticular disease. Ingestion of the recommended therapeutic doses may increase the risk of hypercalcemia in susceptible patients.

Malt Soup Extract. Malt soup extract is obtained from barley.

Indications/Contraindications. Bulk-forming laxatives may be indicated for people on low-residue diets that cannot be corrected, postpartum women, elderly patients, and patients with colostomies, irritable bowel syndrome, or diverticular disease.

Failure to consume sufficient fluid with a bulk laxative decreases drug efficacy and may result in intestinal or esophageal obstruction. Bulk-forming laxatives may be inappropriate for persons who must severely restrict their fluid intake.

Adverse Effects. When taken properly, these agents have few systemic side effects because they are not absorbed. However, esophageal obstruction has occurred in elderly persons, in patients who have difficulty swallowing, and in patients with strictures of the esophagus after they ingested a bulk laxative that had been chewed or taken in dry form. There have been reports of acute bronchospasm associated with the inhalation of dry hydrophilic mucilloid, as well as of hypersensitivity reactions. Diarrhea, abdominal discomfort, flatulence, and excessive loss of fluid can also occur. Because of the danger of fecal impaction or intestinal obstruction, the bulk-forming laxatives should not be taken by individuals with intestinal ulcerations, stenosis, or disabling adhesions.

Usage Considerations. It is important that each dose be taken with a full glass of fluid (at least 240 mL or 8 oz). The powder or granules should be mixed with the fluid. The dose should be adjusted as directed until the required effect has been obtained. Bulk-forming laxatives are appropriate for long-term therapy. The dextrose content of some of the commercial products should be evaluated for usage by diabetic patients and other patients on carbohydrate-restricted diets. Sugar-free bulk-forming agents containing aspartame should be avoided by patients suffering from phenylketonuria.

Emollient Laxatives

Docusate sodium is an anionic surfactant that acts as a stool softener. Other fecal-softening laxatives are docusate calcium and docusate potassium. Docusate does not retard absorption of nutrients from the intestinal tract.

Indications. Orally administered emollient laxatives are best suited to prevent the development of constipation and are of little or no value in treating long-standing constipation. Emollient laxatives may be used for up to 1 week without physician consultation. They are indicated in cases of acute perianal disease to soften and inhibit painful elimination of stool or when avoidance of straining at the stool is desirable (e.g., patients with abdominal hernia or cardiovascular disease, postpartum women, patients who have undergone surgery for anorectal disorders). Fecal-softening emollient laxatives are usually effective in 1–2 days. Liquid formulations may be more palatable if mixed with juices or milk. Fluid intake should be increased to facilitate softening of stools.

Adverse Effects. The surfactant properties of docusate may facilitate transport of other substances across cell membranes. Consequently, a Food and Drug Administration (FDA) advisory panel recommended warning patients not to take these laxatives while taking a prescription drug or mineral oil.

Lubricant Laxatives

Liquid petrolatum (mineral oil) and certain digestible plant oils such as olive oil soften fecal contents by coating them, thus preventing colonic absorption of fecal water.

Indications. Liquid petrolatum is beneficial when used in cases requiring the maintenance of a soft stool to avoid straining. Routine use of liquid laxatives in these cases is probably not indicated; stool softeners are preferred.

Adverse Effects. The adverse effects and toxicity of mineral oil are associated with repeated and prolonged use. Because aspiration into the lungs is possible, mineral oil should not be administered at bedtime or to very young, elderly, or debilitated patients.

The role of mineral oil in impairing the absorption of fat-soluble nutrients is uncertain. Mineral oil should not be taken with meals because it may delay gastric emptying. It should not be given to pregnant patients and should be used with caution in patients taking oral anticoagulants because of its potential to decrease absorption of vitamin K.

When large doses of mineral oil are taken, the oil may leak through the anal sphincter and produce anal pruritus. This leakage can be avoided by reducing or dividing the dose, or by using a stable emulsion of mineral oil. Mineral oil should not be taken with emollient fecal softeners. Prolonged use should be avoided.

Saline Laxatives

The active constituents of saline laxatives are relatively nonabsorbable cations and anions such as magnesium and sulfate ions whose osmotic and possible other effects increase intestinal motility.

Indications. Saline laxatives are indicated for use only when acute evacuation of the bowel is required. They have no place in the long-term management of constipation. In some cases of food or drug poisoning, saline laxatives are used in purging doses.

Adverse Effects. If renal function is markedly impaired, or if the patient is a newborn or is elderly, toxic concentrations of magnesium ion from a magnesium laxative could accumulate, resulting in hypotension, muscle weakness, and electrocardiographic changes. Other adverse effects include abdominal cramping, excessive diuresis, nausea, vomiting, and dehydration.

Precautions. Phosphate salts contain sodium and should be administered with caution to patients on sodium-restricted diets. Cathartics containing sodium may be toxic to individuals with edema, congestive heart disease, or renal failure; phosphates will accumulate with impaired renal function and should be avoided in such patients. The use of phosphate salts in children under 2 years of age can result in hypocalcemia, tetany, hypernatremia, dehydration, and hyperphosphatemia. Phosphate salts should not be used by those who cannot tolerate fluid loss. In patients who are not fluid restricted, oral phosphate salts should be followed by at least one full glass of water to prevent dehydration.

Hyperosmotic Laxatives

Use of glycerin suppositories in infants and adults usually produces a bowel movement within 30 minutes. Adverse reactions and side effects from glycerin suppositories are minimal.

Stimulant Laxatives

Anthraquinone Stimulants. The drugs of choice in this group are the cascara, casanthranol, and senna compounds. Preparations of senna are more potent than those of cascara and can produce considerably more abdominal cramping. Rhubarb, aloe, and aloin should not be recommended. Anthraquinones usually produce their action 8–12 hours after administration.

The active principles of anthraquinones are absorbed from the GI tract and subsequently appear in body secretions, including human milk. The practical significance of this event in nursing infants is poorly defined.

The liquid preparations of cascara sagrada are more reliable than the solid forms.

Diphenylmethane Stimulants. The most commonly used diphenylmethane laxatives are bisacodyl and phenolphthalein.

Bisacodyl has been recommended for cleaning the colon before GI surgery, endoscopy, or radiography. Bisacodyl may reduce or eliminate the need for irrigations in patients with colostomies.

A stool is usually produced 6–10 hours after oral administration and 15–60 minutes after rectal administration.

Adverse effects with chronic use include metabolic acidosis or alkalosis, hypocalcemia, tetany, loss of enteric protein, and malabsorption. The suppository form may produce a burning sensation in the rectum.

Enteric-coated bisacodyl tablets prevent irritation of the gastric mucosa and therefore should not be broken, crushed, chewed, or administered with agents that increase gastric pH such as antacids, histamine$_2$-receptor antagonists, or proton pump inhibitors.

Phenolphthalein exerts its stimulating effect primarily on the colon. It is usually active 6–8 hours after administration.

Phenolphthalein is usually nontoxic. However, at least two types of allergic reactions may follow its use. In susceptible individuals, a large dose may cause diarrhea, colic, cardiac and respiratory distress, or circulatory collapse. The other reaction is a pink to deep purple rash. Patients should be advised to report any rash to the physician or the pharmacist. Osteomalacia has been attributed to excessive phenolphthalein ingestion.

The patient should be forewarned that phenolphthalein can cause pink-to-red discoloration of the urine or red coloration of the feces.

Castor Oil. Castor oil is used in situations requiring a thorough evacuation of the GI tract; it is seldom used routinely for constipation. Prolonged use may result in excessive loss of fluid, electrolytes, and nutrients.

Castor oil is most effective when administered on an empty stomach, and it produces an evacuation within 2–6 hours. Because a laxative effect occurs quickly, the drug should not be given at bedtime. It may be administered with fruit juice or a carbonated beverage to mask its unpleasant taste.

Adverse Effects. Major hazards of stimulant laxative use are severe cramping, electrolyte and fluid deficiencies, enteric loss of protein, malabsorption resulting from excessive hypermotility and catharsis, and hypokalemia. Nevertheless, these laxatives are frequently used by those who self-medicate for constipation. Such abuse can lead to "cathartic colon," a poorly functioning colon.

Precautions. Stimulant laxatives should be used with caution when symptoms of appendicitis (abdominal pain, nausea, and vomiting) are present.

Dosage Forms

Laxative products are available in a wide array of dosage forms. Laxatives available as chewing gum, wafers, effervescent granules, and chocolate tablets may not be thought of as drug products and thus are more likely to be misused and abused. Enemas and suppositories are dosage forms often used.

Enemas. Enemas are used routinely to prepare patients for surgery, child delivery, and GI radiologic or endoscopic examination and to treat certain cases of constipation. The following considerations should be borne in mind:

- Soapsuds enemas are not recommended because of prolonged rectal irritation and possible other complications.
- Sodium phosphate–sodium biphosphate enemas (e.g., Fleet) are saline laxatives. They are more efficient and effective than tap water, soapsuds, or saline enemas; however, chronic use is not warranted.

Proper administration of an enema requires that:

- The patient is lying on the left side with knees bent or in the knee-to-chest position;
- The solution (≤500 mL or 16 oz) is allowed to flow into the rectum slowly; and
- The fluid is retained until definite cramping is felt in the lower abdomen.

Suppositories. Suppositories containing bisacodyl are promoted for postoperative, antepartum, and postpartum care and in preparation for proctosigmoidoscopy.

Therapeutic Considerations in Special Populations

Pediatric Laxative Use

Parents should observe their child for frequency of bowel movements, difficulty in passing stools, pain during bowel movements, and withholding of stools. Any deviation from the usual pattern should be noted. Infants and children appear to show a decreasing frequency of bowel movements with increasing age.

A number of factors can alter a child's bowel habits, including emotional distress, febrile illness, family conflict, dietary changes, or environmental changes. The pharmacist must consider such factors when determining whether constipation exists.

Increasing both fluids and the bulk content of the child's diet may decrease frequency of constipation. Simply increasing the amount of fluid or sugar in the formula may be corrective in the first few months of life. The child should be encouraged to drink water, and excessive milk intake should not be considered a substitute. Unbuttered popcorn is a good bulk-containing snack for children.

If medications are indicated in children under 5 years of age, glycerin suppositories may initiate the defecation reflex. Malt soup extract is relatively safe for infants under 2 months of age. Dark corn syrup (1–2 tsp per feeding) or milk of magnesia (beginning with 1/2 tsp) may be useful for fecal impaction. Bisacodyl may be used for moderate to severe constipation. Stimulants should probably be avoided, as should excessive use of enemas. Enemas are not usually recommended for children under 2 years of age. Senna and mineral oil should be administered only on the advice of a physician. When successful bowel evacuation cannot be achieved with oral supplementation or enemas, pediatricians may prescribe a balanced polyethylene glycol–electrolyte solution (e.g., Golytely, Colyte) to be administered orally.

Geriatric Laxative Use

For geriatric patients without a history of constipation, a thorough investigation should be conducted to determine whether acute cases of constipation have resulted from new or old diseases or from the use of medications. Recommendations of laxative use in this population should be patient specific because the elderly have complicating pathology and multiple disease states and are often vulnerable to medications.

Constipation in elderly persons can result from a number of factors, including failure to establish a time habit, insufficient fluid and/or bulk intake, abuse of stimulant laxatives, and immobility. If any of these factors exist, the pharmacist should consider corrective action in the patient's lifestyle or current drug therapy before recommending a laxative. Elderly patients are particularly sensitive to shifts in fluid and electrolytes. Use of any laxative that alters the fluid and electrolyte balance, particularly saline-type laxatives, may be inappropriate.

An acute episode of constipation can be treated with plain water or saline enemas. For elderly patients requiring laxatives, bulk-forming agents are generally preferred; onset is usually in 2–3 days. Sugar-free products (e.g., Konsyl, Serutan, and various Metamucil products) are recommended for diabetic patients. Glycerin suppositories and orally administered lactulose are safe and have been used successfully in elderly patients; lactulose may be of particular benefit to those who are bedridden. Chronic stimulant laxatives should not be generally recommended. The pharmacist should exercise caution when recommending magnesium-containing products to patients with renal failure or when recommending sodium-containing products to patients with cardiovascular disease.

Laxative Use in Pregnancy

Constipation is common in pregnancy. Pregnant women should be counseled on proper diet, adequate fluid intake, and reasonable exercise. If these measures do not alleviate or prevent the development of constipation, a laxative preparation may be appropriate. In some instances, the pharmacist should consult with the woman's health care provider, especially if any doubt exists regarding the provider's desire for the patient to have a laxative. Laxatives may also have to be administered postpartum to reestablish normal bowel function.

Pregnant women should probably use only bulk-forming or emollient laxatives. Senna and related anthraquinones have been used during breast-feeding despite a lack of information regarding their concentration in breast milk. Bisacodyl appears in breast milk in trace amounts. If these products are used, the infant should be carefully observed for diarrhea. Saline cathartics should be avoided during pregnancy and lactation.

Laxative Abuse

Chronic use of laxative preparations is considered laxative abuse. Excessive use of laxatives can cause diarrhea and vomiting, leading to fluid and electrolyte losses, especially hypokalemia, which may result in a general loss of tone of smooth and striated muscle. Clinical features of laxative abuse include:

- Factitious diarrhea;
- Electrolyte imbalance (e.g., hypokalemia, hypocalcemia, and hypermagnesemia);
- Osteomalacia;
- Protein-losing enteropathy;
- Steatorrhea;
- Cathartic colon; and
- Liver disease.

Laxative abuse can usually be classified as either habitual or surreptitious. The habitual abuser often believes that a daily bowel movement is a necessity and uses a laxative to accomplish this end. Such patients may freely admit to this practice. Some adolescents, college students, and young adults (especially women) use laxatives for weight control. Such abuse, which is virtually always surreptitious, is often part of a pattern of "purging behavior," which also may include self-induced vomiting. These persons may suffer from bulimia nervosa or anorexia nervosa. Surreptitious abusers tend to manifest various psychiatric disturbances. Psychiatric intervention should be encouraged.

Once the abuse has been adequately substantiated by laboratory tests, it may be possible to wean the patient off the laxative before permanent bowel damage occurs and to regularize the patient's bowel habits with a high-fiber diet supplemented by bulk-forming laxatives as needed. Several months may be required to retrain the bowel to work in regular, unaided function. Affected patients should be educated about laxative abuse.

Product Selection Guidelines

- The recommended initial choice for constipation is most often a bulk-forming product.
- A physician should supervise the use of laxatives in patients being treated for perianal disease, persons with conditions in which straining is undesirable (e.g., postoperative patients, patients who have had a myocardial infarct), and patients with chronic constipation.
- Laxatives are not recommended to treat constipation associated with intestinal pathology or constipation secondary to laxative abuse, unless bowel training has been successful.
- Laxative products whose maximum daily dose contains more than 15 mEq (345 mg) of sodium, 25 mEq (975 mg) of potassium, 50 mEq (600 mg) of magnesium, or 90 mEq (1800 mg) of calcium should not be used in patients with kidney or liver disease, heart failure, hypertension, or other conditions requiring restriction of these elements.
- Dextrose-containing products should be used with caution in labile diabetic patients.
- Patients with phenylketonuria should avoid products containing aspartame.

Patient Counseling

When counseling the patient on laxative use, the pharmacist should stress the following points:

- Laxative products should not be used regularly. More natural methods, such as diet, exercise, and fluid intake, should be used to foster regular bowel movements.
- The use of a laxative to treat constipation should be only a temporary measure; once regularity has returned, laxative use should be discontinued.
- If a laxative is not effective after 1 week, a physician should be consulted.
- If a skin rash appears after the patient has taken a laxative containing phenolphthalein, the product should be discontinued and a physician should be contacted.
- Saline laxatives should not be used daily, nor should they be administered orally to children under 6 years of age or rectally to infants under 2 years of age.
- The dose of a stimulant product should be individualized for appropriate effect.
- Mineral oil should be avoided in children under 6 years of age, and it should not be used in conjunction with emollient laxatives, during pregnancy, in elderly patients, and in patients taking anticoagulants.

- Castor oil should not be used to treat constipation.
- Enemas and suppositories must be administered properly to be effective.
- Laxatives should not be used in the presence of abdominal pain, perianal lesions, nausea, vomiting, bloating, or cramping without consulting a physician.
- Laxatives containing phenolphthalein or senna may discolor urine; laxatives containing phenolphthalein may discolor feces and urine pink to red.

CHAPTER 13

Antidiarrheal Products

Questions to ask in patient assessment and counseling

- *How long have you had diarrhea?*
- *Was the onset of diarrhea sudden?*
- *How often do the episodes of diarrhea occur?*
- *What is the character of the stool (i.e., consistency, odor, and color)?*
- *Do your stools contain blood or mucus?*
- *Is the diarrhea associated with other symptoms such as fever, weakness, loss of appetite, vomiting, dizziness, rapid heart rate, gas, or abdominal pain?*
- *Have you tried any antidiarrheal treatments or products? Which ones? Were they effective?*
- *How old are you?*
- *How often do you normally have a bowel movement?*
- *Have other family members experienced similar symptoms recently?*
- *Have you changed your diet recently?*
- *Can you relate the onset of diarrhea to a specific cause such as a particular meal or food (e.g., milk product) or drug?*
- *Have you recently traveled to a foreign country or a border area of the United States?*
- *Have you recently consumed nonchlorinated water such as that from a river, pond, or lake?*
- *Are you taking or have you recently taken any prescription or nonprescription medications? Which ones?*
- *Do you have diabetes, heart or blood vessel disease, or any other chronic medical condition?*

Diarrhea is a symptom that is characterized by abnormal frequency or consistency of stools. It may be acute or chronic. Its presence may signal either a gastrointestinal (GI) or non-GI disease. The approach to treatment depends on the cause of diarrhea.

Diarrhea

A complete medical assessment, including clinical laboratory evaluation, may be required to determine the cause of diarrhea. The etiology may be psychogenic, neurogenic, surgical, endocrine, irritative, osmotic, dietary, allergenic, malabsorptive, infectious, or inflammatory. Table 1 summarizes the types of diarrhea on the basis of physiologic mechanism. The most common clinical types of diarrhea are osmotic and secretory.

Editor's Note: This chapter is adapted from R. Leon Longe, "Antidiarrheal Products," in Covington, T.R., ed., *Handbook of Nonprescription Drugs*, 11th edition. For a more extensive discussion of the physiology of the intestine, diarrhea, and antidiarrheal products, readers are encouraged to consult Chapter 13 of the *Handbook*.

TABLE 1	Clinical classification of diarrhea	
Type	**Mechanism**	**Typical causes**
Osmotic	Unabsorbed solute	Lactase deficit, magnesium antacid excess
Secretory	Increased secretion of electrolytes	*Escherichia coli* infection, ileal resection, thyroid cancer
Exudative	Defective colonic absorption, outpouring of mucus and/ or blood	Ulcerative colitis, Crohn's disease, shigellosis, leukemia
Motility disorder	Decreased contact time	Irritable bowel syndrome, diabetic neuropathy

Types of Diarrhea

Acute Diarrhea

Acute diarrhea is characterized by a sudden onset of abnormally frequent, watery stools accompanied by weakness, flatulence, pain, and possibly fever or vomiting. It may be infectious, toxic, drug induced, or dietary in origin. It may occur as the result of various acute or chronic illnesses. In the United States, infectious diarrhea is usually viral in origin.

Food-Borne Diarrhea. Pathogens most commonly responsible for producing diarrhea in the United States are *Shigella* sp, *Salmonella* sp, *Campylobacter* sp, *Staphylococcus* sp, *Bacillus cereus*, and Norwalk viruses. A thorough history regarding food intake during the week prior to the onset of diarrhea is essential in identifying a probable cause.

The acute diarrhea that may develop among tourists visiting foreign countries or U.S. border areas with warm climates and poor sanitation is usually caused by bacterial enteropathogens, most commonly enterotoxigenic *Escherichia coli,* which is acquired via contaminated food or water. Symptoms generally subside over 3–5 days. Table 2 summarizes the various causes of infectious diarrheas and their treatment.

Infectious diarrhea may be treated with fluid and electrolytes. Often the illness is self-limiting, and normal function of the alimentary tract is restored with or without treatment in 24–72 hours. If the patient has a persistent case of infectious diarrhea, a specific anti-infective may be indicated.

Food-Induced Diarrhea. Food intolerance can provoke diarrhea. Such intolerance may be the result of a food allergy or of ingestion of foods that are excessively fatty or spicy or that contain a high amount of roughage or many seeds.

Acute viral diarrhea may cause a temporary milk intolerance at all ages. Infants born with a lactase deficiency and adults who develop one are intolerant of whole milk and milk-based products (e.g., ice cream), ingestion of which may result in diarrhea.

Viral Gastroenteritis. Diarrhea and vomiting are common in infants and young children. Although the etiology may be difficult to determine, the illness is often caused by a viral infection of the intestinal tract.

TABLE 2 Infectious diarrheas and their treatment

Type	History	Symptoms	Treatment
Bacterial			
Salmonella sp	Ingestion of improperly cooked or refrigerated poultry and dairy products, immuno-compromised host	Onset of 24–48 hours, diarrhea, fever, and chills	Fluid and electrolytes; no antibiotics
Shigella sp	Ingestion of con-taminated vegetables or water, immunocom-promised host	Onset of 24–48 hours, nausea, vomiting, diarrhea	Fluid and electrolytes; antibiotics (cotrimox-azole, ampicillin, ciprofloxacin/ norfloxacin)
Enterotoxigenic *Escherichia coli* (traveler's diarrhea)	Ingestion of contaminated food or water, recent travel outside the United States or to a US border area	Onset of 8–72 hours, watery diarrhea, fever, abdominal cramps	Fluid and electrolytes; in moderate or severe cases, antibiotics (cotrimoxazole, fluoroquinolones)
Campylobacter jejuni	Ingestion of contami-nated water, fecal–oral route, immuno-compromised host	Nausea, vomiting, headache, malaise, fever, watery diarrhea	Fluid and electrolytes; in severe or persis-tent diarrhea, antibiotics (erythromycin, fluoroquinolones)
Clostridium difficile	Antibiotic-associ-ated diarrhea	Watery or mucoid diarrhea, high fever, cramping	Water and electro-lytes; discontinuation of offending agent; oral metronidazole, oral vancomycin, bacitracin, cholestyramine

Continued on next page

Rotaviruses have been implicated as the cause of approximately 50% of all infantile gastroenteritis. Respiratory illnesses such as otitis media or tonsillitis may occur concurrently. The peak infectious period is winter. The illness tends to be self-limiting, lasting 5–8 days, and treatment is usually restricted to symptomatic therapy.

Norwalk viruses have also been implicated in children and adults. The diarrhea usually lasts 2–3 days. Most outbreaks occur in the winter months. The virus is usually transmitted by contaminated water or food (Table 2).

Moderate to severe diarrhea in infants requires prompt evaluation by a health care provider, because severe and possibly dangerous dehydration and electrolyte imbalance may occur relatively quickly.

Protozoal Diarrhea. Giardia lamblia and *Entamoeba histolytica* are protozoa associated with acute diarrhea. Giardiasis is an infection of the small intestine most commonly involving children, travelers, institutionalized patients, and hikers who drink from streams

TABLE 2 *continued*

Type	History	Symptoms	Treatment
Staphylococcus aureus	Ingestion of improperly cooked or stored food	Nausea, vomiting, watery diarrhea	Fluid and electrolytes; no antibiotics
Protozoal			
Giardia lamblia	Ingestion of water contaminated with human or animal feces, travel outside the United States, immuno-compromised host	Chronic watery diarrhea	Metronidazole, quinacrine, furazoli-done
Cryptosporidia	Travel outside the United States, AIDS, immunocompromised host	Chronic watery diarrhea	Fluid and electrolytes
Entamoeba histolytica	Travel outside the United States, fecal-soiled food or water, immunocompromised host	Chronic watery diarrhea	Fluid and electrolytes; metronidazole; iodoquinol
Viruses			
Rotaviruses	Infects infants, fecal–oral spread	Vomiting, fever, nausea, acute watery diarrhea	Vigorous fluid and electrolyte replace-ment; no antibiotics
Norwalk	Infects all ages	"24-hour flu," vomiting, nausea, headache, myalgia, fever, watery diarrhea	Fluid and electrolytes; no antibiotics; bismuth subsalicylate; loperamide

or ponds. Symptoms may be absent or mild. Quinacrine and metronidazole are both effective, but the latter is better tolerated (Table 2).

Drug-Induced Diarrhea. Commonly prescribed antibiotics that have a broad spectrum of activity against aerobic and anaerobic organisms can produce diarrhea as a side effect. Antibiotic-associated diarrhea (AAD) may be caused by an overgrowth of an antibiotic-resistant bacterial or fungal strain or of toxin-producing *Clostridium difficile.* It may begin during or several weeks after treatment. AAD may be self-limiting with antibiotic discontinuation.

C difficile produces toxins that may cause antibiotic-associated pseudomembranous colitis. The diagnosis is suggested by a test for the toxins in the stool. Enteric isolation precautions are recommended because *C difficile* can be spread to other persons. The offending antibiotic must be discontinued and *C difficile* eradicated by treatment with oral metronidazole or oral vancomycin in adults. Metronidazole is preferred because it is less expensive and patients do not develop vancomycin-resistant *Enterococcus.* Treatment in children is less well defined.

Other drugs that can cause diarrhea include:

■ Agents that cause retention of electrolytes and water in the intestinal lumen (e.g., mannitol, sorbitol, lactulose);

■ Magnesium-containing laxatives and antacids;

■ Drugs that affect autonomic control of intestinal motility (e.g., guanethidine, methyldopa, reserpine);

■ Prokinetic agents (e.g., bethanechol, metoclopramide, cisapride); and

■ Other agents (e.g., laxatives, misoprostol, olsalazine, anticancer agents, quinidine, colchicine).

AIDS-Associated Diarrhea. Patients with acquired immunodeficiency syndrome (AIDS) and individuals infected with human immunodeficiency virus (HIV) are susceptible to many intestinal infections that produce diarrhea as one of their manifestations.

Chronic Diarrhea

Chronic diarrhea is the long-term (i.e., lasting more than 4 weeks), abnormally frequent passage of poorly formed or watery stools. Chronic diarrhea may be caused by a disease of the small or large intestine or the stomach, or it may be a secondary manifestation of a systemic disease. The pharmacist should refer patients with persistent or recurrent diarrhea for medical care.

Laxative abuse is a common cause of chronic diarrhea of unknown origin. To identify the laxative abuser, the practitioner must take a thorough drug history and monitor the frequency of laxative purchases. Recovery requires laxative withdrawal, bowel training, psychologic counseling, and, on rare occasions, hospitalization. Screening tests for laxatives may sometimes be the only way to detect laxative abuse.

Psychogenic factors are also associated with chronic diarrhea (e.g., stress-related diarrhea).

Patient Assessment

Evaluation of the patient's responses to the questions presented at the beginning of this chapter should enable the pharmacist to assess the patient's condition and begin to decide on a proper course of action. This triage function requires the pharmacist to differentiate symptoms and make clinical judgments. Figure 1 is a decision tree for managing diarrhea.

The pharmacist should acquire a history of the patient's present illness. The following four groups of patients with either acute or chronic diarrhea should be referred to a health care provider for a complete diagnostic evaluation:

■ Children under 3 years of age;

■ Persons who have multiple medical conditions;

■ Persons with chronic illness such as AIDS, diabetes mellitus, or heart disease; and

■ Pregnant women.

Other conditions that suggest the need for health care provider referral include:

■ Bloody or mucoid stools;

■ Moderate to severe abdominal tenderness or cramping;

■ Temperature ≥101°F or 38°C;

■ Evidence of moderate or severe dehydration (Table 3);

■ Loss of greater than 5% of total body weight; or

■ Diarrhea that has lasted 2 or more days.

TABLE 3   Diarrhea treatment chart

Degree of dehydration (fluid deficit)	Signs[a]	Rehydration therapy (within 4 h)	Replacement of stool fluid losses	Dietary therapy[b]
Mild (3%–5%)	Slightly dry buccal mucous membranes; increased thirst	ORS[c] 50 mL/kg	10 mL/kg or 1/2–1 cup of ORS for each diarrheal stool	Human milk feeding, half- or full-strength lactose-containing milk, or undiluted lactose-free formula
Moderate (6%–9%)	Sunken eyes; sunken fontanelle; loss of skin turgor; dry buccal mucous membranes	ORS 100 mL/kg	Same as above	Same as above
Severe (≥10%)	Signs of moderate dehydration with one of the following: rapid thready pulse, cyanosis, cold extremities, rapid breathing, lethargy, coma	Intravenous fluids (lactated Ringer's solution); 20 mL/kg per hour until pulse, perfusion, and mental status return to normal; then 50–100 mL/kg of ORS	Same as above	Same as above

[a]If no signs of dehydration are present, rehydration therapy is not required. Maintenance therapy and replacement of stool losses should be undertaken.

[b]Infants and children who receive solid food can continue their usual diet, but foods high in simple sugars and fats should be avoided.

[c]Oral rehydration solution (ORS).

Reprinted from Centers for Disease Control and Prevention. The management of acute diarrhea in children: oral rehydration, maintenance, and nutritional therapy. *MMWR*. 1992; 41(RR-16): 14.

Temporary self-treatment may be sometimes needed until a medical appointment can be arranged.

A medication history may help detect drug-induced diarrhea. When a drug is implicated as a cause of diarrhea, the pharmacist should refer the patient to a health care provider who can assess the need to continue the drug or consider alternatives. Patients with a history of chronic GI disease should also be referred to a health care provider.

The patient needs to be monitored for signs of volume depletion. The most accurate assessment of fluid balance is body weight; however, the premorbid weight is seldom known. Signs and symptoms of dehydration are summarized in Table 3. Findings associated with moderate to severe volume depletion also include dizziness, fainting or near fainting, and postural (orthostatic) hypotension. Postural hypotension is defined as a drop in the systolic and/or diastolic pressure by greater than 15–20 mm Hg upon moving from a lying to an upright position. It warrants referral for medical care.

Stool character gives valuable information about diarrhea. For example, undigested food particles suggest small-bowel irritation. Black, tarry stools may indicate upper GI bleeding. Red stools suggest possible lower bowel or hemorrhoidal bleeding (or simply the recent ingestion of red foods such as beets or of a drug such as rifampin). Yellow stools may indicate the presence of bilirubin and a potentially serious liver pathology.

Treatment

Treatment goals are to (1) prevent excessive fluid and electrolyte loss and acid-base disturbance; (2) manage secondary conditions causing diarrhea; (3) provide symptomatic relief; and (4) identify and treat the cause, if possible.

Many nonprescription products are available to assist in managing diarrhea. The pharmacist should exercise caution in recommending them because certain diarrhea-producing diseases might be serious or treated more effectively with agents specific for the underlying cause. Pregnant women and the frail elderly with diarrhea should be referred to their physician for fluid and electrolyte management.

Prophylaxis and Management of Infectious Diarrhea

Prophylaxis of traveler's (infectious) diarrhea is controversial. Many infectious disease experts do not recommend drug prophylaxis but tell travelers to begin treatment when signs or symptoms first appear. If a prophylactic drug is used, it should be started on the day of arrival and taken continuously, including 1–2 additional days after the person's return to the United States. Prophylaxis should not continue for more than 3 weeks, even if travel is still in progress.

Antibiotics are the most effective prophylactic drugs available. Travelers likely to be exposed to excessive sun should be advised to use sunscreen if they are prescribed antibiotics that may produce photosensitivity reactions (e.g., sulfonamides, tetracyclines).

Traveler's diarrhea may be managed with fluid and electrolyte replacement. Loperamide (Diar-Aid, Imodium A-D) is effective for symptomatic managment. Bismuth subsalicylate (Pepto-Bismol) has also been shown to be effective in both preventing and treating symptoms of traveler's diarrhea. The adult prophylactic dosage is 30 mL or two tablets taken four times a day with meals and at bedtime during the first 2 weeks of travel. During bouts of acute diarrhea, the adult treatment dose is 30 mL or two tablets and should be taken every 30 minutes for five doses. No more than eight doses should be taken in any 24-hour period. Package labeling should be consulted with regard to dosing pediatric patients.

Fluid and Electrolyte Replacement

Correction of fluid loss and electrolyte imbalance is very important. Rehydration replaces lost water and electrolytes to restore the normal body composition. After rehydration, electrolyte solutions are given to maintain the normal body composition. If the patient is not volume depleted, only maintenance of fluid and electrolytes is needed.

In mild to moderate diarrhea, oral fluids can be safely prescribed if the patient is not vomiting. Administering fluids without electrolytes is potentially dangerous because of the risk of inducing hyponatremia or causing osmotic diarrhea. If liquids with a very high sugar content (e.g., cola, ginger ale, apple juice) are used for rehydration or maintenance therapy, they should be diluted to one-half strength to avoid osmotic diarrhea.

Commercial oral rehydration solution (ORS) products (Pedialyte, Rehydralyte, Infalyte, Resol) are convenient and safe because they are premixed. These products are either for rehydration or maintenance/preventive management. They can be used for maintenance therapy if water, lactose-free infant formula, breast milk, or low-carbohydrate juice is also given to prevent hypernatremia. Rehydralyte is the only product meeting the American Academy of Pediatrics (AAP) recommendation for rehydration; all others are preventive/maintenance solutions.

Management of Diarrhea in Infants and Children

After the degree of volume depletion has been determined, management is carried out in two phases: rehydration and maintenance with nutritional support. Table 3 outlines guidelines for dietary management of fluid and electrolytes by degree of dehydration, as recommended by the Centers for Disease Control and Prevention (CDC). For severe dehydration, intravenous rehydration should be administered. For mild or moderate dehydration, an ORS with 50–90 mEq/L of sodium should be used for rehydration. After the rehydration phase, fluid losses must be replaced to maintain normal balance. A maintenance ORS should have 40–60 mEq/L of sodium.

Once rehydration is complete, food may be reintroduced while oral solutions are given for maintenance. In older infants and children, the AAP recommends that feeding be reintroduced within the first 24 hours. The AAP recommends gradual reintroduction of milk-based bottle feeding, but breast-feeding should resume immediately after rehydration.

In infants and children, antimotility and adsorbent drugs have not been shown to alter the outcomes of acute nonspecific diarrhea.

Pharmacologic Agents

With the exception of loperamide and bismuth subsalicylate in traveler's diarrhea, scientific evidence is lacking to prove that pharmacologic agents reduce stool frequency or duration of acute nonspecific diarrhea. Nevertheless, when used according to labeling, non-prescription antidiarrheals may provide relief and usually do no harm. Fluid, electrolyte, and nutritional therapies are the most important components to managing diarrhea.

Antiperistaltic Agents

- Include diphenoxylate, loperamide, and opiate derivatives (e.g., paregoric);
- Are effective in relieving cramps and stool frequency;
- Should be used for no more than 48 hours in acute diarrhea;
- May worsen the effects of invasive bacterial infection and may cause toxic megacolon;
- Should be used with caution in patients with fecal leukocytes, fever or recent history of antibiotic use, or acute ulcerative colitis.

Loperamide is an effective antidiarrheal agent in traveler's diarrhea, nonspecific acute diarrhea, and chronic diarrhea associated with inflammatory bowel disease. Like other antiperistaltic drugs, it should be used for no more than 48 hours. The usual nonprescription adult dosage is 4 mg initially and then 2 mg after each loose bowel movement, not to exceed 8 mg per day. Loperamide should never be recommended for children under 2 years of age.

Opiates (e.g., paregoric) and opiate-like agents, once used for diarrhea, have been removed from the nonprescription market because of the risks of physical dependency and excessive sedation.

Adsorbents

- Include attapulgite, kaolin, and pectin;
- May adsorb nutrients, digestive enzymes, and drugs as well as toxins, bacteria, and

various noxious materials in the GI tract (depending on the medication involved, a change in dose, dosage interval, or route of administration may be required until the diarrheal episode is over and the adsorbent drug is discontinued);

■ Following initial treatment, are taken after each loose bowel movement until diarrhea is controlled or maximum daily dose is reached.

Polycarbophil

■ Used for both diarrhea and constipation (absorbs up to 60 times its original weight in water);

■ Adult dose is 4–6 g/day in divided doses;

■ Use in children ≤3 years of age is not recommended without the advice of a health care provider.

Bismuth Subsalicylate

■ Adult dose is 30 mL every 30–60 minutes as needed, to a maximum of eight doses in a 24-hour period;

■ Should not be taken by children <2 years of age; patients with aspirin sensitivity; children and teenagers with or recovering from chicken pox or flu (risk of aspirin-induced Reye's syndrome); nursing or pregnant women (without medical advice);

■ May cause harmless black-stained stool or darkening of the tongue;

■ Subject to same potential drug interactions as aspirin;

■ May increase risk of salicylate toxicity if taken concomitantly with aspirin or other salicylate-containing drugs;

■ May interfere with radiographic intestinal studies.

Digestive Enzymes

■ Lactase enzyme preparations (e.g., SureLac, Lactaid, Dairy Ease, Lactrase) are available for patients with lactase enzymatic deficiency;

■ May be added to milk products or taken with milk at mealtimes to prevent osmotic diarrhea.

Product Selection Guidelines

A complete history must be obtained. The most important data to evaluate are the presence of high fever, duration of illness, presence of blood in the stool, and fluid-electrolyte status.

Criteria for diarrhea evaluation and decision making are summarized in Figure 1. If the patient meets the criteria for self-medication, the pharmacist should assess the degree of dehydration and select either an ORS or a maintenance product on the basis of that assessment (Table 3). If no signs of dehydration are present, preventive therapy with a maintenance ORS may be all that is necessary. For families with infants, the CDC recommends a home supply of ORS.

Nonspecific antidiarrheals have limited value and lack scientific evidence in acute diarrheal illnesses. With suspected infectious diarrhea, antibiotics may be indicated and should be managed by a health care provider.

Uncomplicated acute diarrhea usually improves within 24–48 hours. If the condition remains the same or worsens, the pharmacist should recommend that the patient seek medical care. Moderately or severely volume-depleted patients (especially infants and children) need medical care. Immediate referral to a health care provider is also required if the patient is severely dehydrated, has a high fever, has protracted vomiting, has blood in the stool, is chronically ill, or is immunocompromised.

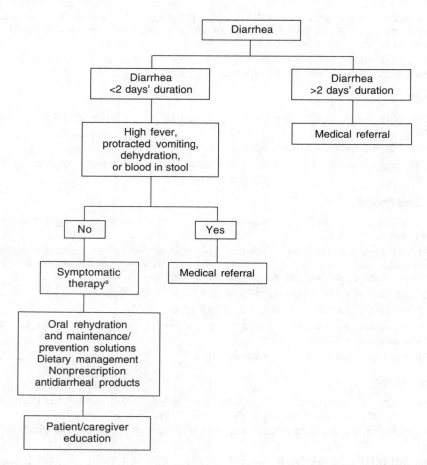

aIf diarrhea is not resolved in 2 days of therapy or if condition worsens, patient should seek medical care.

FIGURE 1 Diarrhea evaluation and decision making.

CHAPTER 14

Hemorrhoidal Products

Questions to ask in patient assessment and counseling

- *What are your symptoms?*
- *How long have your symptoms been present? Do they recur?*
- *Are your symptoms associated with straining at a bowel movement?*
- *Have you noticed any bleeding? Describe it.*
- *What improves or worsens your symptoms?*
- *Have you treated your symptoms without the use of medication? What nondrug measures have you used?*
- *Have you previously used any nonprescription or prescription drugs for these symptoms?*
- *Do you take laxatives? If so, which ones and how often?*
- *Do you take any other medications?*
- *Have you recently changed your diet or amount of fluid intake?*
- *Are you now or have you recently been pregnant?*
- *Do you often experience constipation or diarrhea?*
- *Do you have any other medical conditions such as heart failure, liver disease, inflammatory disease of the intestine, or varicose veins?*

Anorectal Disorders

Hemorrhoids

Hemorrhoids (piles) are abnormally large, bulging, symptomatic conglomerates of hemorrhoidal vessels, supporting tissues, and overlying mucous membranes or skin of the anorectal area.

Etiologic factors associated with hemorrhoidal disease include heredity, erect posture, pregnancy, prolonged standing or sitting, lack of dietary bulk, heavy lifting with straining, constipation, and diarrhea. Pregnancy is the most common cause of hemorrhoids in young women.

Hemorrhoids can be classified according to their location as internal, external, and internal-external.

Internal Hemorrhoids

Internal hemorrhoids occur above the anorectal line. Internal hemorrhoids are sometimes classified according to a four-degree system. First-degree hemorrhoids do not move from

---

Editor's Note: This chapter is adapted from Benjamin Hodes, "Hemorrhoidal Products," in Covington, T.R., ed., *Handbook of Nonprescription Drugs,* 11th edition. For a more extensive discussion of the physiology of the anorectal area, types of anorectal disorders, and signs and symptoms of anorectal disease and its treatment, readers are encouraged to consult Chapter 14 of the *Handbook.*

the anal canal. Second-degree hemorrhoids can descend into the anal canal and return spontaneously. Hemorrhoids that can be returned manually into the anus are referred to as third degree. Fourth-degree hemorrhoids are prolapsed and cannot be reintroduced into the anus.

External Hemorrhoids

External hemorrhoids are recognized as a swelling of the skin and associated blood vessels around the rim of the anus. There are two types of external hemorrhoids, thrombosed and cutaneous. Both occur below the anorectal line. External hemorrhoids are covered by highly innervated skin, and when it is stretched by a thrombosis, sudden and severe pain can result.

Internal-External Hemorrhoids

Internal and external hemorrhoids can occur together and are known as mixed hemorrhoids. There are three types of mixed hemorrhoids. Prolapsed hemorrhoids are characterized by pain, with or without blood. Hemorrhoids without prolapse are characterized by bleeding but no pain. Strangulated hemorrhoids are painful and usually thrombosed; the blood supply is occluded by the anal sphincter.

Acute external hemorrhoids are accompanied by a steady, aching pain that is usually worsened by standing or defecating. Chronic external hemorrhoids often cause no pain. Similarly, uncomplicated internal hemorrhoids rarely cause pain. However, when strangulation, thrombosis, or ulceration occurs, pain may be severe. Patients with severe or persistent pain should be referred to a physician.

Other Anorectal Disorders

Some potentially serious anorectal disorders may present hemorrhoidal-like symptoms. Patients should be promptly referred to a physician if any of the following conditions are suspected:

- *Abscess:* a painful swelling in the perianal or anal canal area caused by a bacterial infection and resulting in the formation of a localized area of pus.

- *Anal fistula:* a channel-like lesion near the anus, associated with swelling, pain, intermittent discharge, and itching.

- *Anal fissure:* a slitlike ulcer in the anal canal lining that may be painful, may exist alone or in conjunction with hemorrhoids, and often causes bleeding, evidenced by bright-red blood on toilet tissue.

- *Condyloma latum:* a firm, wartlike, usually painless lesion that is one of the secondary lesions of syphilis.

- *Condyloma acuminata:* venereal warts, usually sexually transmitted, that appear as multiple, painless lesions in the genital or perianal region.

- *Cryptitis:* inflammation and hypertrophy of the anal crypts, a condition that is primarily characterized by pain aggravated by defecation.

- *Malignant neoplasm:* a serious disease, often characterized by constipation, in which bleeding and pain may be associated with malignant anal tumors that are usually unnoticeable.

- *Polyps:* benign or malignant rectal tumors that are most commonly characterized by bleeding.

Signs and Symptoms of Anorectal Disorders

Itching, burning, inflammation, pain, and swelling are the most common signs and symptoms of minor anorectal disease. Discomfort, a vague and generalized uneasiness, may result from any or all of these symptoms. If these symptoms are caused by hemorrhoids rather than by a more serious anorectal disease, they may be relieved by self-treatment. Bleeding, seepage, protrusion, prolapse, and thrombosis should not be self-treated, both because they may mask a more serious disorder and because no appropriate nonprescription therapy is available.

Itching

Itching (pruritus) is a manifestation of the mild inflammation associated with many anorectal disorders. It may be secondary to swelling, irritation caused by dietary factors, parasitic diseases (e.g., pinworms), or moisture in the anal area.

Sensitivity to fabrics, dyes and perfumes in toilet tissue, detergents, local treatment (including products used to treat hemorrhoidal symptoms), and fecal contents are also common causes of itching.

Burning

Burning suggests a somewhat greater degree of irritation than that associated with itching. The burning sensation may range from a feeling of warmth to a feeling of intense heat and may be constant or associated with defecation.

Inflammation

Inflammation, a tissue reaction distinguished by heat, redness, pain, and swelling, is often caused by trauma, allergy, or infection. The inflammation, but not the underlying cause, may be relieved by self-treatment.

Bleeding

Painless bleeding during defecation is the most common symptom of hemorrhoids. The amount of bleeding varies and is not necessarily related to the amount of hemorrhoidal tissue present. Blood from hemorrhoids is usually bright red and covers the fecal matter or toilet paper. Bleeding may also indicate serious anorectal disease (e.g., abscess, fistula, cancer, colitis, or diverticulitis). In rare cases, chronic blood loss associated with hemorrhoids may produce severe anemia. Bleeding hemorrhoids should not be self-treated.

Seepage

Seepage, the involuntary passing of fecal material or mucus, is caused by an anal sphincter that does not close completely. Such patients should be referred to a health care provider.

Protrusion

Protrusion is defined as the projection of hemorrhoidal or rectal tissue outside the anal canal. The protrusion may vary in size and usually appears after defecation, prolonged standing, or unusual physical exertion. Self-treatment is not appropriate.

Thrombosis

Thrombosis within a hemorrhoid is common. Abrupt onset of severe, constant pain in the anal area, accompanied by a grape-sized lump, is a sign that thrombosis may have occurred. If untreated, the burning pain persists for about 5–7 days, diminishing in intensity after the first day. A hard, tender lump typically appears at the site of the pain; after the second day, the lump slowly dissipates and eventually leaves a skin tag.

If a thrombosed hemorrhoid persists, gangrene and ulcers may develop. If the clot remains exposed, infection may occur and an abscess or fistula may result.

If the thrombosed hemorrhoid resides entirely above the anorectal line, pain may be minimal. Patients are likely to be unaware that such a hemorrhoid is present unless they experience sudden changes in bowel habits.

Assessment

The first step in assessment is to determine the nature of the signs and symptoms. If the patient has not used any medication, the pharmacist should determine if there are any contributing factors such as diarrhea or constipation, obesity, cardiovascular disease, hepatic disease, pregnancy, and chronic cough. The pharmacist should also determine causative factors, such as bowel habits, physical exertion, prolonged sitting or standing, insufficient fiber or liquids in the diet, constipating medications, and laxative abuse.

On the basis of this information, the pharmacist may either recommend a nonprescription product for the temporary relief of minor symptoms or refer the patient to a health care provider.

Nonpharmacologic Treatment

Nondrug Measures

Cleansing the anorectal area with mild, unscented soap and water regularly and after each bowel movement helps relieve hemorrhoidal symptoms and may prevent itching. Practical means of cleansing after a bowel movement include hygienic and lubricated wipes or pads. Patients should be advised to blot or pat rather than rub the perianal area. Toilet tissue should be unscented, uncolored, and soft.

Sitz baths often relieve hemorrhoidal symptoms. Patients should sit in warm water (110°–115°F [43.3°–46.1°C]) two to three times a day for 15 minutes.

Surgical and Nonsurgical Treatments

Large and prolapsed hemorrhoids are often treated with surgery. Nonsurgical treatments include injection of sclerosing agents, rubber-band ligation, dilation of the anal canal and lower rectum, cryosurgery, electrocoagulation, infrared photocoagulation, and bipolar diathermy.

Pharmacologic Treatment

Choice of Agents

The nonprescription pharmacologic agents recommended to relieve symptoms of anorectal disease include local anesthetics, vasoconstrictors, protectants, astringents, wound-healing agents, antiseptics, keratolytics, and anticholinergics, as well as analgesics, anesthetics, and antipruritics (Table 1). Products containing an excessive number of agents may not be optimally effective because of potential interaction among ingredients.

TABLE 1 Indications for the use of nonprescription anorectal pharmacologic agents

Signs/ Symptoms	Analgesic/ Anesthetic/ Antipruritic	Vaso- con- strictor	Pro- tectant	Astringent	Local anesthetic	Kerato- lytic	Cortico- steroid
Discomfort	yes	yes	yes	yes	yes	yes	no
Irritation	no	yes	yes	yes	no	no	no
Itching	yes	yes	yes	yes	yes	yes	yes
Pain	yes	no	no	no	yes	no	no
Swelling	no	yes	no	no	no	no	no
Burning	yes	no	yes	yes	yes	no	no

Local Anesthetics

Local, topical anesthetics temporarily relieve pain, burning, itching, and discomfort by preventing the transmission of nerve impulses. The following local anesthetics have met the Food and Drug Administration (FDA) safety and efficacy standards for use in hemorrhoidal preparations. All are applied externally to the perianal or lower anal canal regions.

■ Benzocaine is safe and effective in concentrations of 5%–20% applied up to six times a day.

■ Benzyl alcohol is effective in concentrations of 5%–20% and may be applied up to six times a day.

■ Dibucaine and dibucaine hydrochloride are considered equivalent in concentrations of 0.25%–1% applied up to three or four times a day.

■ Dyclonine hydrochloride is effective in concentrations of 0.5%–1% and may be applied up to six times a day.

■ Lidocaine is effective in concentrations of 2%–5% and may be applied up to six times a day.

■ Pramoxine hydrochloride 1% may be used as a topical aerosol foam, ointment, cream, or jelly. Adverse effects are rare. Pramoxine hydrochloride exhibits less cross-sensitivity than do most other local anesthetics because it is not chemically derived from lidocaine or procaine. Pramoxine-containing anorectal products may be applied up to five times a day.

■ Tetracaine and tetracaine hydrochloride are effective in concentrations of 0.5%–1% and may be applied up to six times a day.

Local anesthetics may produce local and systemic allergic reactions. Such reactions may cause burning and itching that are indistinguishable from symptoms of the anorectal disease being treated. If symptoms return after cessation of therapy, a health care provider should be contacted.

Vasoconstrictors

Applied locally in the anorectal area, vasoconstrictors stimulate the alpha-adrenergic receptors in the vascular beds, causing constriction of the arterioles and a modest and transient reduction of swelling. They also relieve itching, discomfort, and irritation. The FDA does not recognize or approve the use of these products to control bleeding.

Because of the slight possibility of systemic adverse reactions from topical application, these products should be avoided in patients who have diabetes, hyperthyroidism, hypertension, and difficulty urinating because of an enlarged prostate. Vasoconstrictors should also be avoided by patients taking monoamine oxidase inhibitors, tricyclic antidepressants, or a prescription drug for high blood pressure.

Four vasoconstrictors are approved for external use for itching, discomfort, swelling, and irritation: ephedrine sulfate, epinephrine hydrochloride, epinephrine base, and phenylephrine hydrochloride. Ephedrine sulfate and phenylephrine hydrochloride are also recommended for intrarectal use.

- Ephedrine sulfate has a more prolonged effect than epinephrine. Applied topically, it has an onset of action ranging from a few seconds to 1 minute. Duration of action is 2–3 hours. The recommended concentration, in the final dosage form, is 0.1%–1.25% applied up to four times a day.

- Epinephrine hydrochloride and epinephrine base are effective only when used externally, because epinephrine is inactivated at the pH of the rectum. The recommended concentration is 0.005%–0.01%, and it may be applied up to four times a day.

- Phenylephrine hydrochloride is believed to relieve itching caused by histamine release and to reduce congestion in the anorectal area. The recommended dosage is 0.25% applied up to four times a day.

Protectants

Protectants prevent irritation of the anorectal area and water loss from the stratum corneum by forming a barrier on the skin.

Absorbents, adsorbents, demulcents, and emollients are included in the protectant classification. Many substances classified as protectants are also used as vehicles, bases, and carriers of pharmacologically active substances (e.g., vasoconstrictors, local anesthetics). Recommended protectants are aluminum hydroxide gel (in moist conditions only), cocoa butter, glycerin in aqueous solution, hard fat (cocoa butter substitutes, hydrogenated cocoglycerides, and hydrogenated palm kernel glycerides), kaolin, lanolin, mineral oil, white petrolatum, petrolatum, and topical starch. All are recommended for external and intrarectal use with the exception of glycerin, which is recommended for external use only. Protectants recommended only when used in combination with one, two, or three other protectants and subject to limitations are calamine, zinc oxide, cod liver oil, and shark liver oil. Protectants may be applied up to six times a day or after each bowel movement.

Adverse reactions to protectants are minimal. Wool alcohols (lanolin) may cause allergic reactions. Bismuth salts are considered safe and effective as protectants.

Astringents

Appropriately used, astringents contribute to drying by lessening mucous and other secretions. This drying effect helps relieve local anorectal irritation, discomfort. itching, and burning.

Calamine and zinc oxide in concentrations of 5%–25% are recommended as astringents for both external and internal use when applied up to six times a day. Witch hazel (hamamelis water) in a concentration of 10%–50% is recommended as an astringent for external use up to six times a day in anorectal disorders; its effectiveness is due primarily to its alcohol content. Recommended products should be limited to those containing the appropriate concentration of an astringent ingredient.

Keratolytics

By fostering cell turnover and loosening surface cells, keratolytics may help expose underlying tissue to therapeutic agents. Used externally, they are somewhat useful in reducing itching and discomfort.

The two keratolytics recommended for external use in hemorrhoidal products are aluminum chlorhydroxy allantoinate (alcloxa) and resorcinol. The dosage ranges established by the FDA are up to six 2-g applications per day of a 0.2%–2% ointment for alcloxa and of a 1%–3% ointment for resorcinol.

Analgesics, Anesthetics, and Antipruritics

Menthol (0.1%–1%), juniper tar (1%–5%), and camphor (0.1%–3%) are safe and effective for external use in the anorectal area and may be applied up to six times a day. Camphor (greater than 3%–11%), turpentine oil (rectified) (6%–50%), and menthol (1.25%–16%) are not considered safe and effective for anorectal use.

Corticosteroids

Nonprescription topical corticosteroid-containing products are indicated for temporary relief of minor external anal itching due to minor irritation or rash. There are no approved nonprescription combinations of a corticosteroid with another active ingredient for anorectal use.

Bulk-Forming Laxatives

Because constipation is a precipitating factor in hemorrhoidal disease, patients may be advised to consider using bulk-forming or emollient laxatives (see Chapter 12). Adequate fluid intake should be encouraged.

Miscellaneous Pharmacologic Agents

Indications for nonprescription anorectal pharmacologic agents are summarized in Table 1.

Dosage Forms

Drugs for the treatment of anorectal symptoms are available in many dosage forms. For intrarectal use, suppositories, creams, ointments, gels, and foams are available. Creams, ointments, gels, pastes, wipes, pads, liquids, and foam are used externally. Although there are considerable pharmaceutical differences among ointments, creams, pastes, and gels, the therapeutic differences are not significant.

When used externally, ointments should be applied as a thin covering to the perianal area and the anal canal. For intrarectal use, ointments can be inserted with the fingers or with an applicator called a pile pipe. Pile pipes allow the patient to introduce the ointment into the rectal mucosa, where the potential for systemic absorption is greatest. The pile pipe should have lateral openings, as well as a hole in the end, to allow the drug product to cover the greatest area of rectal mucosa. The pile pipe should be lubricated before insertion by spreading the ointment around the tip.

Suppositories are not generally recommended as a dosage form in treating anorectal disease symptoms. In prone patients, suppositories may leave the affected region and ascend into the rectum and lower colon. If the patient remains prone after inserting a suppository or an ointment, the active ingredients may not be evenly distributed over the rectal mucosa. Suppositories and ointments are relatively slow-acting because they must melt to release the active ingredient.

Foam products present no proven advantage over ointments.

Product Selection Guidelines

After determining that the patient has signs and symptoms amenable to self-treatment, the pharmacist should decide on a suitable anorectal product, if any, taking into account product-specific factors such as ingredients and dosage form. Knowledge of a patient's present medical condition, medical history, medication profile, diet, and socioeconomic factors is necessary to determine how an individual may respond to self-treatment.

Pregnant and nursing women should use only products recommended for external use except for the recommended protectants, which may be used internally. Children with hemorrhoids or other anorectal disease should be referred to a health care provider.

Products containing the least number of recommended ingredients should be suggested. Those with one or a few specific ingredients are most likely to minimize undesirable interactions and maximize effectiveness. Scented and tinted products should be avoided. Symptoms should be managed as specifically as possible.

Patient Counseling

The pharmacist should emphasize the importance of good health care, consumption of sufficient fiber and liquids, and proper hygiene of the anorectal area in helping to prevent and alleviate symptoms of anorectal disease. Specific advice should include the following:

- Before any nonprescription anorectal product is applied, the anorectal area should be washed with mild soap and warm water, rinsed thoroughly, and gently dried by patting or blotting with toilet tissue or a soft cloth.

- Nonprescription anorectal products should be used after, rather than before, bowel movements.

- Products designed only for external anorectal use should not be inserted into the rectum.

- Products used externally in the anorectal area should be applied sparingly.

- Patients should be advised on how to insert a pile pipe or a suppository and how to apply a foam dosage form. If insertion of a product into the rectum causes pain, use of the product should be discontinued and a health care provider consulted promptly.

- If redness, irritation, swelling, pain, or other signs and symptoms develop or worsen, use of the product should be discontinued and a health care provider consulted.

- If seepage, bleeding, black tarry stools, protrusion, or severe pain occurs, a health care provider should be contacted as soon as possible.

- Patients with cardiovascular disease, diabetes, hypertension, or hyperthyroidism, or patients experiencing difficulty urinating, should not use a topical anorectal product containing a vasoconstrictor.

- Patients taking prescription drugs to treat hypertension or depression should not use an anorectal product containing a vasoconstrictor without consulting a health care provider.

- Products containing ephedrine sulfate may cause nervousness, tremor, sleeplessness, nausea, and loss of appetite.

- If bleeding occurs, or if symptoms worsen or do not improve after 7 days of self-treatment, a health care provider should be consulted promptly.

- Sitz baths are an alternative nondrug approach for managing mild symptoms of uncomplicated anorectal disease.

■ Cleansing the anorectal area after defecation with moistened, unscented, and uncolored toilet tissue or a wipe is recommended.

■ The importance of maintaining normal bowel function by eating a well-balanced diet that includes roughage, drinking adequate amounts of fluid, and avoiding excessive laxative use should be emphasized as a means of preventing anorectal disease. A diet high in fiber and fluid will promote the formation of easily passed stools, thereby preventing constipation and the accompanying straining.

■ Bulk laxatives or stool softeners may prevent the straining that can lead to or aggravate hemorrhoids. Patients with symptomatic hemorrhoids may experience a significant reduction in bleeding and pain within a few weeks after beginning the regular use of a bulk laxative. If possible, prescription and nonprescription drugs that may cause constipation should be avoided.

Chapter 15

Anthelmintic Products

Questions to ask in patient assessment and counseling

- *Why do you think you (or your child) might have worms?*
- *Are other members of your family or close contacts also affected?*
- *Have you seen any worms in stools?*
- *Describe your symptoms. Have you had nausea, diarrhea, abdominal pain, rectal itching, or weight loss? Do you become fatigued easily?*
- *How long have the symptoms been present?*
- *Have you seen a physician for this problem?*
- *Has the problem occurred in the past? How was it treated? Did the treatment work?*
- *If the patient is a child, what is his or her age and approximate weight?*
- *If the patient is female, is she pregnant or breast-feeding?*
- *Have you recently traveled out of the country? If so, where and when?*

Helminthic (worm) infections can be serious, but their impact is not generally widespread in the United States. The use of immunosuppressive drugs and the spread of acquired immunodeficiency syndrome (AIDS), however, are resulting in infections by previously unfamiliar parasites in various settings. Increases in international travel and immigration have also escalated the spread of helminthic infections.

Patient Assessment

The use of nonprescription medications in the treatment of helminthic infections is limited, given that only one nonprescription anthelmintic—pyrantel pamoate—is on the market and that this product is indicated only for pinworms. Nonetheless, pharmacists should be aware of the signs, symptoms, and preferred treatment of common helminthic infections in order to counsel patients and refer them to a physician if necessary. See Table 1.

The first indication of a helminthic infection may be a worm passed with a stool. Patients should be advised to place a suspected worm in a container with tap water and take it to a health care provider or laboratory for identification.

Symptoms of intestinal parasitic infection during pregnancy require special attention. Parasitic infections during pregnancy may injure the mother's health, injure the fetus, induce premature labor and/or delivery, and infect the neonate. Care requires risk-and-benefit considerations for the mother and fetus.

Table 1 lists selected human helminthic infections and agents, their sources, and common signs and symptoms. In all cases, the health care provider must be both factual and sensitive, since most people find the thought of a worm infection very disturbing.

Editor's Note: This chapter is adapted from Kathryn K. Bucci, "Anthelmintic Products," in Covington, T.R., ed., *Handbook of Nonprescription Drugs,* 11th edition, which is based, in part, on the chapter with the same title that appeared in the 9th edition but was written by John M. Kinsella. For a more extensive discussion of helminthic infections and their treatment, readers are encouraged to consult Chapter 15 of the *Handbook.*

TABLE 1 Common human helminthic infections in the United States

Class/Genus and species	Common name	Source of infection	Signs and symptoms
Nematoda			
Ancylostoma duodenale, Necator americanus	Hookworm	Contact with contaminated soil; larvae are ingested or penetrate the skin on contact	Anemia caused by blood loss (0.15 mL per worm per day); indigestion, anorexia, headache, cough, vomiting, diarrhea, weakness, urticaria at the site of entry into the skin
Ascaris lumbricoides, Ascaris suum	Roundworm	Ingestion of eggs through contact with fecally contaminated soil	Mild cases may be asymptomatic; GI discomfort, pain, diarrhea; intestinal obstruction in severe cases; occasionally, bile or pancreatic duct may be obstructed; allergic reactions
Enterobius vermicularis	Pinworm, seatworm, threadworm, oxyurid	Ingestion of eggs by fecal contamination of hands, food, clothing, and bedding; reinfection is common; the most common worm infestation in the United States, especially in schoolchildren	Indigestion; intense perianal itching, especially at night, resulting in loss of sleep, irritability and fatigue in children; scratching may cause infection
Trichuris trichiura	Whipworm	Ingestion of eggs through contact with fecally contaminated soil	Mild cases may be asymptomatic; insomnia, loss of appetite, diarrhea, anemia; in severe cases, colitis, proctitis, prolapsed rectum
Anisakis, Pseudoterranova	None	Eating raw or poorly cooked fish	Tingling throat, abdominal pain, fever, nausea, vomiting, diarrhea
Cestoidea			
Taenia saginata	Beef tapeworm	Eating poorly cooked infected beef	No characteristic symptoms; digestive upset, diarrhea, anemia, dizziness vary with the degree of infestation
Taenia solium	Pork tapeworm	Eating poorly cooked infected pork	Similar to beef tapeworm infestation; self-infection with eggs may lead to cysts in eye, brain, heart, other organs
Diphyllobothrium latum	Fish tapeworm	Eating raw or inadequately cooked fish	Similar to beef tapeworm infestation
Hymenolepis nana	Dwarf tapeworm	Eating food contaminated with human feces	Similar to beef tapeworm infestation

Enterobiasis

Enterobiasis, or oxyuriasis, is commonly called pinworm, seatworm, or threadworm infection. It occurs in urban communities as well as in rural and poverty-stricken areas and infects individuals from all socioeconomic strata. Pinworm infection is the most common helminthic infection in the United States.

The most common ways of transmitting pinworm infection in children are direct anus-to-mouth transfer of eggs by contaminated fingers and ingestion of food that has been handled by soiled hands. Eggs may also be spread by house dust, on the coats of pets, or by contaminated objects such as bedding, cups, toothpaste, and doorknobs.

Signs and Symptoms

Signs and symptoms are summarized in Table 1. Perianal itching is a symptom of many conditions and is often mistakenly attributed to pinworm infection; thus, careful investigation of other possible causes is essential. Patients need to be assured that pinworms are common and that no social stigma is attached to this infection. Patients with minor infections may be asymptomatic.

Treatment

The presence of pinworms can be determined by either of two methods. One method is to cover the end of a cotton swab or tongue depressor with tape (sticky side out) and apply this end to the perianal area. The presence or absence of eggs is confirmed by examining the tape under the microscope. Collection of eggs can be done at home, but inspection and evaluation must be done in a laboratory or health care provider's office. Another method used frequently by parents is visual inspection of the anal area with a flashlight an hour or so after the child has gone to bed. Female pinworms can be seen emerging from the anus.

Pyrantel pamoate for the treatment of pinworms has been approved by the Food and Drug Administration (FDA) for nonprescription use. Side effects are uncommon. Helminthic infections other than those caused by pinworms should be diagnosed and treated by a physician.

Guidelines for the use of pyrantel pamoate are as follows:

- If a patient experiences persistent abdominal cramps, nausea, vomiting, anorexia, diarrhea, headache, drowsiness, or dizziness after taking this medication, a physician should be consulted.
- Patients who are pregnant or nursing or who have liver disease should not take this product unless directed by a physician.
- For adults and children, a single dose of 11 mg/kg is recommended, not to exceed 1 g.
- The drug may be taken at any time of the day, with or without meals.
- When one individual in a household has pinworms, the entire household should be treated at the same time. However, infants under 2 years of age or children who weigh less than 25 lb should not be treated before consulting a physician.
- The liquid formulation should be shaken well before the dose is measured. The measuring device provided with the package should be used.
- A repeat course of therapy may be undertaken under the direction of a physician.
- If any worms other than pinworms are present before or after treatment, a physician should be consulted.

The following nondrug measures are recommended to prevent reinfections:

- The bed linens, bedclothes, towels, and underwear of the infected individual and the entire family should be washed. Such items should not be shaken because this can spread eggs into the air. A daily morning shower is encouraged to remove eggs deposited in the perianal region during the night.
- Disinfectants should be used daily on toilet seats and bathtubs.
- The bedroom should be vacuumed frequently.
- Close-fitting shorts should be worn under one-piece pajamas at night to prevent migration of worms and harm from scratching.
- Hands should be washed frequently, especially before meals and after using the toilet. After an infected child goes to the bathroom, the child's fingers should be scrubbed with soap and a brush. The child's nails should be trimmed regularly to prevent hand-to-mouth reinfection.

Ascariasis

Ascariasis is caused by *Ascaris lumbricoides,* also referred to as giant roundworm. This species is most prevalent in warm, moist areas such as some parts of the southeast United States.

Swine ascaris, *Ascaris suum,* which usually occurs in northern states such as New Hampshire, Washington, and Montana, is also infective to humans. Because of the possible presence of *A suum,* the use of pig manure in home gardens should be discouraged. Pharmacists should consider that this type of infection is present if a patient mentions that a large worm has been passed.

Signs and Symptoms

Children characteristically have fever and may lose weight or fail to grow. See Table 1 for additional information.

Treatment

Nutritional supplementation is the first step in treatment. The drug of choice for treating ascarid infections is mebendazole (100 mg taken twice a day for 3 days) or pyrantel pamoate (11 mg/kg in a single dose, not to exceed 1 g). Treatment of swine ascariasis is unnecessary if the worm has already been passed.

Hookworm Infection

In the United States, hookworm infection in humans is caused by *Necator americanus.* When prospective hosts walk barefoot over contaminated soil, the infective larvae rapidly penetrate the intact skin and enter the bloodstream, eventually reaching the small intestine.

Signs and Symptoms

Once the hookworm larvae penetrate exposed skin, an erythematous maculopapular rash and edema with severe itching may persist for several days. The lesions most commonly occur on the feet. If the infection is severe, larvae may migrate to the lungs and produce dyspnea, cough, fever, or congestive heart failure. A major clinical manifestation of hookworm infection is iron-deficiency anemia, which results from the loss of blood that the adult worm extracts while attached to the intestinal mucosa. Other signs and symptoms are summarized in Table 1.

Treatment

Mebendazole (100 mg taken twice a day for 3 days) or pyrantel pamoate (11 mg/kg, not to exceed 1 g, for 3 days) may be used to treat hookworm infections. Anemia may be treated with oral iron supplements.

Whipworm

Whipworms (*Trichuris trichiura*) are acquired through ingestion of feces-contaminated food or water.

Signs and Symptoms

See Table 1. Trauma to the intestinal epithelium and submucosa caused by these worms can cause chronic blood in the stool, resulting in anemia.

Treatment

Mebendazole (100 mg taken twice daily for 3 days) is the preferred treatment for adults and children. No nonprescription drugs are available for treating this infection.

Anisakiasis

This parasite is acquired by ingesting raw, lightly salted or pickled, or inadequately cooked saltwater fish containing infected larvae. Because of the recent popularity of raw fish dishes such as sushi, these previously rare infections have become a growing problem in the United States.

Signs and Symptoms

Larvae of some anisakid species wander into the oropharynx or esophagus, causing a tingling sensation. These larvae, which are up to 3 mm long, are often coughed up within 48 hours of ingestion, causing the patient considerable anxiety. Other species penetrate the wall of the stomach or intestine, producing symptoms that mimic acute appendicitis, ulcer, or cancer. Because no eggs are produced, stool examination is of no use. Diagnosis may require endoscopy or laparotomy.

Treatment

Anthelmintics are apparently ineffective in killing anisakid larvae. The only definitive treatment in severe cases is surgical resection of the inflamed intestine. Patients should be warned of the dangers of eating raw or poorly cooked fish, especially fish from areas where marine mammals are prevalent. Freezing fish at 1.4°F (-17°C) for 24 hours will kill any larvae present.

Cercarial Dermatitis

Cercarial dermatitis, or swimmers' itch, is caused by flukes of the genera *Trichobilharzia* and *Ornithobilharzia,* which are normally blood parasites of ducks and muskrats. Cercariae are capable of penetrating human skin, where they are rapidly killed by an immune reaction.

Signs and Symptoms

Inflammation resulting from the cercariae produces a local erythema, a minute macule at the site of penetration, and intense itching. Because hundreds of cercariae may penetrate, the result is a generalized fiery rash. Cases usually occur in spring and summer in freshwater and saltwater areas where migratory waterfowl and large snail populations are present. Swimmers' itch generally subsides in 24–48 hours.

Treatment

Treatment is symptomatic. Antihistamines and topical corticosteroids reduce the local immune response, and warm baths may relieve the itching.

CHAPTER 16

Emetic and Antiemetic Products

Questions to ask in patient assessment and counseling

Emetics

- Do you want the emetic for immediate or possible future emergency use?
- If for immediate use, have you spoken to a poison control center?
- For whom is the medication? Is the patient a child?
- What substance was taken? How much? When did the ingestion occur?
- Has the patient already been given something for the ingestion?
- What symptoms is the patient showing? Is the patient conscious and alert?
- Does the patient have any chronic or acute illnesses?
- Is the patient taking any nonprescription or prescription medications?

Antiemetics

- Do you know what caused the nausea and vomiting?
- For whom is the medication? How old is the patient?
- Is the patient pregnant?
- Is the patient diabetic?
- How long has the nausea or vomiting been present?
- Have you noted blood in the vomitus? Is the blood red or does it resemble coffee grounds?
- Have you noted other signs or symptoms such as abdominal pain, headache, or diarrhea?
- Is the patient currently taking any medications?
- Is the patient receiving or has the patient recently received radiation therapy or cancer chemotherapy?
- Does the patient have other medical problems?

Vomiting (emesis) is an important defense mechanism by which the body attempts to rid itself of toxins and poisons. It can also be caused by motion sickness, pregnancy, or a variety of serious conditions. Most oral medications and some parenteral and topical drugs can cause nausea and vomiting; consequently, knowledge of the patient's drug history is important. Nausea and vomiting may also be associated with radiation therapy; cancer chemotherapy; and serious metabolic, central nervous system (CNS), gastrointestinal (GI), and endocrine disorders. These conditions are not covered in this chapter because they are not appropriate for self-medication.

Editor's Note: This chapter is adapted from Gary M. Oderda and Jenifer C. Jennings, "Emetic and Antiemetic Products," in Covington, T.R., ed., *Handbook of Nonprescription Drugs*, 11th edition. For a more extensive discussion of this topic, readers are encouraged to consult Chapter 16 of the *Handbook*.

Frequent vomiting, particularly in young women, may indicate an eating disorder that may be associated with ipecac abuse. Such patients should be evaluated by a health care provider. Vomiting may produce complications that include dehydration, aspiration, malnutrition, electrolyte and acid-base abnormalities, and Mallory-Weiss syndrome tears of the esophagus resulting in blood in the vomitus.

Nonprescription emetic medications are used to induce vomiting, primarily in the treatment of a poisoning. Nonprescription antiemetics are used to prevent or control the symptoms of nausea and vomiting that are primarily due to motion sickness, pregnancy, and mild infectious diseases. Some nonprescription antiemetics are promoted for the relief of such vague symptoms as "upset stomach," indigestion, and distention associated with food overindulgence. Their value in treating these complaints is not well documented. The practitioner should be aware that patients may use nonprescription antiemetics to self-treat the early stages of a serious illness.

Emetics

Emetics induce vomiting and are used to remove potentially toxic agents from the stomach. Emetics are used most commonly to treat poisoning.

Baseline Information for Poison Management

All ingestions in which moderate to severe toxicity is possible must be referred to an emergency treatment facility. Knowing the telephone number of the nearest poison control center is essential. A list of the names, addresses, and phone numbers of major poison control centers nationwide appears on pages 294–299 of the *Handbook*.

To assess whether a nonprescription emetic should be administered in the home or referral to a health care facility is warranted, the pharmacist should obtain the following information:

Patient's Name and Location

If talking with the patient or caretaker by phone, the practitioner should first ask for the caregiver's and the patient's name, location, and telephone number.

Name of Product Ingested

The product label or container, if available, may list ingredients as well as the name of the manufacturer or distributor. The potential toxicity of each ingredient must be considered.

Amount Ingested

The amount ingested is often difficult to determine. Patients often underestimate the amount consumed or provide unreliable information.

Time since Ingestion

An emetic is useful only if a substantial amount of the ingested substance remains in the stomach. An emetic is not recommended if several hours have elapsed after ingestion of quickly absorbed agents such as alcohols, yet it may be appropriate several hours after ingestion of agents that are slow to leave the stomach, such as salicylates. Drugs that slow gastric emptying and GI motility include opiates and drugs that have anticholinergic activity (e.g., atropine, scopolamine, antidepressants, phenothiazines).

Signs and Symptoms

If CNS depression, lethargy, somnolence, ataxia, hallucinations, or seizures are present, an emetic should not be used. These patients must be referred for immediate medical evaluation and treatment.

Other Illnesses or Medication Use

The pharmacist must consider the impact of preexisting illnesses or medication use when recommending therapy. Patients with a seizure disorder, particularly one that is not well controlled, are not good candidates for home emetic use. Patients who chronically take theophylline would be at higher risk from an additional theophylline ingestion than those who do not; for this reason, they should be referred to an emergency department.

Patient's Age and Weight

Information on the toxicity of an agent is generally provided on a dose-per-body weight (mg/kg) basis. Thus, one must often need to know the patient's weight to determine appropriate treatment. The patient's age may also help determine the appropriateness and dose of an emetic.

Prior Treatment

The practitioner must determine if any first aid or other procedure has been performed. Some procedures (e.g., using saltwater as an emetic, sticking the finger down the patient's throat to stimulate gagging) are potentially harmful. Such effects would influence further treatment recommendations.

Treatment of Poisoning

Treatment of poisoning entails prevention of absorption and provision of supportive care. Support of vital functions, especially respiratory and cardiovascular, is critical. Stomach contents may be removed by mechanical lavage or administration of an emetic such as ipecac syrup.

Gastric Lavage

Gastric lavage is a procedure in which a tube is placed into the stomach through the mouth or nose. Fluid is instilled into the tube, allowed to mix with stomach contents, and removed by suction.

Ipecac Syrup

Ipecac syrup is the emetic of choice. When a patient asks to purchase ipecac syrup, the pharmacist should determine whether it is to be used immediately or kept in the home as a first-aid measure. If the purchase is for immediate use, the pharmacist should determine whether that use is appropriate and proceed with the line of questioning described at the beginning of this chapter.

If ipecac is purchased for a possible future ingestion, the pharmacist should discuss poison prevention, distribute poison prevention materials, and provide the telephone number of the nearest poison control center. The purchaser should be advised that, whenever possible, ipecac syrup should not be given without first consulting a poison control center, pharmacist, or health care provider.

Dosages. For children 1 year of age and older, the recommended dose of ipecac syrup is 15 mL (1 tbsp). This dose can be repeated once if vomiting has not occurred within 20 minutes. Children from 6 months to 1 year of age may be given 5–10 mL (1–2 tsp). Although home use of ipecac in children under 1 year of age is controversial, the product has been shown to be safe and effective. For adolescents and adults, the initial dose is 15–30 mL and it can be repeated once, if necessary.

Fluid Administration. Fluid administration is generally recommended immediately after the ipecac dose. Children should be given 4–8 oz of clear fluid (e.g., water, juice, soda); adults should receive 12–16 oz. Patients who are ambulatory seem to vomit more quickly than those who are not; therefore, children should be encouraged to play quietly, and adults should be encouraged to move around.

If the patient is to be brought to an emergency facility or health care provider's office, the patient should vomit into a bucket or other container and that container should be brought to the treatment facility so the vomitus can be inspected for evidence of the poison.

Ipecac Toxicity. Toxicity following ipecac syrup administration is rare. After therapeutic doses, diarrhea and slight CNS depression are common; mild GI upset may last for several hours following emesis. Ipecac is cardiotoxic in large doses. Fluid extract of ipecac is 14 times stronger than ipecac syrup and should no longer be found in any pharmacy.

Pharmacists must be aware that ipecac syrup is used to induce vomiting by some bulimic patients. This practice is particularly dangerous because it brings about a drug-induced fluid and electrolyte imbalance and cardiotoxicity. Pharmacists should question any person buying ipecac syrup regularly to be certain it is being purchased for its appropriate use.

Expiration Date. If an expired container of ipecac syrup is the only ipecac available in an emergency, it may be used.

Activated Charcoal

Activated charcoal is an effective adsorbent for many drugs and chemicals (Table 1). It is usually administered as a slurry of 60–100 g of activated charcoal for adults or 15–30 g of activated charcoal for children in a minimum of 8 oz of water.

When multiple doses of activated charcoal are given, a cathartic should be given only with the first dose. If the activated charcoal does not contain sorbitol, a single dose of a saline cathartic such as magnesium sulfate or magnesium citrate may be administered after charcoal administration if bowel sounds are present. This speeds elimination of the charcoal drug complex.

Activated charcoal should be given as soon as possible after ingestion. However, it has been shown to be effective even when administration has been delayed by several hours. There is no systemic toxicity or maximum dose limit. Repeat doses of activated charcoal are recommended to interrupt enterohepatic recycling by binding agents (e.g., phenobarbital, theophylline). In the home, activated charcoal is not a viable substitute for ipecac syrup in pediatric patients because it is difficult for parents to administer a therapeutic dose to children successfully. Contrary to popular belief, burnt toast is not a substitute for activated charcoal and is not indicated in the treatment of poisoning.

Other Methods to Induce Emesis

Ipecac syrup is the only safe and effective emetic. Emetics other than ipecac (e.g., salt water, dishwashing detergent, mustard water) produce erratic and unpredictable results, are often ineffective, and are sometimes dangerous. Lack of efficacy and potential injury to the patient also make mechanically induced vomiting a poor choice.

TABLE 1 Compounds known to be effectively bound by activated charcoal in humans and animals

Oral-activated charcoal inhibits absorption of the following chemicals from the gastrointestinal tract[a]

Acetaminophen	Ethylene glycol	Phenylbutazone
Aconitine	Glutethimide	Phenylpropanolamine
d-Amphetamine	Hexachlorophene	Phenytoin
Aspirin	Kerosene	Propantheline
Atropine	Malathion	Propoxyphene
Barbital	Mefenamic acid	Quinine
Benzene	Mercuric chloride	Salicylamide
Carbamazepine	Methyl salicylate	Secobarbital
Chlordane	Nadolol	Sodium salicylate
Chloroquine	Nicotine	Sodium valproate
Chlorpheniramine	Nortriptyline	Strychnine
Chlorpromazine	Paraquat	Theophylline
Chlorpropamide	Pentobarbital	Tetracycline
Digoxin	Phencyclidine	Tolbutamide
Doxepin	Phenobarbital	Yohimbine
Ethchlorvynol		

Multiple oral doses of activated charcoal accelerate body clearance of the following drugs[b]

Carbamazepine	Nadolol	Phenylbutazone
Dapsone	Phenobarbital	Theophylline
Digitoxin		

[a]Based on controlled experimental investigations in man or experimental animals.
[b]Not necessarily clinically significant.

Adapted with permission from Ellenhorn M, Barceloux D, eds. *Medical Toxicology: Diagnosis and Treatment of Human Poisoning.* 1st ed. New York: Elsevier Science Publishing; 1988: 59.

Contraindications to Emesis

CNS Depression or Seizures

Efforts to induce vomiting should not be attempted in patients who are lethargic, comatose, or experiencing a seizure because they are at high risk of aspirating gastric contents while vomiting. Emetics are not recommended when patients have taken agents that may produce a rapid decrease in the level of consciousness (e.g., antidepressants) or may rapidly produce seizures (e.g., camphor, amphetamines).

Caustic Ingestions

Patients who have ingested a caustic substance should *not* be made to vomit. Caustic agents are strong acids or bases that can severely burn the mucous membranes of the GI tract.

When ingestion of a caustic agent is suspected, the patient, if conscious and able to drink, should immediately be given water or milk to dilute the agent. Most patients who have ingested a caustic agent should be immediately referred to a medical facility.

Controversial Use of Emetics

Antiemetic Drug Ingestion

Use of emetics in cases of acute overdose of antiemetic medications is controversial. If an emetic is given and vomiting does not occur, gastric lavage may be necessary.

Hydrocarbon Ingestion

Patients who have ingested aliphatic hydrocarbons (e.g., kerosene, gasoline, furniture polish) traditionally have not been given emetics because induced vomiting was thought to increase the likelihood of pulmonary aspiration. Studies have since shown that aspiration is not likely to occur when vomiting is induced; however, emptying the stomach of aliphatic hydrocarbons is generally not necessary. However, when a potentially dangerous chemical such as a pesticide is dissolved in a hydrocarbon base, ipecac syrup is generally considered appropriate. In such cases, it should be administered in a hospital.

Antiemetics

Most minor nausea and vomiting are self-limiting symptoms that require minimal therapy. The pharmacist should be cautious about recommending self-medication for these symptoms and should ask appropriate questions to determine whether referral is indicated.

Patient Assessment

In assessing the patient's complaint, the pharmacist should determine:
- The age of the patient;
- The onset and duration of signs and symptoms;
- The nature of precipitating factors;
- A complete history of recent medication use and of food and liquid ingestion;
- Signs and symptoms other than nausea and vomiting (e.g., fever); and
- Chronic or acute medical conditions.

Signs and symptoms or medical conditions associated with nausea and vomiting that necessitate referral include:
- Blood in the vomitus;
- Abdominal pain or distention;
- Prolonged nausea and vomiting (>24–48 hours), especially for children under 1 year of age, or projectile vomiting;
- Dehydration;
- Loss of more than 5% of body weight;
- Fever;
- Severe headache;
- Change in behavior or alertness;
- Pregnancy;

- Diabetes or other medical conditions that may be affected by lack of nutritional intake or missed doses of oral medications;
- Recent trauma, particularly a significant head injury; or
- Suspected poisoning.

Any patient who experiences severe nausea, vomiting and abdominal pain, or forceful, protracted vomiting should receive immediate medical attention.

Children

Regurgitation or spitting up, whereby milk appears to spill gently from the mouth, is common in infants. It generally should not cause concern and does not require medical attention. Vomiting in newborns can result from a number of serious abnormalities. Dehydration and electrolyte disturbances occur more often in children and are potentially life-threatening. Referral to a health care provider is recommended for evaluation of any vomiting in newborns.

One of the more common causes of vomiting in children is acute viral gastroenteritis. Treatment is directed primarily at preventing and correcting dehydration and electrolyte disturbances. Lost fluids should generally be replaced within 24 hours. If severe diarrhea or vomiting persists for more than 24–48 hours, the child should be referred to a health care provider. In addition, the child's health care provider should be contacted if:

- The child is less than 1 year of age;
- The child refuses to drink;
- The child has not urinated in the past 8–12 hours;
- The child appears lethargic or is crying;
- Weight loss or dehydration occurs (signs of dehydration include dry oral mucous membranes, sunken eyes, decreased urine output, absence of tears when crying, decreased skin turgor, listlessness, sleepiness, and fatigue);
- Vomiting occurs with each feeding;
- Vomiting is repeatedly projectile;
- Vomitus contains red, black, or green fluid;
- Vomiting is associated with diarrhea, distended abdomen, fever, or severe headache;
- Vomiting occurs following a head injury; or
- Poisoning is suspected.

If a child is vomiting and referral is not deemed necessary, the following steps can be taken to prevent dehydration:

- Stop all feeding for 1 hour.
- Start clear liquids (i.e., oral rehydration solutions). After 12 hours of well-tolerated clear liquids, start half-strength formula and light solids.
- If half-strength formula or light solids are well tolerated, resume the child's regular diet.
- If the child vomits after any of these steps, start again with clear liquids.

Pregnancy

Nausea, with or without vomiting, may be one of the earliest symptoms of pregnancy. A woman who experiences nausea and vomiting, and who has no other symptoms except a missed menstrual period and perhaps weight gain, should be referred for a pregnancy test.

Women who report nausea and vomiting during pregnancy generally suffer from these symptoms in the early part of the day ("morning sickness"). Some women experience these symptoms in the afternoon or evening, and a small number experience them throughout the day.

These symptoms should be taken seriously and the patient reassured. Because teratogenicity is a major consideration during pregnancy, most health care providers are reluctant to prescribe any medication for a pregnant woman unless it is absolutely necessary. Indications for nonprescription antiemetics approved by the Food and Drug Administration (FDA) do not include the treatment of nausea and vomiting associated with pregnancy. A number of nonpharmacologic approaches can be recommended instead; these include eating small, frequent meals; lowering the fat content of meals; ingesting crackers before arising in the morning; lying down; and avoiding precipitating factors.

Motion Sickness

Motion sickness occurs when visual and vestibular stimuli are not in accord. Symptoms include pallor, yawning, restlessness, nausea, and then vomiting. Susceptibility appears to vary with age. In young children, motion sickness associated with car travel may be minimized by placing the child in a car seat. Antihistamines are the primary nonprescription agents used to prevent or control motion sickness.

Overeating

For nausea associated with excessive or disagreeable food or beverage intake, avoidance or moderation of consumption may prove beneficial. Otherwise, antacids, bismuth-containing products, and H_2-antagonists are indicated for the relief of heartburn, indigestion, and upset stomach associated with dietary overindulgence.

Food Poisoning

Signs and symptoms associated with food poisoning include vomiting in addition to diarrhea, abdominal cramps, and possible fever. Symptomatic treatment is often recommended. This consists of fluid and electrolyte replacement, dietary modification, and antidiarrheal products when appropriate. A diet of clear liquids and simple carbohydrates is recommended for the first 24 hours. If symptoms continue beyond 24 hours, referral to a health care provider is recommended.

Current Medication Use

Many medications (e.g., cancer chemotherapeutic agents, narcotics, antibiotics, estrogens) cause nausea and vomiting as an adverse effect. Other medications, such as digitalis or theophylline, may produce nausea and vomiting as a sign of toxicity. In all such situations, nonprescription antiemetics are not indicated. The patient should be referred to a health care provider.

Other Medical Problems

Bulimia (binge-purge behavior) is a psychologic disorder in which patients attempt to control their weight by repeated vomiting and the chronic use of emetics (most commonly ipecac syrup). These patients should be referred for medical and psychologic management of the underlying problems.

Ingredients in Nonprescription Products

Antacids

Antacids are indicated for the symptomatic relief of upset stomach associated with gastric acidity (e.g., heartburn, dyspepsia, acid indigestion). Because antacids may impair the absorption of many medications, such drugs should not be taken within 1–2 hours of the antacid dose.

H_2-Receptor Antagonists

H_2-receptor antagonists provide symptomatic relief of heartburn, dyspepsia, and indigestion. They are available in lower doses for nonprescription use.

Antihistamines

Antihistamines are the primary nonprescription agents used as antiemetics. Meclizine (Bonine), cyclizine (Marezine), dimenhydrinate (Dramamine), and diphenhydramine (Benadryl) are classified as safe and effective for the prevention and treatment of nausea, vomiting, or dizziness associated with motion sickness. They should be taken at least 30–60 minutes before departure and continued during travel. Meclizine is not recommended for children under 12 years of age, and cyclizine is not recommended for children under 6 years of age.

Drowsiness is the most common side effect of antihistamines. Patients should be warned against engaging in tasks requiring a high degree of mental alertness and physical dexterity. Antihistamines should be used with caution in patients with asthma, narrow-angle glaucoma, obstructive disease of the GI or genitourinary tract, or benign prostatic hypertrophy. Effects of these products are additive with those of other CNS depressants.

Antihistamines appear to have a low risk of teratogenicity; nonetheless, they should be reserved for pregnant women who have severe nausea and vomiting that are unresponsive to nonpharmacologic measures. Patients should be advised to consult their physicians. Many health care providers recommend doxylamine, which is not considered teratogenic, for pregnant women with nausea and vomiting that does not respond to nonpharmacologic measures.

Pyridoxine

Pyridoxine (vitamin B_6) may be effective in treating nausea and vomiting associated with pregnancy. It is not considered teratogenic.

Phosphorated Carbohydrate Solution

Phosphorated carbohydrate solution (Emetrol, Calm-X, Nausetrol) is a mixture of levulose (fructose), dextrose (glucose), and phosphoric acid. It is indicated for nausea and vomiting associated with upset stomach caused by intestinal flu, food indiscretions, and emotional upset. The adult dosage is 15–30 mL at 15-minute intervals until vomiting ceases, to a maximum of five doses in 1 hour. The solution should not be diluted, and the patient should not consume other liquids for 15 minutes after taking a dose. If vomiting does not cease after five doses, a health care provider should be contacted. The high glucose content of these products may cause problems in persons with diabetes.

Bismuth Salts

Bismuth salts are available as a nonprescription suspension and chewable tablet for relief of nausea associated with dyspepsia, heartburn, and gas caused by overindulgence in food or drink. See Chapter 13 of the *Handbook* for a discussion of considerations relating to the use of bismuth salts.

Oral Rehydration Solutions

Signs and symptoms of dehydration include dry mouth, excessive thirst, little or no urination, dizziness, and lightheadedness. Adults should be evaluated for dehydration if they have severe vomiting or diarrhea that persists for more than 48 hours; children should be evaluated if severe diarrhea or vomiting persists for 24 hours.

Oral electrolyte mixtures for rehydration include Pedialyte, Ricelyte, Infalyte, Rehydralyte, Resol, and Naturalyte. Gelatin water, sports drinks, fruit juices, and carbonated beverages may be administered; however, they contain insufficient sodium, potassium, and chloride to produce a rapid therapeutic response to severe dehydration with electrolyte depletion.

In a child with vomiting, the fluid should be given very slowly, starting with 5–10 mL every 10 minutes. The volume may be increased as tolerated.

Acupressure Wristbands

Acupressure wristbands are a nonpharmacologic alternative to the management of nausea and vomiting. They are marketed for the prevention of motion sickness. They have demonstrated a positive response in the suppression of pregnancy-related nausea and vomiting.

Chapter 17

Ostomy Care Products

Questions to ask in patient assessment and counseling

- How long have you had the ostomy?
- Why did you need an ostomy?
- What type of ostomy do you have? Where is it located?
- What is the stoma size?
- Do you irrigate and/or use a pouch?
- What type of appliance are you using?
- Do you have problems with the skin surrounding the stoma?
- Have you noticed any change in the contents of your fecal discharge or urinary output?
- Are you experiencing any problems related to your ostomy, such as diarrhea or odor or gas control?
- Are you taking any prescription or nonprescription medications or vitamins?

An ostomy is the surgical formation of an opening through the abdominal wall for the purpose of eliminating waste. It is usually made by passing the colon, small intestine, or ureters through the abdominal wall. The opening of the ostomy is called the stoma. Ostomies may be permanent or temporary and are performed in individuals of all ages. Reasons for performing ostomies include congenital anomalies, acquired conditions (e.g., inflammatory bowel disease, cancer, radiation damage), and trauma. The particular problems associated with each type of ostomy are directly related to the phase of digestion that is interrupted.

Ostomy surgery necessitates the use of an appliance designed to collect the waste material normally eliminated through the bowel or bladder. The ostomy patient should know how to apply and fit an appliance that affords maximum benefit. Appliance needs may change over time.

Types of Ostomies

The most common types of ostomies are ileostomy, in which the entire colon and possibly part of the ileum are removed; colostomy (ascending, transverse, descending, and sigmoid), in which the colon is partially removed; and urostomy, or urinary diversion, in which the bladder may be removed.

Editor's Note: This chapter is adapted from Michael L. Kleinberg, "Ostomy Care Products," in Covington, T.R., ed., *Handbook of Nonprescription Drugs,* 11th edition, which is based, in part, on the chapter with a similar title that appeared in the 10th edition but was written by Michael L. Kleinberg and Moya J. Vazquez. For a more extensive discussion of ostomies, ostomy appliances and accessories, and other issues related to ostomy care, readers are encouraged to consult Chapter 17 of the *Handbook.*

Ileostomy

An ileostomy is a surgically created opening between the ileum and the abdominal wall. Reasons to have ileostomy surgery include ulcerative colitis, Crohn's disease, trauma, familial polyposis, and necrotizing enterocolitis.

An ileostomy usually begins functioning within 36–72 hours after surgery. The discharge is liquid to semisoft because it contains fluid that normally would be absorbed from the large bowel.

When the colon is removed, as it is in an ileostomy, the body loses the capacity to reabsorb water. Ileostomates (persons with ileostomies) must maintain adequate fluid intake to compensate for this water loss, especially during the initial postoperative period.

Excoriation of the skin is a common problem for ileostomates. Diligent hygiene and special protective measures can help prevent these problems. Because patients with standard ileostomies are never continent, an appliance must be worn at all times.

Colostomy

A colostomy entails the creation of an artificial opening using part of the large intestine or colon. Major indications for a colostomy include obstruction of the colon or rectum, cancer of the colon or rectum, genetic malformation, diverticular disease, trauma, radiation colitis, and loss of anal muscular control. The three types of colostomies are named for the portion of the bowel that is brought to the outside of the body to form the stoma, as described below.

Ascending Colostomy

In an ascending colostomy, the ascending colon is retained but the rest of the large bowel is removed or bypassed. This ostomy usually appears on the right side of the abdomen. Its discharge is semiliquid because the fluid has not been reabsorbed. The patient must wear an appliance continuously.

Transverse Colostomy

In a transverse colostomy, an opening is usually created on the right side of the transverse colon. There are two principal types of transverse colostomy: loop and double-barrel, in which two openings are created. Discharge is semisoft. An appliance must be worn continuously.

Descending and Sigmoid Colostomies

Descending and sigmoid colostomies usually are on the left side of the abdomen. They can be made as double- or single-barrel openings. Because these patients produce a fecal discharge that is usually firm, they may be managed with irrigation and not require a pouch. Ostomates using this method instill an irrigating solution into the ostomy site with an irrigation set. Many patients, however, prefer appliances to irrigation. Loss of bowel tonicity is a long-term complication of routine bowel irrigation in some patients. If this occurs, the bowel is unable to function without irrigation.

Factors to be considered in the decision to irrigate include:

■ The patient's ability to handle the irrigation procedure;

■ The patient's prognosis;

■ The presence of stomal stenosis or peristomal hernia; and

■ The presence of radiation enteritis.

Urinary Diversions

Urinary diversions (urostomies) are performed as a result of bladder loss or dysfunction usually caused by cancer, neurogenic bladder, or genetic malformation. In the most common procedure, an ileal or colon conduit is created by implanting the ureters into an isolated loop of bowel, the distal end of which is brought to the surface of the abdomen. An appliance must be worn continuously.

Continent Diversions

The objective of a continent diversion is to construct a reservoir inside the body, usually from a section of intestinal, urinary, or gastric mucosa, to accommodate fecal or urinary discharge. There are three main types of continent diversions:

Continent Ileostomy

Continent ileostomy entails creation of an internal pouch, made from 35–50 cm of ileum, and a "nipple" that renders the patient continent for stool and flatus. The pouch is emptied three to four times a day by inserting a catheter through the nipple into the pouch.

Restorative Proctocolectomy

Restorative proctocolectomy involves sparing the rectum. An internal pouch is created from the small bowel, but without a nipple valve. The distal end of the ileum is pulled through the rectum and attached. The sphincter is preserved, and no ostomy is necessary. Because of the different ways the internal pouch can be constructed, one may hear this operation described as an "S" or "J" pouch. Recipients of this procedure have frequent bowel movements and may experience perianal skin irritation.

Continent Urostomy

Continent urostomy is much like the continent ileostomy. One difference is that an additional nipple valve is created at the proximal opening of the pouch to keep the urine from refluxing into the kidneys. Other continent urinary operations, such as the Indiana pouch, have been devised; in each case, however, the pouch is drained by a catheter.

The Stoma

The normal stoma is shiny, wet, and dark pink or red. The stoma does not contain nerve fibers, so it does not transmit pain or other sensations. It may bleed slightly if irritated or rubbed, such as during cleaning; however, the bleeding should not be prolonged, nor should the discharge be bloody. In the adult, the stoma is usually ¾–2 inches in size. The stoma gradually shrinks after surgery and reaches its permanent size within several months. Measuring the stoma to ensure proper fit of the appliance is an important aspect of patient care.

Appliances and Accessories

The type of appliance depends on the type of surgery performed. Patients with regulated colostomies (those who irrigate routinely with no output from the stoma between irrigations) may wear closed-end appliances, a stoma cover or cap, or a gauze square. Those with unregulated colostomies and ileostomies usually wear open-end appliances to allow frequent emptying.

The ostomy system is composed of a pouch that is secured to the skin by an adhesive skin barrier. The ideal ostomy system should be leakproof, odorproof, comfortable, easily manipulated, inconspicuous, inexpensive, and safe. No one appliance meets all of these criteria.

Patients must be taught all the self-care skills required to maintain the stoma, including sizing the stoma, cutting a pouch or skin barrier to fit the stoma, applying paste or powder, cleaning the skin, applying the pouch, removing the pouch, and emptying the pouch. The patient must be prepared for stoma functioning at any time during the pouch-changing procedure. For several weeks after the ostomy, patients often need assistance in changing the pouch. If the stoma is poorly placed, there are complications, or the patient is debilitated, routine assistance may be required.

Pouching Equipment

Although reusable appliances have distinct advantages for certain patients, most ostomates are now fitted with odorproof, lightweight, disposable appliances. Most of these appliances incorporate a skin barrier in each flange, eliminating the need for a separate skin barrier. The disposable equipment is available in one- and two-piece systems. Reusable and disposable appliances are available in transparent and opaque styles and in various sizes.

One-piece convexity pouches are available with oval openings that fit flush with the skin, allowing the contents to flow into the pouch without leaking onto the skin. Flushable one-piece pouches are available for use by patients with colostomies. They are not practical for patients with ileostomies or urostomies.

The pouch should be emptied when it is one-third to one-half full. The flange and skin barrier may be left in place for 3–7 days, depending on the condition of the skin and skin barrier. Although activities such as swimming or playing tennis may decrease the wear time of the pouch, this should not discourage participation in sports.

Belts

Special belts attached to various appliances give additional support. Indications for use are a deeply convex faceplate, poor wearing time, activity (especially in children), heavy perspiration, and personal preference. Belts may cause ulcers if worn too tight.

Skin Barriers

Skin barriers are intended to protect the skin immediately adjacent to the stoma from the stoma discharge. They also correct imperfections in the skin surface, allowing the appliance to fit securely. Skin barriers, powders, and pastes are available for special skin problems. The powder is used on weeping skin. The paste is used to seal around the stoma and to fill in creases in the skin.

Solid wafer skin barriers are preattached to the pouch or provided separately and may be custom cut or precut. To apply a skin barrier, the patient should place a bead of skin barrier paste around the stoma or directly to the edge of the skin barrier wafer, apply the skin barrier wafer to wrinkle-free skin, and press the skin barrier around the stoma. Solid wafer skin barriers may melt if exposed to high temperatures. Therefore, during the summer, especially when traveling, the solid wafer skin barrier should be put in an insulated box (ice is not required).

Skin Protective Dressings

A waterproof dressing leaves a thin protective layer on the skin that aids in the removal of adhesive tape and absorbs the stress normally applied to the top layers of the skin when the appliance is removed. These dressings do not replace skin barriers. When the skin is reddened but unbroken, these preparations briefly protect the skin from the contact agent causing the redness. They also can help protect the skin around a draining wound. These dressings come in varying forms: gel, bottle (with brush), spray can, roll-on, and wipe-on packets.

Transparent, semipermeable dressings come in many sizes. They are transparent, sterile materials that are sticky on one side. They can be used as a dressing, as a second skin to which appliances are affixed, or as a prophylactic for preventing skin irritation. They take some dexterity to apply, however, and two persons may be needed to apply larger pieces.

Cleansing and Special Skin Care Products

The stoma and surrounding skin are best cleansed with plain water. If soap is used, it should be rinsed off thoroughly and the skin dried before a new pouching system is applied. Moisturizers and lanolin-containing products should be avoided. Several companies manufacture products especially for the incontinent patient or others at high risk of excoriation.

Tape

Hypoallergenic tape, applied to the skin and faceplate, supports appliances. Waterproof tape may be used during swimming or bathing.

Irrigating Sets

In patients who are candidates for irrigation, control can be maintained without a pouch. A good candidate for irrigation is an adult with a colostomy distal to the splenic flexure who does not have a history of irritable bowel or a disabling handicap. A colostomy irrigation set should be used. This set consists of a reservoir for the irrigating fluid, a tube, a graduated clamp, a soft catheter, and a dam or cone. Perforation of the bowel is a serious complication of irrigation, but it has almost been eliminated by use of a cone, which is inserted ½–1 inch into the colostomy. In patients who are not able to use a cone, the catheter should not be inserted more than 2 inches past the dam. Although introducing water into the bowel stimulates peristalsis, control (i.e., at least 24 hours without any output) is rarely achieved unless the colostomate instills and holds in a prescribed amount of water. Therefore, the dam takes the place of the absent sphincter, allowing the patient to hold in the water.

Frequency of irrigation depends somewhat on the colostomate's normal bowel habits. After control is achieved, the patient may wear a security pouch or a piece of gauze, stoma cover, or cap over the stoma. Irrigation is not necessary for health; it is merely one method of management.

Deodorizers

With properly fitted, disposable, odorproof pouches, deodorizers are not required as often as they are with the reusable systems. Regular changing of the appliance is generally sufficient to prevent odor. Oral deodorizers (internal or systemic) or those inserted into the pouch can be used to reduce stool odor. Liquid concentrates are available as companion products of most ostomy devices; they can be placed directly into the pouch. A common household remedy is to add a capful of mouthwash to the pouch. Ostomates sometimes place aspirin tablets in the pouch to control odor. This practice should be discouraged because aspirin may irritate the stoma. In addition to local methods, devices are available that fit directly on the pouch to filter and control gas and odors.

Potential Complications

Ostomates may experience both physical and psychological complications. The pharmacist should be prepared to handle these complications or refer patients to an enterostomal therapy (ET) nurse.

Physical Complications

Stenosis

Stenosis (narrowing) of the stoma is caused by the formation of scar tissue. The only cure is revision of the stoma.

Fistula

The formation of an opening, or fistula tract, from inside the body to the skin most often is a manifestation of inflammatory bowel disease. Other causes of fistula are cancer, abscess formation, foreign body retention, radiation, tuberculosis, and trauma. Treatment entails hyperalimentation, surgery, or both.

Prolapse

Prolapse, the telescoping of the bowel through the stoma, frequently results when the opening in the abdominal wall is too large. Women with ileostomies occasionally experience prolapse during pregnancy. The prolapse may be reduced by lying on the back and applying continuous pressure against the most distal part of the stoma. Once the prolapse is reduced, rigid ring appliances should be avoided because of the risk of strangulation. The appliance may need to be resized. In some cases, surgical correction is required.

Retraction

Retraction is the recession of the stoma to a subnormal length. If it is not severe, a convex pouching system may be all that is required. In other cases, treatment is surgical correction.

Peristomal Hernia

Peristomal hernia is the protrusion of the colon or ileum into the subcutaneous layers of the skin around the stoma. It can be managed by modification of the pouching equipment or technique, modification of clothing, dietary changes, or surgery.

Skin Irritation

Output Excoriation. Excoriation occurs when an improper pouch is worn, the lumen in the faceplate is too big, or the pouch has leaked and has not been promptly replaced. These problems can allow fecal or urinary output to come in contact with the skin. After diagnosis and treatment, a skin barrier and pouch may be applied. The pouch should be changed as infrequently as possible to lessen irritation. Treatment should be continued until the skin is clear.

Sensitivity. Patch testing of patients with a history of allergy, adhesive tape reaction, eczema, or psoriasis and those with very fair skin can help prevent skin irritation caused by sensitivity to a product. Patch testing can easily be done by the physician or ET nurse and checked by the patient at home.

Hyperplasia. Hyperplasia occurs when the faceplate opening is too large. The affected skin cells multiply and eventually cause agonizing pain. Treatment entails ensuring that the pouch opening is the correct size and that the seal is secure. A mild case of hyperplasia generally resolves in 1 week; severe cases may take from 4–6 weeks to heal. Other treatment methods are cauterization and surgical removal.

Alkaline Dermatitis. Many patients with urinary diversions have problems with alkaline urine. It is a major cause of frank blood in the pouch because it renders the stoma extremely friable.

The treatment is to acidify the urine. The patient should avoid alkaline ash foods, especially citrus fruits and juices, which, although originally acidic, are excreted in alkaline form. Ascorbic acid or cranberry juice acidifies the urine.

To minimize the risk of irritation due to alkaline urine, a cloth soaked with a solution of one-third white vinegar to two-thirds water can be applied for 5–10 minutes to the stoma at least once weekly before putting on the appliance. The frequency of application is determined by the severity of the case.

Infection. Skin infections are generally not a problem in ostomates; however, an infection under the faceplate can be a problem. If the skin is indurated, swollen, and red, it may need incision and draining. The appropriate antibiotic can be prescribed topically, systemically, or both.

Monilial infection may be a problem in patients who wear appliances continuously. The primary symptom is itching. If the condition is diagnosed early, nystatin powder or 2% miconazole powder is useful.

In treating monilial infections, it is also important to ascertain whether the ostomate is taking antibiotics. Any antibiotic, but especially a broad-spectrum agent, changes the flora of the skin, and the entrenched monilia can become difficult to eradicate. For ostomy patients taking antibiotics, nystatin powder or 2% miconazole powder should be continued for 1 month after the monilial infection is gone.

Excessive Sweating. Sweating under the faceplate can decrease wearing time and cause monilial infection. Discomfort from perspiration underneath the collection pouch can be alleviated by purchasing or making a cover or bib to keep the pouch material from touching the skin.

Diarrhea Resulting in Dehydration. Ileostomates and ascending colostomates are at risk of severe diarrhea. The only way to replace the loss may be to administer intravenous fluids. Patients must be aware of the risk of diarrhea so that they can seek medical treatment before dehydration results.

Psychologic Complications

After ostomy surgery, patients may be psychologically depressed. They may fear not being able to engage in former work, participate in sports, perform sexually, or have children. The pharmacist should reassure the patient that the ability to carry out these activities generally remains unchanged. However, the pharmacist should be aware that most men who have a radical resection of the rectum or bladder are rendered organically impotent. Penile implants or other erection aids could enable a man to regain part or all of this function. If the patient is concerned about impotence, referral to a urologist is appropriate. Adverse effects on sexual function also have been reported in women.

The United Ostomy Association comprises various ostomy organizations in the United States whose main purpose is to help ostomy patients by giving moral support and supplying information. Its address is 36 Executive Park, Suite 120, Irvine, CA 92714. Its telephone number is 800-826-0826.

Diet

Most patients can eat a liberal diet, including all the foods eaten before surgery, if the foods are chewed well. However, it is wise to remain on a diet low in fiber for the first 6 weeks after surgery. Urostomates may want to avoid asparagus or other foods that cause odor. Irrigating colostomates should avoid any food that causes them to have loose stools. Patients with ileostomies are prone to obstruction from high-roughage foods eaten in large quantities or exclusive of other food. Such potentially troublesome foods include popcorn, nuts, corn on the cob, mushrooms, bran products, citrus fruits, coconut, Chinese vegetables, raw celery, and raw carrots. These patients should chew these foods well and eat them in small amounts and with other food.

Because they have no control over gas passage, fecal ostomates may prefer to cut down on gas-forming foods such as beans, vegetables of the cabbage family (onions, broccoli, cauliflower, cabbage), beer, and carbonated drinks. Stool odor can be minimized by reducing the consumption of fish, eggs, asparagus, garlic, beans, turnips, foods in the cabbage family, and some vitamins or medications.

Patients with a urostomy, ileostomy, or ascending colostomy must drink adequate amounts of fluid to prevent the precipitation of crystals or kidney stones.

Use of Medications

Because part or all of the colon is removed and intestinal transit time may be altered, the ostomate may experience adverse effects from taking prescription or nonprescription medications, or the medications may be ineffective (Table 1).

Coated or sustained-release preparations may pass through the intestinal tract without being absorbed, and the patient may receive a subtherapeutic dose. The ostomate should look for any undissolved drug particles in the pouch. Liquid preparations or preparations that are crushed or chewed before swallowing are best.

The ostomate also must be careful taking antibiotics, diuretics, and laxatives. Antibiotics may alter the normal flora of the intestinal tract, causing diarrhea or fungal infection of the skin surrounding the stoma. If diarrhea occurs, fluid and electrolyte intake should be increased. Antidiarrheal and antimotility drugs may affect ileal excreta.

Sulfa drugs should be used with caution. Crystallization in the kidney may occur more often in patients having difficulty with fluid balance. To minimize this problem, fluid intake should be increased and the urine should not be acidified. Diuretics should be given with care, because additional loss of fluid may cause dehydration and electrolyte imbalance. The ileostomate should be monitored for signs of hyponatremia if salt substitutes are prescribed.

Laxatives may be used by colostomy patients only under close supervision. If the colostomate is constipated, a stool softener may be recommended. Prokinetic agents (e.g., metoclopramide, cisapride) and antacids may cause problems and should be taken with caution. Products containing calcium may cause calcium stones in the urostomate, products containing magnesium may cause diarrhea in the ileostomate, and aluminum products may cause constipation in the colostomate.

To alleviate potential anxiety, the patient should be counseled about medications that may discolor the feces. Some of these medications and the discoloration they cause are listed below:

- *Aluminum antacids*: whitish color or speckling;
- *Antibiotics (oral)*: greenish gray;
- *Anticoagulants (excess)*: pink to red to black (bleeding);
- *Bismuth salts*: black;
- *Charcoal*: black;

- *Chlorophyll:* green;
- *Ferrous salts*: black;
- *Heparin*: pink to red to black (bleeding);
- *Indomethacin (Indocin)*: green;
- *Oxphenbutazone (Tandearil)*: pink to red to black (bleeding);
- *Phenazopyridine (Pyridium)*: orange red;
- *Phenolphthalein*: red;
- *Salicylates*: pink to red to black (bleeding); and
- *Senna (and other anthraquinone derivatives)*: yellow-green to brown.

TABLE 1   Effects of certain medications on the ostomate

	Colostomate	Ileostomate	Urostomate
Dosage Forms			
Chewable tablets	1	1	1
Enteric-coated tablets	1	3	1
Sustained-release medication	1	3	1
Liquid medication	1	1	1
Gelatin capsules	1	1	1
Compounds			
Alcohol	1	1	1
Antibiotics (poorly absorbed)	1	2,3	1,2
Antidiarrheal agents	1,2	1	1
Calcium-containing antacids	2	2	2
Corticosteroids	1	2	1
Diuretics	1	2	2
Magnesium-containing antacids	2	2	1
Opiates	1,2	1	1
Salicylates	1	1	1
Salt substitutes	1	2	1
Stool softeners	1	2	1
Sulfa drugs	1	1	2
Vitamins	1	2	1

Key:
1 means medication probably has no adverse effects.
2 means medication may cause an increase in adverse effects; patient should be monitored.
3 means medication may be ineffective; patient should be monitored.

CHAPTER 18

Diabetes Care Products and Monitoring Devices

Questions to ask in patient assessment and counseling

- Is there a history of diabetes in your family? Please describe this history.
- Have you been tested for diabetes? If so, what were the results?
- If you were diagnosed as having diabetes, what care plan did your caregiver recommend?
- Have you seen a dietitian? What were the dietitian's recommendations?
- When did you last review your care plan with your physician, pharmacist, nurse, dietitian, or physical therapist?
- Describe how you control your diabetes:
  - What medications are you taking? How do you use them? Please include all medications, even for problems other than your diabetes. Are you allergic to any medications, especially sulfa drugs or insulins containing beef or pork?
  - If you use insulin, what brand do you use? How do you inject it? What injection sites do you use? How do you rotate them? How do you dispose of your syringes and needles? Will you demonstrate your injection technique for me?
  - How do you store your insulin at home? When you travel?
  - Do you test your blood for glucose? If so, what monitoring system do you use? How often do you test? How do you record the results? Will you show me your testing technique?
  - Do you test your urine for glucose? For ketones? Please describe your testing procedures. How do you use the test results to control your diabetes?
  - Describe your diet plan for your diabetes. Do you have trouble following the plan?
  - Are you now using, or have you ever used, a "fad" diet? If so, describe it. How did you learn about the plan?
  - What exercise guidelines do you follow? Describe your exercise habits.
  - Do you consume alcoholic beverages? What have you been told about alcohol and diabetes?
- When did you last see an eye specialist?
- When did you last see a dentist? What is your visit schedule? Describe how you care for your teeth.
- Have you ever seen a foot specialist? If so, when and how often? Describe how you care for your feet.

Editor's Note: This chapter is adapted from Condit F. Steil, R. Keith Campbell, and John R. White, Jr., "Diabetes Care Products and Monitoring Devices," in Covington, T.R., ed., *Handbook of Nonprescription Drugs,* 11th edition, which is based, in part, on the chapter with the same title that appeared in the 10th edition but was written by John R. White, Jr, and R. Keith Campbell. Portions of the Foot Care section in this chapter are based on material written by Nicholas G. Popovich and Gail D. Newton for the 11th edition chapter "Foot Care Products." For a more extensive discussion of the symptoms and classification of diabetes, diabetes screening and complications, as well as diabetes therapy, readers are encouraged to consult Chapter 18 of the *Handbook.*

- *Do you carry identification to show you have diabetes?*
- *Are you a member of the American Diabetes Association?*
- *How do you feel about having diabetes? How does your family feel about it? Does your family understand factors that affect diabetes control?*
- *Do you have specific questions about your diabetes care? Is there any problem right now that I can help you with? If so, what is it?*

Classification, Etiology, and Complications of Diabetes Mellitus

Diabetes mellitus is a syndrome composed of several specific diseases, all of which are characterized by hyperglycemia and a tendency toward the development of macro- or microvascular disease and neuropathy. Approximately 8 million persons in the United States are being treated for diabetes, and some 7 million have undiagnosed diabetes (with no symptoms or only mild symptoms).

Approximately half of all persons with diabetes are over the age of 55. Factors other than age associated with the development of diabetes include heredity, obesity, stress, hormonal imbalance, vasculitis of the vessels supplying the beta cells of the pancreas, and viruses affecting the autoimmune responses of the body.

Table 1 classifies the two major clinical types of diabetes. Approximately 10% of persons with diabetes in the United States have Type I, or insulin-dependent diabetes mellitus (IDDM); the remaining 90% have Type II, or non–insulin-dependent diabetes mellitus (NIDDM).

All major physiologic systems are adversely affected by chronic hyperglycemia and complications in diabetes. Potential complications of the disease are summarized in Table 2. Strict control of blood glucose is essential to all types of treatment.

Symptoms of Diabetes

The more common symptoms of diabetes (e.g., polydipsia, polyphagia, polyuria, fatigue, night-time urination, blurred vision, ketosis, dry mouth) may be fairly easy to detect. Other symptoms that pharmacists should evaluate include weight loss, recurrent monilial infections, prolonged wound healing, gout, visual disturbances, and psychologic changes. While nonspecific for diabetes, these symptoms, in combination or with progressive severity, may indicate its development. Pharmacists who detect these symptoms should refer the patient to a physician for a complete physical examination, history, and laboratory analysis.

Screening and Diagnostic Criteria for Diabetes

The pharmacist may take a role in diabetes screening by having patients complete a diabetes survey developed by the American Diabetes Association (Table 3). Adding up the point values of the questions gives a person's relative risk for developing diabetes. Individuals who reveal a high risk for the disease can then be tested by capillary blood glucose (fingerstick). Pharmacists should be familiar with state and federal laws regarding handling of blood and body fluids before they implement a capillary blood glucose screening program.

Diagnostic criteria from the American Diabetes Association for nonpregnant adult diabetes mellitus are as follows:

- A random plasma glucose level of at least 200 mg/dL in addition to classic and overt symptoms such as polydipsia, polyphagia, polyuria, and/or weight loss;
- A fasting plasma glucose level of at least 140 mg/dL on at least two separate occasions;

TABLE 1 Distinguishing features of the two major types of diabetes mellitus

	Insulin-dependent Type I (IDDM)	Non–insulin-dependent Type II (NIDDM)
Age of onset	Usually, but not always, during childhood or adolescence	Frequently >35
Type of onset	Abrupt	Usually gradual
Prevalence	0.5%	2–4%
Incidence	<10%	>75%
Family history of diabetes	Frequently negative	Commonly positive
Primary cause	Pancreatic beta cell deficiency	End organ (insulin receptors) unresponsiveness to insulin action
Nutritional status at time of onset	Usually thin with weight loss	Usually obese
Postglucose plasma or serum insulin[a], mcU/mL	Absent or minimal	Normal or elevated
Symptoms	Polydipsia, polyphagia, and polyuria	Maybe none
Hepatomegaly	Rather common	Uncommon
Stability	Blood sugar fluctuates widely in response to small changes in insulin dose, exercise, and infection	Blood sugar fluctuations are less marked
Possible etiologic factors include:		
Inheritance	Associated with specific HLA[b] tissue types, but only 40–50% concordance in twins	95–100% concordance in twins, but not associated with specific HLA[b] tissue types
Autoimmune disease	50–80% circulating islet cell antibodies	Negative; <10% circulating islet cell antibodies
Viral infections	Coxsackie, mumps, influenza	No evidence
Proneness to ketosis	Frequent, especially if treatment program is insufficient in food and/or insulin	Uncommon except in the presence of unusual stress or moderate to severe sepsis

Continued on next page

TABLE 1 *continued*

	Insulin-dependent Type I (IDDM)	Non–insulin-dependent Type II (NIDDM)
Insulin defect	Defect in secretion; secretion is impaired early in disease; secretion may be totally absent late in disease	Insulin deficiency present in some patients; others are insulin resistant
		Insulin deficiency—in most patients, insulin secretion fails to keep pace with inordinate demands caused by obesity; this defect may appear initially as a failure to respond to glucose alone, suggesting an impairment in the glucoreceptor of the pancreatic beta cell
		Insulin resistance—in some patients, there is a defect in tissue responsiveness to insulin and evidence of hyperinsulinemia; in such patients, insulin resistance may be mediated by a decreased number of insulin receptors in target cells
		Increased hepatic glucose production in response to altered cellular glucose uptake
Plasma insulin (endogenous)	Negligible to zero	Plasma insulin response may be either adequate but delayed, so that postprandial hypoglycemia may be present when diabetes is discovered, or diminished but not absent
Vascular complications of diabetes and degenerative changes	Infrequent until diabetes has been present for ≈5 years	Frequent
Usual causes of death	Degenerative complications in target organs (e.g., renal failure due to diabetic nephropathy)	Accelerated atherosclerosis (e.g., myocardial infarct); to lesser extent, microangiopathic changes in target tissues (e.g., renal failure)
Diet	Mandatory in all patients	If diet is used fully, hypoglycemic therapy may not be needed
Insulin	Necessary for all patients	Necessary for 20–30% of patients
Oral agents	Rarely efficacious	Often efficacious

[a]Normal response is between 50 and 135 mcU/mL at 60 minutes and less than 100 mcU/mL at 120 minutes after 100 g of oral glucose.
[b]Human leukocyte antigen.

TABLE 2 Potential complications of diabetes mellitus

Body location	Description
Eyes	Retinopathy, cataract formation, glaucoma, and periodic visual disturbances due to microvascular disease and other metabolic complications such as increased sorbitol; leading cause of new blindness
Mouth	Gingivitis, increased incidence of dental cavities and periodontal disease
Reproductive system (pregnancy)	Increased incidence of large babies, stillbirths, miscarriages, neonatal deaths, and congenital defects due to metabolic abnormalities
Nervous system	Motor, sensory, and autonomic neuropathy leading to impotence, neurogenic bladder, paresthesias, gangrene, altered gastrointestinal motility, and cardiovascular problems
Vascular system	Large vessel disease resulting in atherosclerosis and microvascular disease leading to retinopathy, nephropathy, and decreased peripheral perfusion
Skin	Numerous infections and specific lesions such as skin spots, diabetic bullae, lipodystrophies, and necrobiosis lipoidica diabeticorum due to small vessel disease, increased lipids in blood, and pruritus
Kidneys	Diabetic glomerulosclerosis causing nephropathy
Reticuloendothelial system (infections)	Cystitis, tuberculosis, skin infections, difficulty in overcoming infections, and moniliasis in diabetic women

Adapted from Pharmaceutical services for patients with diabetes. *Am Pharm* (module 4). 1986 May; NS26 (5): 8.

■ A fasting plasma glucose level below 140 mg/dL plus at least two oral glucose tolerance tests that yield 2-hour plasma glucose levels of at least 200 mg/dL and one intervening value (at 30, 60, or 90 minutes) of at least 200 mg/dL.

Diagnostic criteria for children and pregnant women are also available from the American Diabetes Association.

Treatment

The objectives in the treatment of diabetes, in order of importance, are to:

■ Relieve and prevent diabetic symptoms;

■ Prevent hypoglycemic reactions;

■ Maintain blood glucose levels close to euglycemia (between 80 and 150 mg/dL) to prevent or slow progression of chronic complications;

- Achieve and/or maintain optimal weight;
- Promote normal growth and development in children;
- Eliminate or minimize all other cardiovascular risk factors; and
- Integrate the patient into health care through intensive education and involvement in self-care, using the premise that the patient must become a primary caregiver.

Key elements in the treatment of diabetes can be remembered with the five DEEDS: *D*iet, *E*xercise, *E*ducation, *D*rugs, and *S*elf-monitoring of blood glucose. Caloric planning and increased physical activity are part of the treatment plan for both types of diabetes. Education is crucial to the patient's understanding of the disease and mastery of the skills needed to achieve glycemic control. Sulfonylureas, metformin, or insulin are used to control hyperglycemia. Nonprescription products—in addition to insulin—formulated especially for use by the person with diabetes can be helpful adjuncts. Finally, self-monitoring of blood glucose enables the patient to adjust medication, diet, and exercise carefully to maintain near-normal blood glucose levels.

Insulin Therapy

The prescription drugs used to treat diabetes are discussed in depth in major textbooks on prescription drugs.

Patient access to the medication is unrestricted in many instances. Thus, pharmacists should be knowledgeable about insulin products and the pharmacotherapy of diabetes mellitus. Pharmacists also need to be familiar with drugs that may affect blood glucose control by themselves or by interacting with sulfonylureas, metformin, or insulin. They should recognize which drugs can cause or exacerbate peripheral neuropathy, retinopathy, and nephropathy, as well as which drugs can cause hypoglycemia or hyperglycemia (Tables 4, 5, and 6).

Type I patients must be treated with exogenous insulin. Persons who require insulin initially are generally younger than 30 years of age at diagnosis and are lean, prone to developing ketoacidosis, and markedly hyperglycemic, even in the fasting state. Insulin is indicated for Type II patients who do not respond to diet and exercise therapy alone or to therapy with oral sulfonylureas or metformin, as well as to those who have fasting plasma glucose concentrations of greater than 200 mg/dL. Insulin therapy is also necessary for some Type II patients who are subject to situational stresses such as infection, pregnancy, or surgery.

All persons using insulin should be trained to inject themselves. Most children with diabetes can begin giving themselves their own insulin injections between the ages of 6 and 9, under appropriate parent supervision.

Insulin Preparations

Insulins may be categorized based on the species source, type, strength, and purity.

Commercially available animal-derived insulins are either pure pork or a mixture of beef and pork. Biosynthetic human insulin is now available. Human insulin has a more rapid onset and a shorter duration of action than pork insulin, which has a more rapid onset and a shorter duration of action than beef insulin.

Insulins may be divided into three groups according to promptness of action onset, duration, and intensity of action following subcutaneous (SC) injection. Rapid or short-acting insulin is regular insulin. Neutral protamine Hagedorn (NPH) and lente insulin suspensions are intermediate-acting insulins; ultralente insulin suspension is long-acting.

TABLE 3   Diabetes screening questionnaire

Could you have diabetes and NOT know it?	Point values[a]
1. My weight is equal to or above that listed in the chart below.[b]	Yes 5____
2. I am under 65 years of age, and I get little or no exercise during a usual day.	Yes 5____
3. I am between 45 and 64 years of age.	Yes 5____
4. I am 65 years old or older.	Yes 9____
5. I am a woman who has had a baby weighing more than 9 pounds.	Yes 1____
6. I have a sister or brother with diabetes.	Yes 1____
7. I have a parent with diabetes.	Yes 1____
	Total____

Women		Men	
Height (in.) (w/o shoes)	Weight (lb)[b] (w/o clothing)	Height (in.) (w/o shoes)	Weight (lb)[b] (w/o clothing)
57	127	61	146
58	131	62	151
59	134	63	155
60	138	64	158
61	142	65	163
62	146	66	168
63	151	67	174
64	157	68	179
65	162	69	184
66	167	70	190
67	172	71	196
68	176	72	202
69	181	73	208
70	186	74	214
		75	220

[a]A score of 3–5 indicates a low risk for diabetes; a score higher than 5 points indicates a high risk. Anyone scoring above 5 points should see a physician promptly for evaluation.

[b]Chart lists weights 20% heavier than those recommended for men or women with medium frames.

Adapted with permission from *Diabetes Alert*. Alexandria, VA: American Diabetes Association; 1995.

Regular insulin injected intramuscularly (IM) provides faster absorption with a greater initial drop in plasma glucose levels than does SC injection. Regular insulin injected intravenously (IV) produces the highest pharmacologic level of insulin in the least time.

If more than 60 U of insulin are injected at one site, there is potential for erratic absorption. Patients receiving large doses of insulin should perhaps split the doses and inject in two different sites.

Insulin Regimens

Single-injection regimens are not advocated for any newly diagnosed person. They provide consistent glycemic control in few patients. By using multiple daily injections or an insulin infusion pump, however, intensified regimens can achieve near-euglycemic blood glucose levels. The goal of intensive therapy is to mimic the insulin action of a functioning pancreas. Numerous regimens can be devised to fit the patient's lifestyle.

Insulin Mixtures

As the purity of insulins has improved, the problem of stability in mixing insulins has decreased. Regular insulin may be mixed with NPH insulin in any proportion desired; the resultant combination is stable for approximately 1 month at room temperature and 3 months when refrigerated. Patients mixing regular and lente insulin should either inject the mixture immediately or allow it to stand for 24 hours and then inject it. Lente and ultralente insulins may be combined in any ratio desired at any time. These mixtures are stable in any proportion for 18 months if refrigerated; however, sterility is not guaranteed.

Patients using infusion pumps may use either normal saline or Lilly's Insulin Dilution Fluid to dilute the insulin in the pump. Regular insulin may be mixed in any proportion with normal saline for use in the pump, but the combination should be used within 2–3 hours after mixing. Regular insulin may be mixed with Lilly's Insulin Dilution Fluid in any proportion, and it will be stable indefinitely.

TABLE 4 Drugs that can cause peripheral neuropathies

Antimicrobials	Nitrofurantoin, ethambutol, isoniazid, colistin, strepto-mycin, metronidazole, amphotericin B
Anticonvulsants	Phenytoin, carbamazepine
Antirheumatics	Indomethacin, colchicine, penicillamine, gold compounds
Cytotoxics	Vincristine, procarbazine, cytarabine, chlorambucil
Cardiovascular drugs[a]	Hydralzine, clofibrate, disopyramide
Miscellaneous agents	Cimetidine, ergotamine, methysergide, amitriptyline, amphetamines

[a]Nitroglycerin can cause postural hypotension in diabetic patients with autonomic neuropathy.

Adapted from Pharmaceutical services for patients with diabetes. *Am Pharm* (module 4). 1986 May; NS26 (5): 5.

TABLE 5   Drugs that can cause nephropathy

Penicillamine, gold salts, nonsteroidal analgesics (large doses over time)

Aminoglycoside antibiotics (neomycin, kanamycin, gentamicin, tobramycin)

Cephaloridine, rifampin, cyclophosphamide, heroin, methotrexate, and methysergide

Adapted from Pharmaceutical services for patients with diabetes. *Am Pharm* (module 4). 1986 May; NS26 (5): 5.

Storage of Insulin

Insulin is heat labile and should normally be kept under refrigeration (36°–46°F [2°–8°C]). Patients need not refrigerate vials of insulin currently in use because they contain bacteriostatic agents. However, the insulin should be used within 1–2 months and should be stored away from heaters, radiators, or sunny windows.

Freezing insulin does not necessarily affect potency, but insulin action may be altered. Patients who are traveling can ensure the stability and potency of their insulin by storing it in an insulated container with ice or a cooling agent.

Preparation of Insulin Dose

Pharmacists should instruct patients in the following technique:

- Inspect vials for signs of contamination or degradation.
- Wash hands with soap and water.
- Make sure the proper insulin is used—that is, the correct insulin in the correct strength from the source normally used.
- Agitate the insulin gently but thoroughly.
- Wait until any foam that has formed from agitation subsides. Then gently roll the vial between the palms of the hands or repeatedly invert it until the suspension is evenly distributed. To avoid generating air bubbles in the insulin, do not shake the bottle.
- Wipe off the top of the vial with an alcohol swab or a cotton ball moistened with alcohol. Be sure that no cotton or cloth fibers remain on the rubber stopper.
- Remove a clean syringe from storage. Touch only the hub of the plunger and the barrel of the syringe; avoid touching the hub of the needle.
- Inject into the intermediate-acting insulin vial an amount of air equivalent to the needed insulin dose.
- Inject into the regular insulin vial an amount of air equivalent to the needed insulin dose.
- Invert the vial and syringe and withdraw the appropriate number of units of insulin from the regular insulin vial.
- Repeat the above step with the vial of intermediate-acting insulin.
- When the correct number of units of insulin (without air bubbles) has been measured, withdraw the needle.

TABLE 6 Drugs that may cause hypoglycemia or hyperglycemia

Hypoglycemia	Hyperglycemia
Acetaminophen	Acetazolamide
Alcohol (acute)	Alcohol (chronic)
Amitriptyline	Amiodarone
Anabolic steroids	Antimicrobial (pentamidine, rifampin,
Beta blockers	sulfasalazine, nalidixic acid)
Biguanides	Asparaginase
Chloroquine	Beta-agonists
Clofibrate	Caffeine
Disopyramide	Calcium channel blockers
Fenfluramine	Chlorpromazine
Fluphenazine	Chlorthalidone
Guanethidine	Corticosteroids
Haloperidol	Cyclosporine
Imipramine	Diazoxide
Insulin	Encainide
Lithium	Estrogens
Monoamine oxidase inhibitors	Ethacrynic acid
Norfloxacin	Fentanyl/Furosemide
Pentamidine	Indapamide
Perphenazine/Amitriptyline	Interferon alpha
Phenobarbital	Lactulose
Prazosin	Niacin and nicotinic acid
Propoxyphene	Oral contraceptives
Quinine	Phenytoin
Salicylates in large doses	Probenecid
Sulfonamide antibiotics	Sugars (dextrose, fructose, mannitol,
Sulfonylurea agents	sorbitol, sucrose)
Tetrahydrocannabinol	Sympathomimetic amines
	Thiazide diuretics
	Thyroid preparations
	Tricyclic antidepressants

■ Holding the syringe with the needle upright, draw an air bubble into the syringe, invert the syringe, and roll the bubble through to mix.

■ Tap the barrel of the syringe briskly two or three times to remove any air bubbles.

■ Expel the air bubble and recap the needle, or lay the syringe on a flat surface such as a table or shelf with the needle over the edge to avoid contamination.

Injection Technique

The following procedure is recommended:

■ Check the record to confirm where the insulin was injected previously. Rotate injection sites.

■ Clean the injection site with an alcohol swab or a cotton ball moistened with alcohol.

- Pinch a fold of skin with one hand. With the other hand, hold the syringe like a pencil, place the needle on the skin with the beveled edge up, and push the needle quickly through the fold of skin at a 45°–90° angle. Before injecting the insulin, draw back slightly on the plunger to be sure a blood vessel has not been penetrated. If blood appears in the syringe barrel, withdraw the needle and repeat the injection in another spot on the body.
- Inject the insulin by pressing the plunger in as far as it will go.
- Withdraw the needle quickly and press on the injection site with the swab or cotton ball moistened with alcohol.
- When injection is completed, dispose of the syringe and needle properly.
- Record the injection site.

Patients should be taught that insulin is to be injected deep into SC tissue. The technique for injection may need to be altered with each individual, depending on the amount of SC fat present. For persons with a substantial amount of fat, a 60° angle or more with the skin stretched will accomplish the deep SC injection needed. For a thin person, a 45° angle with the skin pinched up may be required. The purpose of pinching the skin is to lift the fat off the muscle and thus avoid IM or IV injection, which may result in a more rapid onset of action and severe hypoglycemia. Properly injected insulin leaves only the needle puncture dot to show the injection site.

Pharmacists should stress the importance of rotating injection sites to limit irritation. Fever, exercise, extremely hot weather, or a sauna or Jacuzzi can increase peripheral blood flow, which also speeds insulin absorption. Conversely, cold packs, cold extremities, or a hypothermal blanket may slow the onset of action because the absorption rate is decreased.

Patients must learn the proper technique to prevent skin damage. Several devices are available to assist the patient in self-administration of insulin.

Adverse Reactions Associated with Insulin Therapy

Adverse reactions to insulin include insulin resistance, insulin allergy, lipodystrophies, and hypoglycemia—the most common complication of insulin therapy.

Hypoglycemia. Symptoms of hypoglycemia include a parasympathetic response (nausea, hunger, and flatulence), diminished cerebral function (confusion, irritability, agitation, lethargy, and personality changes), sympathetic responses (tachycardia, sweating, and tremor), coma, and convulsions. Ataxia and blurred vision are common. The profile of the hypoglycemic patient is summarized by pale moist skin, nervousness, excitability, irritability, mental confusion, hunger, headache, normal to rapid breathing, and a numb or tingling tongue. Morning hyperglycemia may be a result of asymptomatic nocturnal hypoglycemia in patients who are otherwise well controlled on intensive insulin regimens. These patients may describe symptoms of confusion or may even become unconscious without any other signs or symptoms of hypoglycemia. Patients with these symptoms must monitor their blood glucose levels between 2:00 am and 3:00 am to determine if the glucose is low (Somogyi phenomenon) or normal/high (dawn reaction). They should be assisted in interpreting the results and adjusting their therapy.

All manifestations of hypoglycemia are relieved rapidly by glucose administration. Because of the potential danger of insulin reactions progressing to hypoglycemic coma, persons with diabetes should always carry packets or cubes of table sugar, a candy roll, or glucose tablets, and should eat 2 tsp (10 g) or two cubes of sugar, five to six Lifesavers, or two glucose tablets at the onset of mild hypoglycemic symptoms (e.g., sweating, hunger, weakness, nausea, dizziness, mood changes). Alternatively, they may drink at least one-half cup of orange juice, one-third cup of apple juice, or 6–12 oz of any sugar-containing carbonated beverage. If the glucose concentration remains below 60 mg/dL, the treatment may be repeated in 15 minutes and the carbohydrate dose may be increased to 15 g. A snack consisting of one to two cups of milk, a piece of fruit, or cheese and soda crackers is generally enough to treat mild hypoglycemia if mealtime is not imminent. Blood glucose should be monitored frequently.

If symptoms are intermediate (e.g., confusion, poor coordination, headache, double vision), more aggressive administration of glucose and a sugar load may be required. A glucagon emergency kit containing an ampule of glucagon (1 mg), a syringe of diluent, and clear directions should be provided to every Type I patient in case of hypoglycemia-associated unconsciousness. Family members and other caregivers and coworkers should be taught to mix and administer glucagon. The usual dose for adults and children weighing more than 20 kg is 1.0 mg administered in a similar manner as insulin; for children weighing less than 20 kg, the usual dose is 0.5 mg. Normally, the patient will regain consciousness within 5–10 minutes and be able to swallow some sweetened water. If there is no response after 5–10 minutes, a second injection may be given. If the response is still insufficient, the patient should be taken to an emergency room or a physician immediately. When there is doubt about whether a patient is hypoglycemic or hyperglycemic, sugar should be given initially until the condition can be accurately evaluated.

Patients who demonstrate a sensitivity to animal insulin usually develop redness at the injection site. The reactions may be treated with diphenhydramine or hydroxyzine. The long-term solution may be changing to human insulin, to which hypersensitivity reactions are very rare.

Insulin Resistance. Insulin resistance is a rare condition in which a patient requires more than 200 units of insulin a day for more than 2 days in the absence of ketoacidosis or acute infection. True insulin resistance can be managed by switching to a human source insulin or administering systemic glucocorticoids.

Insulin Lipodystrophy and Allergy. Lipodystrophy occurs in two forms: lipoatrophy (the breakdown of SC fatty tissue, leaving hollowed areas under the skin) and lipohypertrophy (the hyperdevelopment of fatty tissue, causing bulges under the skin). Lipoatrophy improves in most patients when human insulin is substituted. Lipohypertrophy is generally seen in patients who use the same sites for repeated insulin injection. The pharmacist should investigate the patient's injection technique and rotation schedule.

Nondrug Therapy

The pharmacist should stress the importance of maintaining normal weight. Proper exercise and diet are essential. Patients who need help adhering to their prescribed exercise program or adjusting their diet should be referred to a physical therapist or dietitian who deals with persons with diabetes.

Exercise

Patients are encouraged to participate in exercise that uses the large muscle groups at submaximal levels (e.g., swimming, running, biking). Activities that require heavy straining, such as weight lifting, are discouraged. Daily aerobic exercise helps lower blood glucose levels by allowing glucose to penetrate the muscle cells for metabolism without the assistance of insulin. Exercise improves circulatory function; aids in breathing, digestion, and metabolism; and improves cardiovascular endurance.

Exercise may cause hyperglycemia if there is inadequate insulin available when the patient begins the activity. It may cause hypoglycemia if the patient's blood glucose concentration is normal or low just before exercise and proper precautions are not observed. Consistency with exercise is important.

Patients must be trained to monitor their blood glucose levels before, during, and after exercise and to adjust their diet and insulin injections accordingly. An exercise log may help the patient maintain a regular schedule.

If a problem arises, the pharmacist should check to ensure that the patient is ingesting carbohydrates before exercise, injecting preexercise insulin at nonexercised sites, and participating in prescribed physical activities at the appropriate time of day with regard to peak insulin activity and food intake. The pharmacist should also determine that the patient recognizes the symptoms of hypoglycemia, carries a sugar source as well as a glucagon emergency kit, and wears a medical identification necklace or bracelet.

Diet

Diet therapy is a cornerstone of diabetes management. This is especially true for patients with Type II diabetes. The pharmacist can offer dietary counseling and refer the patient to a registered dietitian for detailed education and training.

Diabetes patients were taught for many years to avoid simple sugars. However, there is little evidence that the assumed rapid absorption and increase in glucose actually occurs when some sugar is part of the basic meal plan. Rather than being concerned about the type of carbohydrate source, one should address the total amount of carbohydrates consumed.

To help patients modify their eating behaviors, pharmacists should encourage them to keep a diet log similar to the exercise log. Dietary guidelines are available from the American Diabetes Association.

Alternative Sweeteners. When special foods are being prepared, sucrose should be omitted and alternative sweetening agents substituted.

The Food and Drug Administration (FDA) classifies sweeteners as nonnutritive or nutritive. *Nonnutritive* refers to sweeteners without calories, such as saccharin or cyclamates. *Nutritive* refers to sweeteners with calories, such as aspartame, fructose, sorbitol, and mannitol.

Pharmacists should encourage patients to read the labels of all foods marked "dietetic" because such labeling does not mean "diabetic." Pharmacists should be familiar with all products directed at diet therapy.

Precautions

Reading the label on all food and drug products is essential to maintaining glycemic control.

Alcohol and Alcohol-Containing Products

Precautions that apply to the general public regarding the use of alcohol apply to persons with diabetes as well. Because avoidance of alcohol is not always possible or desired, patients should be assessed individually to determine if ingesting alcohol to reduce emotional tension, relieve anxiety, or stimulate appetite outweighs the potential adverse effects on blood glucose control. There is little evidence to support concern over the consumption of small amounts of alcohol (e.g., 4 oz of wine, 12 oz of beer, 1.5 oz of distilled spirits). Alcoholic beverages should always be consumed with food. Either hyper- or hypoglycemia may develop in diabetic patients who ingest alcohol. Hypoglycemia is the most common effect, especially when alcohol is consumed on an empty stomach.

Additional guidelines for alcohol use in patients include:

- Discussing the use of alcohol with a physician to ensure that no other contraindications exist;
- Eating first and spacing drinks;
- Not drinking if overweight or if diabetic control is unstable;
- Avoiding mixes that contain sugar;
- Calculating the alcohol in the diet schedule and decreasing fat intake; and
- Considering that alcohol promotes hypoglycemia the following day.

Caffeine

Response to caffeine is highly variable among diabetic patients. Caffeine intake may need to be considered in patients who tend toward hyperglycemic episodes at specific times of the day.

Sugar-Containing Products

A list of sucrose-free pharmaceutical preparations is useful so that the pharmacist may suggest a suitable product for patient use. Cough preparations that contain simple syrup may have a clinically significant effect on a brittle insulinopenic diabetic patient. However, the amount of extra sugar ingested to relieve a cough would not be significant in most well-controlled cases of diabetes.

Sympathomimetic Amines

Ephedrine, pseudoephedrine, phenylpropanolamine, phenylephrine, and epinephrine increase blood glucose and cause increased blood pressure by vasoconstriction. They should be used cautiously in persons with diabetes. Sympathomimetic amines do not have as potent an effect on blood glucose as does epinephrine.

Salicylates

Aspirin products can cause hypoglycemia in diabetes patients; however, the clinical significance of aspirin is questionable if the patient is monitoring for diabetes control. Other nonprescription choices for analgesia can pose problems with adverse effects on renal function. Patients should be counseled to use these products with caution.

Preventing Complications

General Hygiene

Persons with diabetes are more susceptible to bacterial infection and less able to fight infections, particularly monilial infections, than is the general population. The most easily infected part of the body is the skin. Minor cuts and scratches should be promptly cleansed thoroughly with soap and water. Any patient with a serious cut, burn, or puncture wound should see a physician immediately.

Daily bathing with mild soap and thorough drying is recommended. Patients should inspect their bodies daily, starting at the top of the head and working down to the feet and toes. They should check for any signs of dry or cracked skin, chafing or irritation, infection, injury, and areas with visible changes from increased pressure by clothing or shoes. Any new lesions or old lesions not resolving properly should be brought to the attention of a physician as soon as possible.

The pharmacist should discuss the appropriate use of nonprescription topical antimicrobial products and should refer the patient to a physician when medical attention is indicated.

Foot Care

Approximately 25% of persons with diabetes develop severe foot or leg problems. Approximately 50% of leg amputations are performed on patients with diabetes.

Predisposing Factors for Foot Infections

Any constant irritation of the diabetic foot can cause an ulceration within 24 hours. Repeated and unrelieved pressure on a callus site can encourage ischemia and ulceration. This situation may go unnoticed until bleeding becomes significant or an odor is noticed from the wound. Factors that predispose diabetes patients to foot infections include angiopathy, peripheral neuropathy, peripheral vascular disease, and a weakened immune system.

Preventive Foot Care

Daily Inspection. With the aid of a mirror, patients should daily inspect their feet and lower legs (especially between toes and pressure areas) for cuts, blisters, calluses, scratches, cracks, evidence of pressure, changes in color, excessive dryness, and excessive moisture. Some clinicians train family members to perform the daily inspection for patients who cannot easily see their foot skin surface.

Proper Hygiene. Patients must wash their feet every day with mild soap and lukewarm water, after which the feet should be thoroughly dried, especially between the toes.

Shoes and socks should be changed a couple of times every day, depending on the patient's tendency to retain moisture on the feet and in the shoes.

Prevention of Vasoconstriction. To prevent vasoconstriction, patients should massage their feet every day, rubbing upward toward the tips of their toes. If patients have varicose veins, the feet should be massaged gently but the legs should not.

It is wise to remove the shoes for a time during prolonged travel.

Constricting clothing (e.g., elastic hosiery with a tight top band) decreases blood flow to the feet and should be avoided by diabetic patients. Patients should not cross their legs when sitting. If the weight of the bedclothes is uncomfortable, it helps to place a pillow under the covers at the foot of the bed. Since components of tobacco can cause vasoconstriction in the extremities, patients should abstain from using tobacco products.

Recommendations for Footwear. Patients should wear soft, comfortable, professionally fitted leather shoes.

If lower-extremity edema is a complicating condition, the patient should purchase shoes at the end of the day. Shoes should then be "broken in"; that is, new shoes should be worn no longer than a half hour the first day, and that time should be increased by an hour each subsequent day.

Pharmacist's Role in Preventive Care. The pharmacist can play a role in preventive foot care by asking persons at risk for diabetic foot ulcers about neuropathic symptoms, history of claudication or resting pain, history of prior orthopedic foot problems or surgeries, and current or previous smoking habits and alcohol intake. Overweight individuals also have a higher risk of foot pathology. Patients with any of the above risk factors should be instructed in the care of their feet and monitored closely.

Treatment of Foot Conditions

First Aid for Minor Injuries. Patients should avoid using strong antiseptics (e.g., tincture of iodine) to treat infection because they can irritate and dry the skin. A mild disinfectant might be preferable, but not without medical supervision. If it is necessary to cover the wound with a gauze bandage, only fine paper tape or cellophane tape (Scotch Tape) should be used to secure the bandage to the skin. Adhesive tape can make the skin soggy, encourage the growth of microorganisms, and irritate the skin when removed. Any redness, blistering, pain, or swelling should be brought to the attention of the physician.

Corns and Calluses. Corns and calluses occur as a result of friction, usually from improperly fitting footwear. A common problem is the development of a callus under the ball of the foot. Curling and stretching the toes several times during the day helps prevent this problem, as does finishing each step on the toes rather than on the ball of the foot.

To remove a callus or corn, the patient should soak the foot with mild soap in lukewarm water for about 15 minutes. The excess tissue can then be gently rubbed off with a towel, a file, medium sandpaper, or pumice stone. The excess skin should *never* be allowed to become irritated. Corns and calluses should *not* be cut or trimmed with razor blades or paring knives. The patient should *not* use a nonprescription topical corn or callus remover, whose primary active ingredient is salicylic acid. Patients should also avoid corn medications, which contain keratolytic agents. If the corn or callus is particularly discomforting, a podiatrist should be consulted.

Athlete's Foot. Athlete's foot in the diabetic patient should never be treated with acidic or astringent preparations. A specific antifungal drug should be used, and the patient should immediately contact a physician or podiatrist.

Foot Ulcers. When counseling a patient about a possible foot ulcer, the pharmacist should err on the side of safety and suggest that the patient consult a physician or podiatrist.

An important nondrug measure is to have the patient keep weight off the foot, especially if the foot is swollen or shows signs of a deep infection. As long as the patient keeps walking, even for as little as 10 minutes a day, an infected lesion may not heal.

Dental Care

Gingivitis and dental caries occur at an increased rate in diabetic patients. Patients should have their teeth checked at least twice each year; they should brush and floss their teeth at least twice daily and massage their gums with a brush, a Water Pik, or their fingers. They should consult a dentist at the first sign of abnormal conditions of the gums, inform their dentist that they have diabetes, and discuss dental care products.

Pharmacists should ensure that patients use sugar- and alcohol-free dental products, know which toothbrush has been recommended, and know how to floss correctly. Patients should be monitored for changes in oral health and referred to their dentist when appropriate.

Eye Care

Diabetes is the leading cause of blindness in the United States. Pharmacists should encourage patients to have their eyes examined at least once each year. Pharmacists can educate patients concerning the relationship of good vision and good blood glucose control. Patients should be discouraged from using topical ophthalmic preparations unless they are recommended or prescribed. Patients who note any change in vision or develop any irritation of the eye should see their doctor immediately.

Product Selection Guidelines

Syringes and Needles

Two types of syringes are available: glass (reusable) and plastic (disposable). Almost all patients use plastic insulin syringes. The advantages of disposable syringes and needles include ensured sterility and ease of penetration, a wide bore, and a 25% smaller angle in the needle bevel. The needles are finer (27, 28, and 29 gauge), sharper, and silicone coated for ease of insertion. There is less pain associated with the smaller needles, and there is virtually no "dead space" (i.e., the measurable space in the needle and at the hub of the needle and syringe that contains drug that is not injected). Dead space is a potential source of error when two different fluids are drawn, measured, and mixed in the same syringe. Needles are available in 1/2- and 5/8-inch lengths; the longer needle is used for obese patients and when back leakage of insulin occurs.

Disposable U-100 syringes with the capacity of 0.3 cc (30 U) and 0.5 cc (50 U), called low-dose syringes, and those with the capacity of 1.0 cc (100 U) may be used with U-100 insulin only. The low-dose syringes have a smaller-caliber barrel so that the U-100 insulin can be measured in 1-U increments, yielding a more accurate dose. Thus, patients who require less than 30–50 U of U-100 insulin per injection may use the low-dose syringes to measure the dose more accurately. The low-dose syringe barrels are also easier to read.

Reuse of disposable plastic syringes is not generally recommended, although patients who have been following this practice without problems for several years should not be discouraged. Syringes that are to be reused over a few days may be stored at room temperature. It is important to ensure that any patient who reuses a syringe and needle pay close attention to aseptic technique to avoid touch contamination. The needles should probably not be cleaned with alcohol because this removes the silicon coating.

Injection Aids

A variety of products are available for the visually impaired. There are "dose gauges" that allow doses to be dialed in, have audible dose selectors, come in Braille, or have prefilled syringes that are disposable after multiple dose use.

There are also several types of insulin injection devices or automatic injectors for patients who have an aversion to self-injection. The injected insulin disperses into a very thin spray as it enters the SC tissue. Patients using a jet injector for the first time may have to adjust the insulin dose because the increased tissue contact may cause the insulin to be absorbed faster than when it is injected with a needle. Patients who do not have enough fat tissue may inject insulin into muscle tissue with a jet injector. Jet injector devices cause less lipoatrophy and inflammation than customary needle administration; they also facilitate reaching and rotating the injection sites. The jet injector must be held firmly against the skin. If contact is lost, the dose may not be properly administered.

For patients who use the syringe and needle for injection but dislike sticking themselves, a small flexible catheter (the Button Infuser) can be inserted SC, usually in the abdomen, and anchored at the site. It allows the patient to give multiple doses of insulin by attaching a syringe to a portal and injecting. The catheter can remain in place for 24–72 hours, and the patient may inject insulin several times a day. The Button Infuser is less complicated than an insulin pump and is often more acceptable to patients requiring multiple daily injections than the individual needle and syringe.

Insulin Infusion Pumps

Portable, battery-driven, open-loop, continuous infusion pumps, used to administer insulin to some Type I patients, are programmed to provide an individualized, continuous basal amount of SC insulin throughout a 24-hour period, and to handle fluctuations in blood glucose when the patient is not eating. The patient must self-monitor blood glucose at least four times a day and determine how much insulin should be injected and when. Most patients should change the infusion line and cannula sites every 2 days to prevent soreness and infection. When the syringe or reservoir is empty, it must be replaced.

Patients selected for insulin pump therapy must be highly motivated, capable of being educated, responsible for keeping records, able to follow specific procedures, and willing to perform and log blood tests daily. Type II patients and children with diabetes are not encouraged to use an insulin pump.

Blood and Urine Testing and Record Keeping

Proper blood or urine testing for glucose and urine ketones, as well as maintenance of adequate records of daily control, is an essential part of the diabetic patient's routine.

Blood Glucose Tests

Maintenance of blood glucose control is impossible without measurement. Self-monitoring of blood glucose (SMBG) is the most accurate method a patient can use. Blood glucose tests can be divided into two types. One type uses only reagent strips; the other uses reagent strips and a blood glucose meter.

Reagent Strips. Reagent strips can be read visually to obtain a range of the blood glucose level. The patient places a drop of blood on the strip and waits 30–60 seconds before wiping or washing the blood off. After waiting about a minute longer, the patient compares the color on the strip with the colors on a color meter chart.

Test strips should be stored at room temperature. Bottle caps should be replaced immediately and tightly.

Glucose Meters. Used in conjunction with reagent strips, a glucose meter gives the specific blood glucose level rather than a range. One type uses a photometric measurement based on a dye-related reaction. The patient places a drop of blood on a reagent strip and blots it; the strip is then inserted into a meter and read photometrically or colorimetrically. The other type measures blood glucose through an electronic charge via a chemical reaction.

The blood glucose monitoring method recommended must be flexible and capable of being easily incorporated into the patient's daily routine. Patients should try several meters before selecting one.

Lancets and Other Test Accessories. Patients may need blood lancets and lancet holders, alcohol swabs or cotton balls and alcohol, and other accessories. The patient should be instructed to use the sides of the finger, where there are fewer nerve endings than in the middle and thus less pain. The patient should wash hands just before sticking the finger, preferably with warm water, which will increase blood supply. If this is not possible, alcohol swabs can be used for cleansing. The patient should ensure that the alcohol has evaporated before sticking the finger because alcohol can alter the test results.

Patient Education in SMBG. SMBG is becoming recommended for all types of patients with diabetes. Most insurance companies and managed care organizations, under the provisions of major medical plans, will reimburse patients for all or part of the cost of SMBG.

Patients who should be strongly encouraged to self-test their blood glucose include those

- With an abnormal or unstable renal threshold;
- With renal failure;
- Whose glycemic control is unstable and insulin dependent;
- With impaired color vision;
- Who have trouble with urine testing;
- Who have difficulty recognizing true hypoglycemia;
- Who are pregnant;
- Who are using drug therapy for diabetes control; and
- Who prefer to self-test their blood glucose.

Proper education will encourage more patients to perform SMBG consistently. Return demonstration by the patient is necessary to ensure patient understanding and to correct any errors. Any recommendations on technique made to the patient should be incorporated into the patient profile for follow-up. The pharmacist should document the sale of the device and training on the profile and correspond with the patient's primary physician regarding the training session.

Urine Glucose Tests

Urine glucose testing is recommended for patients who cannot or will not monitor their own blood glucose. Urine glucose testing gives the patient an idea of what blood glucose level has been in the past several hours. There are two chemical reactions for testing for glucose in the urine: copper reduction tests (Clinitest) and glucose oxidase tests (dip-and-read tests).

Patients may be taking drugs that can interfere with urine glucose testing methods and should be instructed to test their urine using both methods. If the test results differ, there is a strong possibility that a drug is interfering with the test results.

Tests for Urinary Ketones

Testing for urine ketones is advised for all patients who use insulin. The urine should be tested whenever blood glucose levels are greater than 200–250 mg/dL and during periods of illness or stress. The presence of ketones on two or more consecutive urine tests should be reported to the physician.

The Role of the Pharmacist

The pharmacist should emphasize the importance of testing for and recording urine and blood glucose levels, and can assist the patient in selecting and using any monitoring products. Diabetes category, patient motivation, and physical handicaps (e.g., poor vision) should be considered when recommending a testing product. Samples of testing products in the pharmacy's diabetes center can be used to help the patient make the selection. The pharmacist should be ready to instruct the patient and should ask the patient to demonstrate his or her ability to perform the test properly. The patient should be encouraged to keep accurate records of the tests and to return with his or her logbook, which should also contain records of body weight, activities, diet, and medication use, so that the pharmacist can determine how well the diabetes is being controlled. The pharmacist should also discuss drug interferences with each urine monitoring method.

The pharmacist can ensure that the patient understands the steps to care and communicate this to the patient's other health care providers via written communication.

The pharmacist may also become the "gatekeeper" for access to others in the medical community, maintaining a ready listing of potential referral sources for different diabetes-related needs (e.g., podiatrist, dietitian, ophthalmologist).

Identification Tags

All persons with diabetes should wear identification bracelets, necklaces, or tags. Patients should also carry identification cards that contain their name, address, and telephone number; the amount and type of medication used; and the name and telephone number of their physician.

Recommendations for Travel

Persons with diabetes should take enough supplies for the entire trip plus 1 week. They should always carry an extra vial of insulin to ensure that they have insulin derived from the same source. Patients traveling abroad should bring an adequate supply of insulin and syringes because the most common type available in most foreign countries is U-40 insulin. They should not travel with prefilled syringes, however, because the syringes may be accidentally jarred and the dose wasted. Patients should also carry one or two glucagon kits and instructions for use.

All patients who travel should carry an identification card and wear an identification bracelet, necklace, or tag that indicates they have diabetes and is written in the country's dominant language. Organizations are available that help locate physicians abroad. It is recommended that patients planning foreign travel prepare cards with key phrases (e.g., "I am diabetic," "Please get me a doctor," and "Sugar or orange juice, please") written in the dominant language of the countries to be visited. They should also carry a letter from a physician stating that they have diabetes and noting other major medical problems, current medications by both brand and generic names, and information concerning medical insurance.

Patients who are traveling should control their diets carefully, allow time for physical activity, and carry candy or sugar to combat possible hypoglycemic attacks. Those who are changing time zones should also recognize that changes of 2 hours or more require adjustments of the insulin dose.

Because patients will probably need to monitor their blood glucose more often, owing to changes in diet, activity, and meal schedules, they should also take extra batteries and strips for the glucose meter, a bottle of strips that can be read visually, alcohol wipes, cotton balls, and lancets. Even if patients do not usually monitor their urine for ketones, it is advisable to do so while traveling.

Patient Education

Patient education is one of the critical keys to success in controlling diabetes. Every diabetic patient should know:

■ What diabetes is and why treatment is necessary;

■ How to test blood for glucose;

■ How to test urine for acetone and perhaps sugar;

■ How to administer and store insulin and correctly take and store oral medications for control and complication therapy;

■ What dose and time are best for administration of oral agents, if appropriate;

■ What the symptoms are of uncontrolled diabetes and ketosis;

- What the symptoms are of hypoglycemia;
- What the emergency treatment is for hypoglycemia;
- How to select the proper foods;
- How to modify treatment for exercise or illness;
- How to care for the feet;
- What precautionary measures to take while traveling;
- How to contact the physician, pharmacist, or emergency department;
- When to return for follow-up.

CHAPTER 19

Nutritional Products

Questions to ask in patient assessment and counseling

- *Why do you think you need a vitamin, mineral, or nutritional supplement?*
- *What are your symptoms? Did they appear suddenly or gradually?*
- *What is your age and weight?*
- *Do you eat meats, vegetables, dairy products, and grain products every day?*
- *Are you dieting or do you have any type of dietary restrictions?*
- *Do you participate regularly in sports? Do you exercise? Do you have a job requiring physical activity?*
- *Do you have any chronic illness (diabetes, peptic ulcer, ulcerative colitis, or epilepsy)?*
- *Are you taking any prescription or nonprescription medications?*
- *Are you taking or have you recently taken any vitamins, minerals, or nutritional supplements?*
- *Do you donate blood? How often? When did you last donate blood?*
- *Do you smoke or are you around smokers daily?*
- *Do you drink alcohol? How often and how much?*
- *Are you pregnant?*
- *Do you take oral contraceptives (birth control pills)?*

Nutrition experts agree that foods, not supplements, are the preferred source of vitamins and minerals, and that most individuals can meet their requirements by eating a balanced diet. Although most Americans probably do receive adequate amounts of vitamins and minerals from their usual diet, some segments of the population (e.g., elderly persons, smokers, nursing home patients, and teenagers) are less likely to consume the recommended dietary allowances (RDAs) of vitamins and minerals. Primary attention should be directed toward improving the diet; under some circumstances, a supplement is appropriate.

Recommended Dietary Allowances

Guidelines for optimum nutrition are provided by two organizations: the Food and Nutrition Board of the National Research Council–National Academy of Sciences and the Food and Drug Administration (FDA). The Food and Nutrition Board has set forth its recommendations in terms of RDAs, the levels of daily intake of essential nutrients that, based on scientific knowledge, the Board judges to be adequate to meet the known nutrient needs of most healthy persons (Table 1). The Food and Nutrition Board has also recommended an "estimated safe and adequate daily dietary intake" of other nutrients for which human requirements are not quantitatively known (Table 2).

Editor's Note: This chapter is adapted from Loyd V. Allen, Jr., "Nutritional Products," in Covington, T.R., ed., *Handbook of Nonprescription Drugs,* 11th edition. For a more extensive discussion of nutrition, vitamins, minerals, and nutritional supplements, readers are encouraged to consult Chapter 19 of the *Handbook.*

TABLE 1 Food and Nutrition Board, National Academy of Sciences–National Research Council recommended dietary allowances (RDA),[a] revised 1989

Category	Age (y) or condition	Weight[b] (kg)	(lb)	Height[b] (cm)	(in)	Protein (g)	Vitamin A (mcg RE)[c]	Fat-soluble vitamins Vitamin D (mcg)[d]	Vitamin E (mg α-TE)[e]	Vitamin K (mcg)
Infants	0.0–0.5	6	13	60	24	13	375	7.5	3	5
	0.5–1.0	9	20	71	28	14	375	10	4	10
Children	1–3	13	29	90	35	16	400	10	6	15
	4–6	20	44	112	44	24	500	10	7	20
	7–10	28	62	132	52	28	700	10	7	30
Males	11–14	45	99	157	62	45	1,000	10	10	45
	15–18	66	145	176	69	59	1,000	10	10	65
	19–24	72	160	177	70	58	1,000	10	10	70
	25–50	79	174	176	70	63	1,000	5	10	80
	51+	77	170	173	68	63	1,000	5	10	80
Females	11–14	46	101	157	62	46	800	10	8	45
	15–18	55	120	163	64	44	800	10	8	55
	19–24	58	128	164	65	46	800	10	8	60
	25–50	63	138	163	64	50	800	5	8	65
	51+	65	143	160	63	50	800	5	8	65
Pregnant						60	800	10	10	65
Lactating	1st 6 months					65	1,300	10	12	65
	2nd 6 months					62	1,200	10	11	65

[a]The allowances, expressed as average daily intakes over time, are intended to provide for individual variations among most normal persons as they live in the United States under usual environmental stresses. Diets should be based on a variety of common foods in order to provide other nutrients for which human requirements have been less well defined.

[b]The use of these figures does not imply that the height-to-weight ratios are ideal.

[c]RE = retinol equivalents. One RE = 1 mcg retinol or 6 mcg beta-carotene. One IU = 0.3 mcg retinol or 0.6 mcg beta-carotene.

[d]As cholecalciferol; 10 mcg cholecalciferol = 400 IU of vitamin D.

Continued on next page

223

TABLE 1 *continued*

Category	Age (y) or condition	Weight[b] (kg)	(lb)	Height[b] (cm)	(in)	Water-soluble vitamins Vita-min C (mg)	Thia-mine (B$_1$) (mg)	Ribo-flavin (B$_2$) (mg)	Nia-cin (B$_3$) (mg NE)[f]	Pyridoxine (vitamin B$_6$) (mg)	Folic acid (folate) (mcg)	Cyano-cobalamin (vitamin B$_{12}$) (mcg)
Infants	0.0–0.5	6	13	60	24	30	0.3	0.4	5	0.3	25	0.3
	0.5–1.0	9	20	71	28	35	0.4	0.5	6	0.6	35	0.5
Children	1–3	13	29	90	35	40	0.7	0.8	9	1.0	50	0.7
	4–6	20	44	112	44	45	0.9	1.1	12	1.1	75	1.0
	7–10	28	62	132	52	45	1.0	1.2	13	1.4	100	1.4
Males	11–14	45	99	157	62	50	1.3	1.5	17	1.7	150	2.0
	15–18	66	145	176	69	60	1.5	1.8	20	2.0	200	2.0
	19–24	72	160	177	70	60	1.5	1.7	19	2.0	200	2.0
	25–50	79	174	176	70	60	1.5	1.7	19	2.0	200	2.0
	51+	77	170	173	68	60	1.2	1.4	15	2.0	200	2.0
Females	11–14	46	101	157	62	50	1.1	1.3	15	1.4	150	2.0
	15–18	55	120	163	64	60	1.1	1.3	15	1.5	180	2.0
	19–24	58	128	164	65	60	1.1	1.3	15	1.6	180	2.0
	25–50	63	138	163	64	60	1.1	1.3	15	1.6	180	2.0
	51+	65	143	160	63	60	1.0	1.2	13	1.6	180	2.0
Pregnant						70	1.5	1.6	17	2.2	400	2.2
Lactating	1st 6 months					95	1.6	1.8	20	2.1	280	2.6
	2nd 6 months					90	1.6	1.7	20	2.1	260	2.6

[e] α-TE = alpha-tocopherol equivalents. 1 mg *d*-alpha-tocopherol = 1 mg α-TE = 1.49 IU.

[f] NE = niacin equivalent, equal to 1 mg of niacin or 60 mg of dietary tryptophan.

TABLE 1 *continued*

Category	Age (y) or condition	Weight (kg)	Weight (lb)	Height (cm)	Height (in)	Calcium (mg)	Phosphorus (mg)	Magnesium (mg)	Iron (mg)	Zinc (mg)	Iodine (mcg)	Selenium (mcg)
Infants	0.0–0.5	6	13	60	24	400	300	40	6	5	40	10
	0.5–1.0	9	20	71	28	600	500	60	10	5	50	15
Children	1–3	13	29	90	35	800	800	80	10	10	70	20
	4–6	20	44	112	44	800	800	120	10	10	90	20
	7–10	28	62	132	52	800	800	170	10	10	120	30
Males	11–14	45	99	157	62	1,200	1,200	270	12	15	150	40
	15–18	66	145	176	69	1,200	1,200	400	12	15	150	50
	19–24	72	160	177	70	1,200	1,200	350	10	15	150	70
	25–50	79	174	176	70	800	800	350	10	15	150	70
	51+	77	170	173	68	800	800	350	10	15	150	70
Females	11–14	46	101	157	62	1,200	1,200	280	15	12	150	45
	15–18	55	120	163	64	1,200	1,200	300	15	12	150	50
	19–24	58	128	164	65	1,200	1,200	280	15	12	150	55
	25–50	63	138	163	64	800	800	280	15	12	150	55
	51+	65	143	160	63	800	800	280	10	12	150	55
Pregnant						1,200	1,200	320	30	15	175	65
Lactating	1st 6 months					1,200	1,200	355	15	19	200	75
	2nd 6 months					1,200	1,200	340	15	16	200	75

Adapted with permission from Food and Nutrition Board, National Research Council–National Academy of Sciences. *Recommended Dietary Allowances.* 10th ed. Washington, DC: National Academy Press; 1989.

TABLE 2 Estimated safe and adequate daily dietary intakes of selected vitamins and minerals[a]

Category	Age (y)	Vitamins		Trace elements[b]				
		Biotin (mcg)	Panto-thenic acid (mg)	Copper (mg)	Manganese (mg)	Fluoride (mg)	Chromium (mcg)	Molybdenum (mcg)
Infants	0–0.5	10	3	0.4–0.6	0.3–0.6	0.1–0.5	10–40	15–30
	0.5–1	15	3	0.6–0.7	0.6–1.0	0.2–1.0	20–60	20–40
Children	1–3	20	3	0.7–1.0	1.0–1.5	0.5–1.5	20–80	25–50
and	4–6	25	3–4	1.0–1.5	1.5–2.0	1.0–2.5	30–120	30–75
adolescents	7–10	30	4–5	1.0–2.0	2.0–3.0	1.5–2.5	50–200	50–150
	11+	30–100	4–7	1.5–2.5	2.0–5.0	1.5–2.5	50–200	75–250
Adults		30–100	4–7	1.5–3.0	2.0–5.0	1.5–4.0	50–200	75–250

[a]Because there is less information on which to base allowances, these figures are not given in Table 1 and are provided here in the form of ranges of recommended intakes.

[b]Because the toxic levels for many trace elements may be only several times the usual intakes, the upper levels for the trace elements given in the table should not be habitually exceeded.

Adapted with permission from Food and Nutrition Board, National Research Council–National Academy of Sciences. *Recommended Dietary Allowances.* 10th ed. Washington, DC: National Academy Press; 1989: 284.

Lack of knowledge prevents RDAs from being set for all known nutrients. Further, the application of RDAs to individuals may require adjustment owing to climate, strenuous physical activity, or the presence of a disease state.

The FDA publishes a less comprehensive set of values to be used for labeling purposes. These values, formerly known as the US recommended daily allowances (US RDAs), appear in Table 3.

Malnutrition

The primary causes of malnutrition include starvation, disease-related factors, eating disorders, alcoholism, and food faddism. Because of pathophysiologic, physiologic, behavioral, or economic situations, certain segments of the population are predisposed to vitamin deficiencies:

- Iatrogenic situations: for example, oral contraceptive and estrogen users, patients on prolonged broad-spectrum antibiotics or parenteral nutrition;
- Inadequate dietary intake: for example, alcoholics, the impoverished, the aged, patients on severe calorie-restricted diets or fad diets, or patients with eating disorders;

TABLE 3   US recommended daily allowances (US RDAs) for labeling purposes

	Unit	Infants	Children under age 4	Adults and children aged 4 or older	Pregnant and lactating women
Vitamin A	IU	1,500	2,500	5,000	8,000
Vitamin D	IU	400	400	400	400
Vitamin E	IU	5	10	30	30
Ascorbic acid	mg	35	40	60	60
Folic acid	mg	0.1	0.2	0.4	0.8
Thiamine	mg	0.5	0.7	1.5	1.7
Riboflavin	mg	0.6	0.8	1.7	2.0
Niacin	mg	8	9	20	20
Pyridoxine	mg	0.4	0.7	2	2.5
Cyanocobalamin	mcg	2	3	6	8
Biotin	mg	0.05	0.15	0.3	0.3
Pantothenic acid	mg	3	5	10	10
Calcium	g	0.6	0.8	1.0	1.3
Phosphorus	g	0.5	0.8	1.0	1.3
Iodine	mcg	45	70	150	150
Iron	mg	15	10	18	18
Magnesium	mg	70	200	400	450
Manganese[a]	mg	0.5	1.0	4.0	4.0
Copper	mg	0.6	1.0	2.0	2.0
Zinc	mg	5	8	15	15
Protein	g	—	20(28)[b]	45(65)[b]	—

[a]Proposed US reference daily intake (RDI).

[b]Values in parentheses are US RDIs when the protein efficiency ratio (PER) is less than that of casein; the other values are used when the PER is equal to or greater than that of casein. No claim may be made for a protein with a PER equal to or less than 20% that of casein.

- Increased metabolic requirements: for example, pregnant or lactating women; women of childbearing age who have regular menstrual blood loss; infants; children undergoing periods of accelerated growth; or patients with major surgery, cancer, severe injury, infection, or trauma;
- Poor absorption: for example, the aged; or patients with such conditions as prolonged diarrhea, severe gastrointestinal (GI) disorders or malignancy, surgical removal of a section of the GI tract, celiac disease, obstructive jaundice, or cystic fibrosis.

Nutritional Assessment

Assessment of nutritional status is difficult in the ambulatory environment. Only severe dietary deficiencies are likely to be reflected physically. For example, a patient's fingernails may lose their luster and become dark at the upper ends. Hair, eyes, mouth, or teeth may reflect nutritional status. Visible goiter, poor skin color and texture, obesity or thinness relative to bone structure, and edema may also be indications of malnutrition. The pharmacist should be able to recognize overt but nonspecific symptoms of vitamin and mineral deficiencies where prompt physician referral may be crucial. Just as nutritional deficiencies may lead to disease, disease may lead to nutritional deficiencies.

The Pharmacist's Role in Vitamin and Mineral Use

Pharmacists should know which population groups tend to be poorly nourished, should exercise good observational skills, and should know which questions yield helpful information. The more specific the information obtained from the patient, the more helpful the pharmacist can be in determining the need for nutritional supplementation.

The average American consuming an average diet does not need vitamin supplementation. Prolonged ingestion of vitamins has not been tested for safety; and some vitamins, such as A, D, niacin, and pyridoxine, are known to be toxic in high doses. Thus, patients should be cautioned against initiating high-dose self-medication with vitamins.

Patients inquiring about vitamin product claims should be educated about the increased potential risk of the nontraditional use of vitamins (e.g., potential adverse effects from alternative doses, drug interactions with prescription or nonprescription drug products).

Multivitamin Therapy

In general, an inexpensive supplemental preparation that supplies close to 100% of the RDA for each vitamin will meet the needs of most patients requiring or desiring supplements.

"Natural" Vitamins

The body cannot distinguish between a vitamin molecule derived from a synthetic source and one derived from a natural source, and synthetic vitamins are absorbed to the same extent as the more expensive natural vitamins.

Fat-Soluble Vitamins

Vitamins A, D, E, and K are the fat-soluble vitamins. These vitamins are stored in body tissues, and when excessive quantities or megadoses are ingested, they may be toxic. Deficiencies of these vitamins occur when fat intake is limited or fat absorption is compromised. Drugs that affect lipid absorption (e.g., cholestyramine, mineral oil) may precipitate such a deficiency. Table 4 lists the food sources, causes of deficiency, signs and symptoms of deficiency, adverse effects of large doses, and drug interactions of the fat-soluble vitamins.

Vitamin A

The designation "vitamin A" refers to a group of compounds essential for vision, growth, reproduction, cellular differentiation and proliferation, and integrity of the immune system.

Vitamin D (Calciferol)

Vitamin D, which has properties of both hormones and vitamins, is necessary for the proper formation of the skeleton and for mineral homeostasis. It is closely involved with parathyroid hormone, phosphate, and calcitonin in the homeostasis of serum calcium.

Vitamin E (Tocopherol)

Vitamin E is present in all cell membranes. It functions primarily as an antioxidant in protecting cellular membranes from oxidative damage. Alpha-tocopherol is the most active of the vitamin E compounds.

Vitamin K

Phytonadione (vitamin K_1) is present in many vegetables. Menaquinone (vitamin K_2) is a product of bacterial metabolism (in the colon). Menadione (vitamin K_3) is a more potent, synthetic compound. Factors II (prothrombin), VII, IX, and X of the plasma clotting cascade depend on vitamin K for hepatic synthesis.

Water-Soluble Vitamins

Ascorbic Acid (Vitamin C)

Ascorbic acid protects the capillary basement membrane, is necessary to form collagen, and serves as an antioxidant.

Ascorbic acid has been promoted for prevention of the common cold and for attenuation of symptoms should a cold occur, but these claims are largely unsupported.

Detailed information on ascorbic acid and water-soluble vitamins appears in Table 5. Recommended doses and RDAs of ascorbic acid appear in Tables 1 and 3.

Cyanocobalamin (Vitamin B_{12})

The term "vitamin B_{12}" refers to all cobalamins that have vitamin activity in humans. Vitamin B_{12} is active in all cells, especially those in the bone marrow, the central nervous system (CNS), and the GI tract. It is involved in fat, protein, and carbohydrate metabolism. Vitamin B_{12} is produced almost exclusively by microorganisms, which accounts for its presence in animal protein. Because vitamin B_{12} is conserved by the body, it requires approximately 3 years for a deficiency to develop; however, it may occur much earlier in patients with malabsorption.

Vegetarians who consume no animal products are at risk for developing a vitamin B_{12} deficiency. They should consider taking vitamin B_{12} supplements or adjust their diet to include fermented foods, such as soy sauce, that contain the vitamin.

Folic Acid (Pteroylglutamic Acid, Folacin)

The function of folic acid is closely related to that of vitamin B_{12}. A folic acid deficiency can occur as a consequence of a vitamin B_{12} deficiency. Folates are present in nearly all natural foods. The diet should include some foods that require little cooking because folates are heat labile.

Increased amounts of folic acid are needed during pregnancy, lactation, and infancy, as well as for infection, hemolytic anemias and blood loss. Because of the potential for folic acid to mask the signs of pernicious anemia, which is caused by a vitamin B_{12} deficiency, products containing more than 0.8 mg of folic acid per dose are available only by

TABLE 4 Fat-soluble vitamins

Vitamin	Food sources	Causes of deficiency	Signs and symptoms of deficiency	Adverse effects of large doses*	Drug interactions**
Vitamin A	Fish, butter, cream, eggs, milk, organ meats, carrots, squash, pumpkin, dark leafy vegetables	Excessive excretion of vitamin A due to cancer, tuberculosis, pneumonia, chronic nephritis, urinary tract infections or prostate disease; OR impairment of vitamin A absorption due to celiac disease, short-gut syndrome, obstructive jaundice, cystic fibrosis, or liver cirrhosis	Night blindness, abnormal conjunctival dryness, photophobia, other ocular changes; permanent vision loss if deficiency is not corrected; drying and hyperkeratinization of the skin	Hypervitaminosis A; headache, diplopia, nausea, vomiting, vertigo, hypercalcemia, drowsiness, fatigue, malaise; teratogenic risk at doses above RDA	Large doses increase hypoprothrombinemic effect of warfarin; oral contraceptives increase vitamin A plasma levels
Vitamin D	Milk and milk products, eggs, animal livers, fish, beef	Dietary; GI disorder (hepatobiliary disease, malabsorption, chronic pancreatitis); acidosis; chronic renal failure; hereditary disorders of vitamin D metabolism; phosphate depletion; renal tubular disorders; poisoning from lead, cadmium, or outdated tetracycline; prolonged parenteral nutrition without vitamin D supplementation	Calcium abnormalities associated with bone formation (rickets, osteomalacia, bone fracture); inhibition of growth in infants; tetany (due to insufficient calcium in muscle tissue); liver disease; myopathy (due to decreased muscle phosphate)	Anorexia, nausea, weakness, weight loss, polyuria, constipation, vague aches, stiffness, soft-tissue calcification, hypercalcemia, hypercalciuria, kidney stones, renal failure, hypertension, anemia	Phosphate lowers calcium level and contributes to vitamin D deficiency; phenytoin or barbiturates may decrease the half-life of vitamin D; magnesium-containing antacids should be avoided in patients with severe renal disease
Vitamin E	Vegetable oils, margarine made from plant oils, green vegetables, nuts, wheat germ, whole grains	Abnormal fat absorption (e.g., in patients with cystic fibrosis); may occur in premature, very-low-birth-weight infants	Premature infants: edema, hemolytic anemia, reticulocytosis, thrombocytosis Adults: reproductive failure, neurologic abnormalities	Relatively nontoxic, even in doses up to 1000 IU/day; hazards of long-term, high dose therapy unknown	May enhance warfarin anticoagulation
Vitamin K	Pork liver, spinach, kale, cabbage, cauliflower	Factors that interfere with bile production or secretion; malabsorption syndromes; bowel resection; breast-feeding; regional enteritis; blind loop syndrome; ulcerative colitis; chronic, broad-spectrum antibiotic therapy	Defective blood coagulation with hemorrhage	None Menadione may cause hemolytic anemia, hyperbilirubinemia, and kernicterus in newborns due to interaction with sulfhydryl groups	Oral anticoagulants are antagonists of vitamin K; broad-spectrum antibiotic therapy may initiate vitamin K deficiency by decreasing gut flora if dietary intake is inadequate; large quantities of vitamins A and E may interfere with vitamin K absorption or metabolism

* Doses several times the RDA.
** Cholestyramine and mineral oil may decrease the absorption of all fat-soluble vitamins.

TABLE 5 Water-soluble vitamins

Vitamin	Food sources	Causes of deficiency	Signs and symptoms of deficiency	Adverse effects of large doses	Drug interactions
Ascorbic acid (Vitamin C)	Green and red peppers, collard greens, broccoli, spinach, tomatoes, potatoes, strawberries, citrus fruits, meats, fish, poultry, eggs, dairy products	Dietary	Malaise, weakness, capillary hemorrhages and petechiae, hyperkeratotic follicles (corkscrew hairs), swollen hemorrhagic gums, bone changes, impaired wound healing Scurvy may develop with profound deficiency	Rare Nephrolithiasis; hemolysis in G6PD-deficient patients	May increase serum levels of estrogens; may reduce anticoagulant action of warfarin; large quantities in the urine interfere with urine glucose tests; megadoses may cause crystalluria with acidic drugs (e.g., sulfonamides) or more rapid excretion of basic drugs (e.g., tricyclic antidepressants, amphetamines); concomitant administration with cholestyramine decreases absorption of vitamin C and activity of the cholestyramine
Cyanocobalamin (Vitamin B₁₂)	Meats, oysters, clams	Poor absorption or utilization; increased requirement or excretion of this vitamin; vegetarian diet	Mimic those of folate deficiency Macrocytic anemia, glossitis, paresthesia, unsteadiness, poor muscular coordination, mental confusion, agitation, hallucinations, overt psychosis	None reported	Neomycin may impair cyanocobalamin absorption
Folic acid	Liver, lean beef, veal, yeast, leafy vegetables, legumes, some fruits, eggs, whole-grain cereals	Alcoholism, malabsorption, food faddism, liver disease, various therapeutic agents	Similar to those of cyanocobalamin deficiency (see above); most common feature is megaloblastic anemia	None reported	Phenytoin may inhibit folic acid absorption; folic acid may decrease serum phenytoin levels; pyrimethamine and methotrexate are folic acid antagonists
Niacin	Lean meats, fish, liver, cold cereals, whole grains, green vegetables, legumes	Dietary; most often occurs in alcoholics, poorly nourished elderly persons, and individuals on bizarre diets	Dermatitis, diarrhea, dementia (the "3 Ds"); also neuropathy, glossitis, stomatitis, proctitis, characteristic rash	Nausea, vomiting, diarrhea, hepatotoxicity, skin lesions, tachycardia, hypertension, flushing or burning sensations, hyperuricemia	Nothing reported

Continued on next page

TABLE 5 *continued*

Vitamin	Food sources	Causes of deficiency	Signs and symptoms of deficiency	Adverse effects of large doses	Drug interactions
Pantothenic acid	Meats, liver, milk, eggs, vegetables, cereal grains, legumes	Malabsorption syndromes	Somnolence, fatigue, headache, paresthesia, hyperreflexia and muscular weakness in the legs, cardiovascular instability, GI complaints, changes in disposition, increased susceptibility to infection	Generally nontoxic Ingestion of >20 g has resulted in diarrhea and water retention Dexpanthenol may prolong bleeding time in hemophiliacs	Nothing reported
Pyridoxine (Vitamin B$_6$)	Meats, cereals, lentils, nuts, bananas, avocados, potatoes	Alcoholism, severe diarrheal syndromes, food faddism, drugs (isoniazid, hydralazine, penicillamine, cyclo-serine), malabsorption syndromes, genetic diseases (cystathi-oninuria and xanthinuric aciduria)	Infants: convulsive disorders, irritability Adults: pellagralike dermatitis; scaliness around the nose, mouth and eyes; oral lesions; peripheral neuropathy; dulling of mentation; convulsions; peripheral neuritis; sideroblastic anemia	Sensory neuropathy; prolactin inhibition	Pyridoxine deficiency may be caused by: isoniazid, cyclos-erine, hydralazine, penicilla-mine, oral contraceptives Pyridoxine may reduce serum levels of phenobarbital and phenytoin, or antagonize therapeutic action of levodopa (but not the combination of levodopa/carbidopa)
Riboflavin (Vitamin B$_2$)	Meats, poultry, fish, green vegetables, dairy products, enriched and fortified grains, cereals, and bakery products	Inadequate diet Marginal deficiencies detected in alcoholics, vegetarians, and women taking oral contracep-tives	Ocular symptoms (eyes are light-sensitive or easily fatigued; blurry vision; itching, watery, sore eyes; bloodshot appearance) Later signs: stomatitis, glossitis, seborrheic dermatitis, magenta tongue	A harmless yellow-orange fluorescence or discolora-tion of the urine	Nothing reported
Thiamine (Vitamin B$_1$)	Hull of rice grains, pork, beef, fresh peas, beans	Inadequate diet, alcoholism, malabsorp-tion syndromes, prolonged diarrhea, pregnancy, food faddism	Peripheral neuropathy, cardiac dysfunction, tachycardia, pain in precordial or epigastric areas, paresthesia of the extremities, weakness, atrophy Severe or prolonged deficiency may result in beriberi (includes Wernicke's encephalopathy and Korsakoff's psychosis)	Large parenteral doses may result in itching, tingling and pain; anaphylactic reactions rare, but possible	Nothing reported

prescription. Pharmacists should refer all patients with suspected anemias for medical consultation.

Niacin (Nicotinic Acid)

Niacin and niacinamide are constituents of the coenzymes that serve as electron transfer agents in the aerobic respiration of body cells. Niacin is unusual as a vitamin in that humans can synthesize it from dietary tryptophan. About 60 mg of tryptophan are equivalent to 1 mg of niacin.

The classic niacin deficiency state is pellagra, which involves dermatitis, diarrhea, dementia, and neurologic changes (e.g., mild tremor, depression, peripheral neuropathy). The characteristic rash in niacin-deficient patients develops on the face and on pressure points. The skin becomes thickened and hyperpigmented or may appear burned.

Niacin requirements are increased during acute illness; during convalescence after a severe injury, infection, or burns; when caloric expenditure or dietary caloric intake is substantially increased; or when the patient has a low tryptophan intake. Treatment of pellagra involves the ingestion of 300–500 mg of niacinamide daily in divided doses. Because other nutritional deficiencies may be present, treatment may include the other B vitamins, vitamin A, and iron. Niacin has been used in daily dosages of 1 to 2 g three times per day, up to 8 g per day, to treat hypercholesterolemia and hyperlipidemia.

Because of the adverse effects on the GI tract, high doses of niacin are contraindicated in patients with gastritis or peptic ulcer disease. Use in patients with asthma should be undertaken carefully because niacin may provoke histamine release.

Patients should be forewarned that niacin may cause flushing and a sensation of warmth, especially around the face, neck, and ears, as well as itching, tingling, and headache. This reaction may be diminished if they take 325 mg of aspirin or 200 mg of ibuprofen 30 minutes before the niacin dose. These effects usually decrease with continued therapy. If niacin causes GI upset, it should be taken with meals.

Niacinamide does not produce the discomforting flushing associated with therapeutic doses of niacin; however, it also does not have a beneficial lowering effect on plasma lipids.

Pantothenic Acid

Pantothenic acid is a precursor of coenzyme A (CoA), a product that is active in many biologic reactions and that plays a primary role in cholesterol, steroid, and fatty acid synthesis. Deficiency states are rare. It is difficult to separate pantothenic acid deficiency symptoms from symptoms of other deficiencies. A safe and adequate daily intake for adults is 4–7 mg.

Pyridoxine (Vitamin B$_6$)

Pyridoxine is a cofactor for more than 60 enzymes. It exists in three forms: pyridoxine (vitamin B$_6$), pyridoxal, and pyridoxamine. The average US diet provides slightly less than the RDA. Infant formulas are required to contain pyridoxine hydrochloride.

Symptoms of pyridoxine deficiency in adults are difficult to distinguish from those of niacin and riboflavin deficiencies.

Treatment of sideroblastic anemia requires 50–200 mg per day of pyridoxine hydrochloride to aid in the production of hemoglobin and erythrocytes. Several pyridoxine-dependent inborn errors of metabolism respond to high doses of pyridoxine.

A pyridoxine dose of 50 mg/day with isoniazid, or a dose of 20 mg per day with cycloserine, is recommended to overcome isoniazid- or cycloserine-induced pyridoxine antagonism, which might otherwise result in peripheral neuropathy. A depressive syndrome occasionally experienced by women taking oral contraceptives has responded to daily pyridoxine supplementation of 20–100 mg.

Riboflavin (Vitamin B$_2$)

Riboflavin is involved in numerous oxidation and reduction reactions, including the cytochrome P-450 reductase enzyme system involved in drug metabolism.

Thiamine (Vitamin B$_1$)

Thiamine is necessary for several functions in carbohydrate metabolism and in neurologic function. Symptoms of thiamine deficiency may become evident in 3 weeks after thiamine intake is stopped. The amount of vitamin required increases with increased caloric consumption. Several genetic diseases, all classified as vitamin-responsible inborn errors of metabolism, respond to the administration of thiamine.

Thiamine deficiency is common among alcoholics. High-dose, parenteral thiamine is commonly given to patients who are admitted to hospitals for alcohol detoxification and treatment. A vitamin supplement containing thiamine is often prescribed for the alcoholic patient.

Vitamin-Like Compounds and Pseudovitamins

Bioflavonoids (Vitamin P)

These flavonoids are widely distributed in plants and are concentrated in the skin, peel, and outer layers of fruits and vegetables. Bioflavonoids have no accepted preventive or therapeutic role in human nutrition.

Biotin (Vitamin H)

Biotin is a member of the B-complex group of vitamins. It plays an important role in fat, amino acid, and carbohydrate metabolism. Sources include liver, egg yolk, cauliflower, salmon, carrots, bananas, soy flour, and yeast.

Deficiency states of biotin are rare but have been associated with nausea, vomiting, lassitude, muscle pain, anorexia, anemia, and depression. Dermatitis, a grayish color of the skin, and glossitis may be among the physical findings. Individuals undergoing a rapid weight loss program with intense caloric restriction may not be obtaining adequate biotin and should receive supplementation. No RDA has been determined for biotin; however, 100–200 mcg per day is generally considered safe and adequate. Side effects and drug interactions have not been reported.

L-Carnitine (DL-Carnitine)

A number of actions are attributed to carnitine. It is required to transport long-chain fatty acids in mitochondria, which is prerequisite to their beta oxidation and to maintenance of energy production. Food sources include dairy products and meat, especially red meat. Newborns have a low capacity for carnitine synthesis.

Carnitine deficiency may be evidenced by muscle weakness, cardiomyopathy, abnormal hepatic function, decreased ketogenesis, and hypoglycemia during fasting. No RDA has been established. Therapy should include a pharmaceutical supplement and a high-carbohydrate, low-fat diet. L-Carnitine is without appreciable adverse effects in normal adults.

Choline

Choline is contained in most living cells. It is a precursor in the biosynthesis of acetylcholine. Although choline is found in egg yolks, cereal, fish, and meat, it is also synthesized in the body. Choline is obtained from the diet as either choline or lecithin. A deficiency state has not been identified in humans.

An average diet will furnish 200–600 mg of choline daily. Most adults tolerate up to 20 g per day with no adverse effects.

Essential Fatty Acids (Vitamin F)

The essential fatty acids are involved in the development of various biomembranes. The typical Western diet, with its heavy polyunsaturated fat and oil content, provides ample essential fatty acids.

Linoleic and linolenic acids are essential in human nutrition. Linoleic acid deficiency symptoms include scaly skin, hair loss, and impaired wound healing.

Inositol

Inositol is widely distributed in nature and is synthesized in the body. It is found in fruits, vegetables, whole grains, meats, and milk. A normal dietary intake is approximately 1 g per day. The value of inositol in human nutrition has not been established.

Laetrile (Amygdalin, Vitamin B_{17})

Laetrile occurs naturally in almond, apricot, and peach pits and in apple seeds. It consists of 6% cyanide by weight. When spelled with a small "l", it refers to amygdalin, marketed by its promoters as a cancer cure and a synonym for cyanogenetic glycosides. Many toxic reactions have been reported worldwide with the ingestion of cyanogenetic glycosides; cyanide poisoning has occurred with some laetrile products.

Although it is called vitamin B_{17}, laetrile contains no vitamin activity and has no nutritional or therapeutic value and no approved medical use. Use may lead to critical delays in seeking and receiving appropriate medical attention.

Taurine (Aminoethanesulfonate)

Taurine is included in human infant formulas, enteral products, and some parenteral nutritional solutions. It is important in many metabolic activities and is normally biosynthesized in adequate amounts. No RDA has been established.

Minerals

Minerals constitute about 4% of body weight. Different body tissues contain different quantities of different elements. For example, bone has a high content of calcium, phosphorus, and magnesium; soft tissue has a higher quantity of potassium. Minerals function as constituents of enzymes, hormones, and vitamins.

A well-balanced diet is required to maintain proper mineral balance. Calcium and iron are two elements that may require particular dietary attention from normal individuals. Optimal mineral intake values for humans are still imprecise, and only estimated ranges are available for some minerals.

Mineral deficiency is often difficult to evaluate. Hair analysis has received attention in recent years, and its noninvasiveness is advantageous.

Calcium

Calcium is a major component of bones and teeth. The calcium content in bone is continuously undergoing resorption and formation. In elderly people, resorption predominates over formation, and a decrease in calcium absorption efficiency results in a gradual loss of bone (osteoporosis).

Rich dietary sources of calcium include milk and other dairy products. Teenagers experiencing rapid growth and bone maturation need to consume adequate calcium via dairy products, especially milk, or nutritional supplements in tablet or capsule form. Adults can meet calcium RDA levels by incorporating dairy products into their diets.

Consequences of decreased calcium levels include convulsions, tetany, behavioral and personality disorders, mental and growth retardation, and bone deformities, the most common of which are rickets in children and osteomalacia in adults.

Causes of hypocalcemia include malabsorption syndromes, hypoparathyroidism, vitamin D deficiency, long-term anticonvulsant therapy, and decreased dietary intake of calcium, especially during growth periods, pregnancy, and lactation and in the elderly. Some suggest that, for women, about 1100 mg per day before menopause and 1500 mg per day after menopause is advantageous; during pregnancy and lactation, 1200 mg per day is recommended. Weight-bearing exercise is also important in maintaining bone mass.

Calcium in doses greater than 2 g per day can lead to high levels of calcium in the urine and to renal stones. Hypercalcemia is associated with anorexia, nausea, vomiting, constipation, and polyuria. High calcium intake levels may inhibit the absorption of iron, zinc, and other essential minerals. Corticosteroids inhibit calcium absorption from the gut and may cause increased bone fractures and osteoporosis. Excessive ingestion of aluminum-containing antacids may result in negative calcium balances. Phosphates, calcitonin, sodium sulfate, furosemide, magnesium, cholestyramine, estrogen, and some anticonvulsants also lower calcium serum levels. Thiazide diuretics increase serum calcium levels.

Iron

Iron is widely available in the US diet. It plays an important role in oxygen and electron transport.

Dietary iron is available in two forms. Heme iron is found in meats and is reasonably well absorbed. Nonheme iron constitutes most of the dietary iron and is poorly absorbed. Therefore, the published values of the iron content of foods are misleading because the amount absorbed depends on the nature of the iron. About 10% of the total iron content (heme plus nonheme) of foods is absorbable if no iron deficiency exists. In the iron-deficient state, about 20% is absorbed.

Iron deficiency results from inadequate diet, malabsorption, pregnancy and lactation, or blood loss. There are three stages of iron deficiency: iron depletion, iron-deficient erythropoiesis, and iron deficiency anemia. Iron deficiency anemia is the most common form of anemia in the United States. Signs of anemia include easy fatigability, weakness, lassitude, pallor, split or "spoon-shaped" nails, sore tongue, angular stomatitis, dyspnea on exertion, palpitation, and a feeling of exhaustion. Coldness and numbness of the extremities may be reported. Small red blood cells and low hemoglobin concentrations (hypochromic, microcytic anemia) characterize iron deficiency.

Iron deficiency remains a problem for certain segments of the population, especially children in poverty and menstruating and pregnant women. Iron supplements are recommended as a component of prenatal care. The four life periods when iron deficiency is most common are from 6 months to 4 years of age, during early adolescence, during the female reproductive years, and during and after pregnancy. The donation of 500 mL (1 pint or unit) of blood produces a loss of approximately 250 mg of iron. This is not a significant problem in healthy, well-nourished adults with adequate iron stores, but those who donate frequently may benefit from short-term iron replacement following blood donation.

Chronic use of drugs such as salicylates, nonsteroidal anti-inflammatory drugs, reserpine, corticosteroids, warfarin, ulcerogenic drugs, antiprothrombinemic drugs, or most drugs used to treat neoplasms might indicate drug-induced blood loss. The differential diagnosis in adults should rule out iron deficiency owing to excess blood loss associated with peptic ulcer disease, hemorrhoids, inflammatory bowel disease, esophageal varices, diverticulitis, intestinal parasites, regional enteritis, or cancer.

A patient who reports blood loss should be referred to a physician immediately. Abnormal blood loss may be indicated by (1) vomiting blood; (2) bright red blood in the stool or black, tarry stools; (3) large clots or an abnormally heavy flow during the menstrual period; or (4) cloudy or pink-red urine (assuming that dyes in drugs that may cause urine discoloration have been ruled out). Blood loss through the stool is not always obvious. Periodic testing using home occult blood test kits may be considered for certain high-risk or at-risk patients.

Most healthy individuals who self-medicate, including menstruating females, will absorb adequate iron from one 325-mg ferrous sulfate tablet (containing 60 mg of elemental iron) per day. The usual therapeutic dose of two to four tablets daily for 3 months is probably reasonable in treating a deficiency. If the patient has an inadequate response after this period, a physician should be consulted.

If iron supplementation is appropriate, the product choice should be based on how well the iron preparation is absorbed and tolerated as well as on its price. Because ferrous salts are more efficiently absorbed than ferric salts, an iron product of the ferrous group is usually appropriate. Ferrous sulfate is the standard against which other iron salts are compared. Ferrous citrate, ferrous tartrate, ferrous pyrophosphate, and some ferric salts are not well absorbed.

Ferrous salts may be given in combination with ascorbic acid to increase absorption; the ratio should be 200 mg of ascorbic acid to 30 mg of elemental iron.

The enteric-coated and delayed-release products are generally more expensive but may cause fewer symptoms of gastric irritation. However, overall iron absorption is decreased by delaying the time of release.

All iron products tend to irritate the GI mucosa and may produce nausea, abdominal pain, and diarrhea. These effects may be minimized by reducing the dose or giving iron with meals. However, food may decrease the amount of iron absorbed by as much as 50%.

Constipation is a frequent side effect of iron therapy. This has prompted the formulation of iron products that also contain a stool softener (e.g., docusate).

During iron therapy, stools may become black and tarry. Black, tarry stools may also indicate GI blood loss and a serious GI problem. Medical referral is indicated if an underlying GI condition is suspected or if the patient has a history of GI disease.

Accidental poisoning is a life-threatening medical emergency. As few as 15 325-mg ferrous sulfate tablets have been lethal to children. The clinical outcome depends on the speed and accuracy of treatment. Treatment of iron toxicity may begin immediately at home by giving ipecac syrup to induce vomiting.

Iron is chelated by many substances. Its interaction with antacids may be clinically significant. Iron appears to chelate with several of the tetracyclines, resulting in decreased tetracycline and iron absorption. Patients should take tetracycline 3 hours after or 2 hours before iron administration. Allopurinol should not be given with iron unless recommended by a physician.

Magnesium

Magnesium is required for normal bone structure formation and the proper functioning of more than 300 enzymes. Extracellular magnesium is critical to the maintenance of nerve and muscle electrical potentials.

All unprocessed foods contain magnesium. Vegetables and whole seeds such as nuts, legumes, and unmilled grains are good sources of magnesium.

Deficiency states are usually due to GI tract abnormalities, renal dysfunction, general malnutrition, alcoholism, and iatrogenic causes. Magnesium deficiencies are rarely noted in the normal adult population. Deficiencies have been observed, however, in individuals with alcoholism, diabetes, chronic diarrhea, and renal tubular damage.

Hypermagnesemia is characterized by muscle weakness, CNS depression, diarrhea, hypotension, bradycardia, and confusion. It can occur with overzealous use of magnesium sulfate (epsom salts) or magnesium hydroxide (milk of magnesia) as a laxative, or even with use of magnesium-containing antacids in patients with severe renal failure.

Phosphorus

Phosphorus is essential for many metabolic processes. There is a reciprocal relationship between calcium and phosphorus; when serum calcium is high, serum phosphate is generally low, and vice versa. Phosphorus is present in nearly all foods, especially protein-rich foods and cereal grains.

Because nearly all foods contain phosphorus, deficiency states do not usually occur unless induced. For example, patients receiving aluminum hydroxide as an antacid for prolonged periods may exhibit weakness, anorexia, malaise, pain, and bone loss. This is because aluminum hydroxide binds phosphorus, making it unavailable for absorption.

Trace Elements

Trace elements (Table 6) are considered essential for numerous physiologic processes. "Ultratrace minerals" have been defined as those elements with an estimated dietary requirement of usually less than 1 mg per day; these include arsenic (E), boron (E), bromine (NE), cadmium (NE), chromium (E), fluorine (NE), lead (NE), lithium (PE), molybdenum (E), nickel (E), selenium (E), silicon (E), tin (NE), and vanadium (PE). The designation "E" represents essential, "PE" means probably essential but further study is required, and "NE" means not essential because the evidence for its necessity is inadequate.

Nutritional Supplements

Supplemental nutritional products should be used as adjuncts to a regular diet, not as substitutes for food. The pharmacist should consult a dietitian or physician concerning nutritional supplementation and refer patients when necessary.

Patients purchasing a nonprescription dietary supplement should be instructed on its proper use and storage, including dilution and preparation techniques (see product table "Enteral Food Supplement Products" in *Nonprescription Products: Formulations & Features*). In addition, the pharmacist should discuss possible adverse effects such as diarrhea.

Enteral Nutrition

Enteral nutrition is the provision of liquid nutrients by tube or by mouth into the GI tract. It is being increasingly used for nutritional support in patients who cannot ingest or digest sufficient amounts of food. Its advantages over parenteral feeding include preservation of the structure and function of the GI tract, more efficient use of nutrients, decreased incidence of infections and metabolic complications, and reduced cost. Enteral foods are not diet foods or health food supplements and are not intended for that purpose.

There are two basic types of enteral feeding devices (tubes): those that enter the GI tract through the nose (nasogastric or nasoenteral tubes) and those that enter through the abdominal wall (gastrostomies, duodenostomies, or jejunostomies). The small diameter of nasogastric tubes often results in clogging, especially when medications are added to the enteral liquids being administered through the tubes. Gastrostomy and jejunostomy tubes, which have larger diameters, allow quicker and easier administration of medications and feeding preparations.

TABLE 6 Trace elements

Element	Dietary sources	Function	Dose/RDA	Signs and symptoms of deficiency	Adverse effects/ Drug interactions	Comments
Chromium	Liver, fish, whole grains, milk	Helps maintain normal glucose use	50–200 mcg/ day	Glucose intolerance, + circulating insulin, glyco- suria, fasting hyperglyce- mia, + serum cholesterol and triglycerides, neuro- pathy, encephalopathy	Trivalent forms nontoxic; hexavalent forms encountered through industrial exposure toxic and carcinogenic	Chromium picolinate has been promoted for cholesterol lower- ing, weight loss, increasing muscle mass, and controlling diabetes; these claims are largely unsubstantiated
Cobalt	—	Essential component of vitamin B_{12}	None established	No deficiency state reported	Goiter, myxedema, conges- tive heart failure; cyanosis and coma in children	Ingested cyanocobalamin metabolized to form the B_{12} coenzymes
Copper	Organ meats, shellfish, chocolate, whole-grain cereals, legumes, nuts	Essential for proper structure and function of the CNS; role in iron metabolism	Adults: 1.5–3 mg; Children: 0.7–2.5 mg	Impaired iron absorption with resultant hypochromic anemia	Emetic action in doses of 250 mg Large amounts of ascorbic acid impair copper absorption	Wilson's disease is an inborn error of metabolism resulting in failure to eliminate copper, resulting in CNS, kidney, and liver damage; symptoms respond to penicillamine
Fluorine	Most municipal water supplies are fluoridated to 1 ppm	Occurs in bones and tooth enamel; reduces tooth decay	See Table 2	No deficiency state reported other than tooth decay	Life-threatening toxicity: salivation, abdominal pain, nausea, vomiting, diarrhea, urticaria, muscle weakness, tremors, seizures Death has occurred after 2 g sodium fluoride in adults and 0.5 g in children Chronic toxicity manifests as changes in structure of bones and teeth	50 mg/day has been used for osteoporosis, but may have adverse effects Supplements recommended for children who consume water low in fluoride ion (e.g., well water) Nonprescription products include topical rinses; also available by prescription for topical or oral administration

Continued on next page

TABLE 6 *continued*

Element	Dietary sources	Function	Dose/RDA	Signs and symptoms of deficiency	Adverse effects/ Drug interactions	Comments
Iodine	Iodized salt, saltwater fish, shellfish	Required to synthesize thyroxine and triiodothyronine, which regulate metabolic rate of cells	See Table 1	Goiter	Hypersensitivity in some individuals Chronic intoxication (iodism): unpleasant taste and burning in mouth or throat, soreness of teeth or gums	Iodine supplements unwarranted for most individuals; content of typical diets is well above the RDA
Manganese	Vegetables, fruits, nuts, legumes, whole-grain cereals	Essential for glucose utilization, cartilage and steroid synthesis	See Table 2	Only one case of deficiency reported	Rare; may occur form inhalation of dust and industrial fumes containing manganese May reduce iron absorption	Sufficient quantities present in the average diet
Molybdenum	Milk, organ meats, beans, breads, cereals	Acts as an electron transfer agent in oxidation-reduction reactions	See Table 2	Parenteral nutrition without molybdenum may result in deficiency, which may be treated with ammonium molybdate	Goutlike symptoms; copper deficiency	Human requirement easily furnished by the average diet
Nickel	Chocolate, nuts, dried beans, peas, grains	Not clearly delineated	None established	Not documented	None reported	—
Selenium	Meats, seafoods, some cereal grains	Present in all tissues; one selenoenzyme is important in the destruction of inflammatory hydroperoxides	See Table 1	Cardiomyopathy, muscle pain, abnormal nail beds Deficiency uncommon in the general population; has been reported in patients with alcoholic cirrhosis	Loss of hair and nails, skin lesions, CNS and teeth involvement	Included in some multivitamin and mineral preparations; doses in excess of 0.2 mg per day not recommended

TABLE 6 *continued*

Element	Dietary sources	Function	Dose/RDA	Signs and symptoms of deficiency	Adverse effects/ Drug interactions	Comments
Silicon	Cereal products, root vegetables, unrefined grains of high fiber content	Development and maintenance of connective tissue	None established	No deficiency state described	Nontoxic	—
Tin	—	May be involved in growth and reproductive functions	None established	No deficiency state described	None reported	Evidence of its necessity lacking; adequate quantities apparently obtained form the diet
Vanadium	Shellfish, mushrooms, parsley, dill seed, black pepper	May be involved in growth and reproductive functions	None established	No deficiency state described	Diarrhea, anorexia, depressed growth, neurotoxicity Toxicity may be diminished by administration of ascorbic acid, EDTA, chromium, protein, ferrous iron, chloride, and possibly aluminum hydroxide	Evidence of its necessity not well established
Zinc	Oysters, liver, beef, lamb, pork, legumes, peanuts, whole-grain cereals	Integral part of 70 metalloenzymes; a cofactor in the synthesis of DNA and RNA; involved in the mobilization of vitamin A from the liver; essential for normal cellular immune functions and for spermatogenesis	See Table 1 Treatment of suspected deficiency: 150 mg elemental zinc daily in three divided doses Only 10%–40% absorbed from the GI tract	Marginally low zinc values associated with growth retardation in children, slow wound healing in adults, birth defects, problems in childbirth Other symptoms: loss of appetite, skin changes, immunologic abnormalities	Vomiting, dehydration, muscle incoordination, dizziness, abdominal pain High intake may decrease copper levels May decrease tetracycline absorption Iron and zinc supplements decrease each other's absorption; less pronounced when taken with a meal	Malabsorption syndromes, GI tract abnormalities, long-term parenteral nutrition, infection, myocardial infarct, major surgery, alcoholism, liver cirrhosis, pregnancy, lactation, and high-fiber diets predispose individuals to a suboptimal zinc status Chronic ingestion of >15 mg elemental zinc per day not recommended without medical supervision

Classification of Enteral Nutrition Products

Many commercial preparations are available for enteral feeding. Some are designed for general nutrition; others are designed for specific metabolic or clinical conditions. They may be classified according to clinical indications or product composition.

Clinical Indications Method

Enteral feeding products are classified as natural foods, polymeric solutions, monomeric solutions, solutions for specific metabolic needs, modular solutions, and hydration solutions.

Product Composition Method

Enteral preparations classified according to composition are either supplemental or complete, with general and specialized applications. Supplemental protein-calorie formula products are to be used only as adjuncts to a regular diet because they are not nutritionally complete. Some products (Mull-Soy and Nutramigen) are milk free and can be used by individuals who have a milk allergy and lactose malabsorption. One product (Controlyte) with a low protein and electrolyte content may be appropriate for patients with acute or chronic renal failure.

Complete formulas can be used orally or as tube feedings. They may be used as sole dietary intake (if the patient's electrolytes are monitored) or as supplementation. These products may contain ingredients that make them appropriate for special needs. Several such products (Instant Breakfast, Sustacal, and Meritene) are milk based; others (Compleat-B and Gerber Meat Base Formula) have a mixed-food base. Another type supplies protein in the form of crystalline amino acids or protein hydrolysate, carbohydrate in the form of oligosaccharides or disaccharides, and vitamins and minerals in the form of individual chemicals. These last products are chemically defined diets, also known as "elemental diets"; examples include Vivonex and Jejunal.

All chemically based products require little or no digestion, are absorbed over a short distance in the small intestine, and have low residue. These attributes mean that the number and volume of the stools are reduced, making these products appropriate for patients who have had ileostomies or colostomies and who wish to decrease fecal output.

Administration and Monitoring Guidelines

Supplemental and complete formulas are available in several forms, including powders that must be diluted with water or milk, liquids that must be diluted, and liquids and puddings that are ready to use. The extent of dilution is based on the amount of nutrients needed and the amount that can be tolerated.

If the preparations are taken orally, 100–150 mL should be ingested at one time. Over the course of a day, 2000 mL of most preparations provide about 2000 calories. If the patient is tube fed, 40–60 mL of the product per hour may be given initially. Once opened, the container should be kept cold to prevent bacterial growth, and all prepared products remaining after 24 hours should be discarded. Tubing should be rinsed three times a day with water. If diarrhea, nausea, or distention occur, the diet should be withheld for 24 hours and then gradually resumed. For elderly or unconscious persons or for patients who recently have had surgery, elevating the head of the bed is advisable to avoid aspiration.

Pharmacists should store supplemental formula products at temperatures under 75°F (23.8°C). Expiration dates should be checked before dispensing.

Patients must be monitored for biochemical abnormalities, electrolyte values, and adequate nutrition and hydration. Urine and blood glucose concentrations can be monitored. Persons with diabetes may require increased insulin doses. Edema may be precipitated or aggravated in patients with protein-calorie malnutrition or cardiac, renal, or hepatic disease because of the relatively high sodium content of the elemental diets. Some commercially available nutritional products are a source of vitamin K supplementation, which may interfere with oral anticoagulant therapy. Tube feedings have been shown to interfere with the absorption of phenytoin administered via the tube. This interaction can be avoided by flushing the tube with saline (or water) before and after phenytoin and waiting 15 minutes both before and after the dose is given.

Information useful in educating and counseling patients is included in Table 7.

TABLE 7 Selected information useful in counseling patients about nutritional supplements

For proper nutrition, foods from all the basic food groups (meats, fruits and vegetables, dairy products, and grains) should be eaten. Vitamin supplements are not a substitute for a well-balanced diet.

Patients should not self-medicate if they suspect a vitamin deficiency but should consult their physician or pharmacist.

Labels on all vitamin or vitamin and mineral preparations should be read carefully before supplements are taken. The contents and the amounts of vitamins and minerals should be compared with those in the RDAs.

Doses of vitamins and minerals higher than the RDAs should be taken with caution. All vitamins and minerals have dose-related adverse effects.

Vitamins or vitamin and mineral supplements should be taken with meals if their use is associated with GI symptoms.

Liquid vitamin and mineral supplements may be mixed with food (fruit juice, milk, baby formula, or cereal).

Some vitamin supplements have a special coating and should be swallowed whole.

Children should be taught that vitamins are drugs and cannot be taken indiscriminately.

Vitamin and combination vitamin and mineral supplements should be stored out of the reach of children, especially if the product contains iron.

Iron supplements or vitamins with iron may turn stool black. This is not a cause for alarm unless it is associated with other GI symptoms.

Niacin-containing products may cause a flushing sensation, which should decrease in intensity with continued therapy.

Riboflavin-containing products may cause a yellow fluorescence in the urine.

CHAPTER 20

Infant Formula Products

Questions to ask in patient assessment and counseling

- What is your baby's age and weight?
- Is your baby under a physician's care?
- Is the baby being breast-fed or receiving an infant formula?
- Does your baby receive other liquids besides breast milk or an infant formula?
- Is your baby receiving any solid foods, including cereal? If so, is the food fed by spoon or added to bottle feedings?
- Is your baby allergic or sensitive to milk? Does your baby have other dietary restrictions? Does your baby have any chronic health problems?
- Are you giving your baby a multivitamin product? Was it recommended by your baby's physician?
- Is your baby receiving fluoride supplementation?
- Does your baby have diarrhea, constipation, or vomiting?
- Does your baby have a fever, loss of appetite, decreased tearing, decreased salivation, or fewer wet diapers?
- Do you understand how your baby's formula should be prepared?

Breast-feeding is the desired method for feeding infants from birth to at least 4–6 months of age. This is because human milk provides a nutritional source that is physiologically sound and because breast-feeding tends to facilitate a close mother–child relationship. Breast-feeding also decreases the incidence of infant allergy and illness.

For women who do not want to breast-feed or are unable to do so, commercially prepared infant formulas are a good alternative in industrially developed nations. Such formulas are less desirable in developing countries, however, where inadequate sanitation, lack of refrigeration, and the inability of illiterate mothers to follow formula preparation instructions increase the risk of infant morbidity and mortality.

Infant Feeding Practice

Advances in uniformity, convenience, nutritional quality, and safety have established infant formulas as an alternative method for feeding infants. The composition of commercial infant formulas conforms with guidelines based on extensive assessments of infant nutritional needs. Variations among formulas allow for product selection that will meet a specific infant's nutritional requirements. However, these variations produce differences in palatability, digestibility, sources of nutrients, and convenience of administration. The pharmacist, in consultation with the infant's parents and physician, should be able to

---

Editor's Note: This chapter is adapted from Rosalie Sagraves, Claudia Kamper, and Judi Doerr, "Infant Formula Products," in Covington, T.R., ed., *Handbook of Nonprescription Drugs,* 11th edition. For a more extensive discussion of infant feeding, infant physiology and growth, the components of a healthy infant diet, content of various milks, breast-feeding, and infant formulas, readers are encouraged to consult Chapter 20 of the *Handbook.*

evaluate indications, advise on the selection of an infant formula, and help ensure its appropriate use. The pharmacist should also be able to help educate women about breast-feeding and refer women with questions about breast-feeding to organizations such as the La Leche League.

Components of a Healthy Infant Diet

Acceptable growth is achieved through an adequate intake of energy, protein, carbohydrates, minerals, and vitamins. The Food and Nutrition Board of the National Research Council established recommended dietary allowances (RDAs) designed to meet the needs of most healthy infants (Table 1). The Food and Drug Administration (FDA) has also issued recommendations for nutrition for infants.

TABLE 1   Recommended dietary allowances of nutrients for full-term infants

Nutrient	RDA 0–6 mo	RDA >6–12 mo	Nutrient	RDA 0–6 mo	RDA >6–12 mo
Energy (kcal/kg/day)	108	98	**Minerals**		
Protein (g/kg/day)	2.2	1.6	Calcium (mg)	400	600
			Phosphorus (mg)	300	500
Essential fatty acids			Magnesium (mg)	40	60
Linoleic acid (% of kcal)[a]	2.7	2.7	Iron (mg)	6	10
			Iodine (mcg)	40	50
Vitamins			Zinc (mg)	5	5
Vitamin A (mcg)[b]	375	375	Copper (mg)[e]	0.4–0.6	0.6–0.7
Vitamin D (mcg)[c]	7.5	10	Manganese (mg)[f]	0.3–0.6	0.6–1
Vitamin E (mg)[d]	3	4	Fluoride (mg)[f]	0.1–0.5	0.2–1
Vitamin K (mcg)	5	10	Chromium (mcg)[f]	10–40	20–60
Vitamin C (mg)	30	35	Selenium (mcg)	10	15
Thiamine (mg)	0.3	0.4	Molybdenum (mcg)[f]	15–30	20–40
Riboflavin (mg)	0.4	0.5			
Vitamin B_6 (mg)	0.3	0.6			
Vitamin B_{12} (mcg)	0.3	0.5			
Niacin (mg)[e]	5	6			
Folate (mcg)	25	35			
Pantothenic acid (mg)[f]	2	3			
Biotin (mcg)[f]	10	15			

[a]No specific recommendations for linolenic acid have been identified by the National Research Council, Food and Drug Administration, or CON/AAP.

[b]Retinol equivalents (REs); 1 RE = 3.33 IU of vitamin A activity from retinol.

[c]Cholecalciferol; 10 mcg of cholecalciferol equals 400 IU of vitamin D.

[d]Alpha-tocopherol equivalents (TEs); 1 mg of delta-alpha-tocopherol = 1 alpha-TE. The activity of alpha-tocopherol is 1.49 IU/mg.

[e]Niacin equivalents (NEs); 1 NE = 1 mg of niacin or 60 mg of dietary tryptophan.

[f]Estimated safe and adequate daily dietary intakes. Because there is less information on which to base allowances, some figures are provided as ranges of recommended intakes.

Reprinted with permission from Food and Nutrition Board, Commission on Life Sciences, National Research Council. *Recommended Dietary Allowances*. 10th ed. Washington, DC: National Academy Press; 1989.

Fluid

Water makes up a larger proportion of the infant's body composition than it does of the older person's. Maintenance water or fluid needs in infancy are estimated to be approximately 100 mL/kg daily for the first 10 kg of body weight plus 50 mL/kg daily for each kilogram between 10 and 20 kg. Additional losses caused by conditions such as diarrhea, fever, and rapid breathing should be offset by fluid intake in excess of maintenance levels.

Carbohydrates

Although there is no RDA for carbohydrates, under normal circumstances an infant can efficiently use 40%–50% of total calories from a carbohydrate source. Lactose is the primary carbohydrate source in human milk and milk-based formulas. Premature infants are relatively lactase deficient and thus are prone to lactose intolerance, which may be manifested by diarrhea, abdominal pain or distention, bloating, gas, and cramping. Secondary lactase deficiency is temporary, while congenital lactase deficiency is not. Formulas with nutrient sources other than cow milk may be used when lactose intolerance or hypersensitivity is suspected.

Protein and Amino Acids

The accepted average daily RDA for protein is 2.2 g/kg from birth to age 6 months and 1.6 g/kg from age 6 months to 1 year. Equally important as the overall protein intake is the amino acid composition of the protein. Histidine, tyrosine, cystine, and taurine may need to be supplemented in preterm infants.

In evaluating the adequacy of an infant's protein intake, one must consider not only the absolute amount of protein ingested, but also the growth rate of the child, the quantity of nonprotein calories and other nutrients necessary for protein synthesis, and the quality of the protein itself. Some authors have suggested that amino acid and protein requirements are more meaningful when expressed in terms of calories; therefore, requirements or supplementation levels may appear in grams per 100 kcal.

Fat and Essential Fatty Acids

The FDA recommends a minimum fat intake of 3.3 g/100 kcal (30% of calories) and a maximum of 6 g/100 kcal (60% of calories) for infants. Children need fats for adequate growth and development; the concern about high fat in the adult diet does not apply to children.

The diet must contain small amounts of linoleic acid, a polyunsaturated fatty acid (PUFA) that has been proven to be an essential nutrient. Linoleic acid deficiency manifests as increased metabolic rate, drying and flaking of the skin, hair loss, and impaired wound healing. The American Academy of Pediatrics (AAP) recommends linoleic acid intakes of 300 mg/100 kcal, or approximately 3% of total calories.

Micronutrients

Infant formulas are generally supplemented with adequate amounts of vitamins and minerals to meet the needs of full-term infants.

Vitamin A

Vitamin A is essential for vision, growth, and cellular function. Deficiency in vitamin A and its precursors is uncommon in the United States. RDA values change little as the growth rate decreases. Toxicity can occur with acute or chronic ingestion of exceedingly high doses, causing headache, vomiting, diplopia, alopecia, desquamation, bone abnormalities, liver damage, and dryness of the mucous membranes.

Vitamin D

Vitamin D is essential in mineral homeostasis and bone mineralization and is particularly important in infancy. Infant formulas should be fortified with 400 IU vitamin D per quart. Intake of as little as five times the RDA in children may result in toxicity, resulting in hypercalcemia, hypercalciuria, soft-tissue calcium deposition, and irreversible calcium deposition in the kidneys and heart.

Vitamin E

Vitamin E serves an important role in muscular and neurologic function. The RDAs are 3 mg per day for infants 0–6 months of age and 4 mg per day for infants older than 6 months.

Preterm infants are born with disproportionately small body stores of vitamin E and a reduced capacity for intestinal vitamin E absorption. It has been suggested that up to 17 mg of vitamin E may be required as an oral supplement in preterm infants until they reach 3 months of age.

Vitamin K

Vitamin K and vitamin K–active compounds are essential in the formation of prothrombin and other proteins responsible for coagulation of the blood. Milk-based formulas contain enough vitamin K to prevent deficiency.

Biotin

The recommended intake of biotin is 10–15 mcg per day. Deficiency manifests as seborrheic dermatitis.

Minerals

Calcium and Phosphorus

Calcium and phosphorus are crucial to the development and maintenance of the human skeleton. In addition, phosphorus is an integral component of many biochemical reactions. The recommended ratio of calcium to phosphorus is 1.3:1 for infants between birth and 6 months of age and 1.2:1 for infants older than 6 months.

Formulas designed for full-term infants are deficient in calcium and phosphorus relative to the needs of low-birthweight (LBW) or preterm infants. These infants need supplementation via special infant formulas.

Iron

The FDA recommends that all formulas contain at least the lower level of iron found in human milk (0.3–0.5 mg/L) and that iron be in a bioavailable form. Infants are at risk for iron deficiency and should be given formulas supplemented with 1–2 mg/100 kcal of iron, or approximately 6–12 mg/L.

Formulas for LBW infants contain less than or equal to 3 mg of iron per liter because iron supplementation in LBW infants up to 2 months of age has been associated with an increased risk of hemolytic anemia. The decision to supplement iron in infants fed LBW formulas should be made by the physician.

Zinc, Copper, and Manganese

The RDA of zinc for formula-fed infants is 5 mg per day. The AAP recommendation for copper in infant formulas is 60 mcg/100 kcal. The requirement for manganese is unknown. Provisional recommendations are shown in Table 1.

Vitamin and Mineral Supplements

There is no evidence that vitamin and mineral supplementation is necessary for formula-fed full-term infants or for normal, breast-fed infants of well-nourished mothers. However, iron and vitamin D supplementation has been recommended for breast-fed full-term infants.

Vitamin and mineral supplementation may be needed for preterm and LBW infants, infants whose mothers are inadequately nourished, and those with other nutritional deficiencies (see Chapter 20 of the *Handbook*).

Breast-Fed Full-Term Infants

Supplementation of vitamin D is recommended for breast-fed infants as a protective measure against the development of rickets. Vitamin A deficiency rarely occurs in breast-fed infants; therefore, vitamin A may be omitted from supplements designed to provide vitamin D for infants.

A malnourished nursing mother and her infant should receive multivitamin supplements containing vitamin B_{12} to prevent megaloblastic anemia.

Breast-fed infants rarely develop iron deficiency anemia before 4–6 months of age because neonatal stores of iron are adequate. After 6 months of age, neonatal stores may be depleted; consequently, in normal, breast-fed full-term infants, the addition of an iron supplement (2 mg/kg of ferrous sulfate daily) may be desirable. An iron supplement is preferable to iron-fortified cereal.

Fluoride supplements may not be necessary if the breast-fed infant lives in an area where the water is fluoridated. Too much fluoride may cause enamel fluorosis.

Formula-Fed Full-Term Infants

Full-term infants who consume adequate amounts of an iron-fortified commercial milk-based formula do not need vitamin and mineral supplementation in the first 6 months of life.

Vitamin and mineral supplements are not needed for infants older than 6 months of age who receive a diet of formula, mixed feedings, and increased amounts of table food. A multivitamin with minerals may be needed if the infant is at special nutritional risk. If a powdered or concentrated formula is used, fluoride supplements should be administered only if the community's drinking water contains less than 0.3 ppm of fluoride. Ready-to-use formulas are manufactured with defluoridated water and contain less than 0.3 ppm of fluoride. Therefore, if an infant fed ready-to-use formula does not drink water or juice or eat solid foods, the physician may recommend a fluoride supplement.

Preterm Infants

All preterm infants need vitamin and mineral supplementation. Until these infants can consume about 300 kcal per day or until they reach a body weight of 2.5 kg, a multivitamin supplement should be administered to provide the equivalent of the RDAs for full-term infants. The supplement should include vitamin E in a form well absorbed by preterm infants. Because of conflicting data from clinical studies, it may be prudent to monitor vitamin E serum concentrations and to maintain them at 1–3 mg/dL.

Folate can be added to a multivitamin preparation to provide the RDA (Table 1). The shelf life of folate is 1 month, and the label should read "shake well."

To minimize the possibility of hemolytic anemia in infants with insufficient vitamin E absorption, iron supplements should be withheld until the preterm infant is several weeks old. Iron is required at a dosage of 2 mg/kg per day starting by at least 2 months of age. Iron-fortified formulas supply sufficient iron to prevent iron deficiency in preterm infants.

Calcium, phosphorus, and vitamin D supplementation in preterm infant formulas is necessary.

Content of Various Milks

Comparison of Human Milk and Whole Cow Milk

Cow milk is the nutrient source for commercially prepared milk-based infant formulas. Both human and cow milk contain more than 200 ingredients in the fat- and water-soluble fractions. Estimates of the concentrations of selected nutrients contained in pooled mature human milk and in cow milk are listed in Table 2. The two types of milk differ significantly in the quantity and availability of nutrients.

Carbohydrates

The carbohydrate percentage in cow milk is lower than that in human milk, and carbohydrate supplementation is necessary for milk-based formulas. Honey and other unrefined foods are not recommended for carbohydrate supplementation because they may contain spores of *Clostridium botulinum.*

Protein

Not only does cow milk contain a higher percentage of protein than human milk, but the protein differs in composition. This difference alters digestibility and can create a milk sensitivity that may induce problems in digesting a milk-based formula or elicit an allergic response to milk protein.

Sensitivity to cow milk differs from milk allergy. Sensitivity may be relieved by altering the casein-to-lactalbumin ratio; however, an allergic reaction requires that all animal milk protein be eliminated from the diet. The amino acid content of cow milk is inappropriate for the neonate's immature enzyme systems.

Fat

Human milk and cow milk have similar total fat contents. Essential fatty acids should provide approximately 3% of the total caloric intake. The cholesterol content varies in both milks, from 20 to 47 mg/100 mL in human milk and from 7 to 25 mg/100 mL in cow milk. Infants fed milk-based formula can efficiently digest fat from vegetable oil because of gastric enzyme activity.

Minerals and Electrolytes

The mineral content of cow milk is several times greater than that of human milk. Cow milk and human milk differ in absolute and proportionate amounts of calcium and phosphorus.

Because iron in human milk is more bioavailable, an infant should be able to absorb approximately 50% of the iron from human milk (versus only 10% of that from cow milk, 10% of that from unfortified milk-based formula, and 4% of that from iron-fortified formula).

The zinc content of human milk is lower than that of cow milk, but it is more bioavailable.

Cow milk contains more sodium, potassium, and chloride than does human milk. These higher electrolyte and mineral concentrations, when combined with the high protein content of cow milk, result in a smaller margin of safety against hyperosmolar dehydration. The larger renal solute load of cow milk, in combination with higher environmental

TABLE 2 Composition of mature human milk and cow milk

Composition	Human milk	Cow milk
Water (mL/100 mL)	87.1%	87.2%
Energy (kcaL/100 mL)	69	66
Protein (g/100 mL)	1.05 ± 0.2	3.1–3.5
Casein (% protein)	40%	80%
Whey (% protein)	60%	20%
Alpha-lactalbumin (g/100 mL)	0.2–0.3	0.1
Beta-lactoglobulin (g/100 mL)	—	0.4
Lactoferrin (g/100 mL)	0.1–0.3	trace
Secretory IgA (g/100 mL)	0.08–0.1	trace
Albumin (g/100 mL)	0.05	0.04
Fat (g/100 mL)	3.9 ± 0.4	3.8
Carbohydrate		
Lactose (g/100 mL)	7.2 ± 0.3	4.9
Electrolytes (per liter)		
Calcium (mg)	280 ± 26	1200
Phosphorus (mg)	140 ± 22	920–940
Calcium/phosphorus ratio	2:1	1.3:1
Sodium (mg)	180 ± 40	506
Potassium (mg)	525 ± 35	1570
Chloride (mg)	420 ± 60	1028–1060
Magnesium (mg)	35 ± 2	120
Sulfur (mg)	140	300
Minerals (per liter)		
Chromium (mcg)	50 ± 5	20
Manganese (mcg)	6 ± 2	20–40
Copper (mcg)	60	110
Zinc (mg)	0.5–1.4	3–5
Iodine (mcg)	110 ± 40	80
Selenium (mcg)	20 ± 5	5–50
Iron (mg)	0.3–0.5	0.5
Vitamins (per liter)		
Vitamin A (IU)	1898	1025
Thiamine (mcg)	150	370
Riboflavin (mcg)	380	1700
Niacin (mcg)	1700	900
Pyridoxine (mcg)	1130	460
Pantothenate (mg)	2.6	3.6
Folic acid (mcg)	85	68
Vitamin B_{12} (mcg)	0.5	4
Vitamin C (mg)	43	17
Vitamin D (IU)	40	14
Vitamin E (mg)	2.3	0.4
Vitamin K (mcg)	2.1	17

Source:

Nutrition in Infancy and Childhood. 5th ed. St Louis: Times Mirror/Mosby College Publishing; 1993: 90.

Williams AF. *Textbook of Paediatric Nutrition.* 3rd ed. London: Churchill Livingstone; 1991: 26–27.

Suskind RM, Lewinter-Suskind L. *Textbook of Pediatric Nutrition.* 2nd ed. New York: Raven Press; 1993: 33–42.

temperatures or the presence of fever, vomiting, or diarrhea, can place an infant at risk for severe dehydration.

Reduced-Fat Cow Milk

The AAP does not recommend skim or 2% milks during the first 12 months of life. Fat restriction is not recommended for young children.

Whole Cow Milk

The current position of the AAP is that iron-fortified infant formula is the only acceptable alternative to breast milk during the first year of life.

Evaporated Milk

Evaporated milk is a sterile, convenient source of cow milk that has standardized concentrations of protein, fat, and carbohydrate. Vitamin D is added to evaporated milk during processing, but evaporated milk formulas fail to meet recommendations for ascorbic acid, vitamin E for preterm infants, and essential fatty acids.

Goat Milk

Unfortified goat milk is deficient in folate and low in iron and vitamin D. The evaporated form of Meyenberg goat milk is supplemented with vitamin D and folic acid. Powdered Meyenberg goat milk is supplemented with folic acid only and is recommended only for infants older than 1 year. Because the powder formulation is not a complete formula for infants, the manufacturer recommends supplementation with vitamins.

Breast-Feeding

Mature breast milk, which develops approximately one month after an infant's birth, is the standard against which most commercially prepared infant formulas are compared.

Human milk provides certain advantages over cow milk, goat milk, and infant formulas; however, normal growth and development are possible without human milk.

Benefits of Breast-Feeding

Reported benefits of breast-feeding include protection against infections such as gastrointestinal (GI) illness and respiratory infection. Conflicting results have been reported regarding breast-feeding and a lower rate of respiratory infection. However, respiratory infections in breast-fed infants are likely to be less severe. Breast milk may also confer protection against otitis media.

Potential Problems with Breast-Feeding

Hyperbilirubinemia

One minor problem associated with human milk is the presence of increased levels of nonesterified fatty acid in the breast milk of some women. This condition leads to a prolonged unconjugated hyperbilirubinemia in infants. Breast-feeding need not be stopped in most cases of breast-milk jaundice. If the infant appears in danger from hyperbilirubinemia itself, a temporary pause in breast-feeding for 1–3 days usually reduces the bilirubin to a safe level. Breast-feeding can then be resumed. No detrimental effects have been reported in infants as a result of breast-milk jaundice.

Human Immunodeficiency Virus

Although the risk of transmitting the human immunodeficiency virus (HIV) in breast milk appears to be low, there have been reports of such transmission. The Committee on Infectious Diseases of the AAP recommends that women in the United States who are infected with HIV should not breast-feed, nor should they donate breast milk to milk banks.

Medications in Breast Milk

Oral Contraceptives. It is debatable whether maternal use of an oral contraceptive while breast-feeding significantly affects lactation. Some studies have found decreased milk production. AAP recommendations state that low-dose combination oral contraceptives or progestogen-only contraceptives are not contraindicated during breast-feeding as long as milk production has been established.

Transfer of Medications to Breast Milk. Most medications are transferred from maternal blood to breast milk via passive diffusion. This transfer depends on a variety of factors. Maternal factors include the dose of medication, the frequency and route of administration, and the pharmacokinetics of the drug, which may change dramatically in the weeks following pregnancy. Factors relating to the quality of the breast milk, certain characteristics of the drug, and the infant also affect the ability of the drug to pass into the breast milk. Medications of concern to breast-feeding women are listed in Table 3.

TABLE 3 Medications of concern to breast-feeding women

Medications that are contraindicated in breast-feeding women[a]

Bromocriptine	Ergotamine
Cimetidine	Gold salts
Cyclophosphamide	Lithium
Cyclosporine	Methotrexate
Doxorubicin	Phenindione

Medications that require cautious use and medical supervision

Aspirin	Salicylazosulfapyridine
Phenobarbital	

Medications that require temporary stopping of breast-feeding

Metronidazole	Radiopharmaceuticals

[a]Drugs of abuse (e.g., amphetamines, cocaine, heroin, marijuana, nicotine, and phencyclidine) are contraindicated for use during breast-feeding.

Source:

Briggs GG, Freeman RK, Yaffe SJ. *Drugs in Pregnancy and Lactation.* 4th ed. Baltimore: Williams & Wilkins; 1994.

Briggs GG. Drugs in pregnancy and lactation. In: Young YL, Koda-Kimble MA, eds. *Applied Therapeutics: The Clinical Use of Drugs.* 5th ed. Vancouver, Wash: Applied Therapeutics Inc; 1992: 1–33.

To help minimize an infant's intake of a medication via breast milk, the following strategies should be followed when possible:

■ A drug should be selected from a class of drugs that is the least likely to be distributed into breast milk.

■ A *nonoral* route that minimizes systemic absorption should be selected when the option exists (e.g., inhaled beta-agonists, topical corticosteroids).

■ A drug that can be taken once daily may be recommended.

■ When multiple doses are needed, infant feedings should coincide with trough rather than peak drug concentrations.

■ If there is concern about toxicity to the infant, the infant should be monitored. If possible, serum or urine drug concentrations should be obtained.

■ If the mother needs a short course of a drug that is not recommended during breast-feeding, breast-feeding may be interrupted for four to five half-lives. During this time, the infant should be given previously expressed breast milk or an infant formula, and the woman should pump her breasts to prevent engorgement.

■ If the breast-feeding infant is to be weaned soon, the mother could delay beginning a medication if this option is medically acceptable.

Commercial Infant Formulas

Caloric Density

The RDA for energy is 108 kcal/kg for infants from birth to 6 months of age and 98 kcal/kg from age 6 months to 1 year. A full-term infant should have no difficulty consuming enough diluted formula (20 kcal/oz or 67 kcal/100 mL) to meet these caloric needs, but a preterm or LBW (<2500 g) infant has a higher caloric need and may require as much as 130 kcal/kg daily. An infant recovering from illness or malnutrition also requires more calories. Infant formulas with caloric densities significantly lower or higher than 67 kcal/100 mL are regarded as therapeutic formulas to be used for the management of special clinical conditions and only under medical supervision.

Osmolarity and Osmolality

There is no meaningful difference in the osmolalities of the commonly used ready-to-use formulas that provide 67 kcal/100 mL. Directions for diluting concentrated formulas must be followed exactly to prevent harmful hyperosmolar states, such as diarrhea and dehydration.

Renal Solute Load

The renal solute load is important because it determines the quantity of water that is excreted by the kidneys. Infants are less able to concentrate their urine than are older children and adults. Feeding an infant a formula that is too concentrated may produce a hypertonic urine that may cause dehydration.

Types, Uses, and Selection of Commercial Infant Formulas

Formulas for full-term infants are milk-based or milk-based with added whey protein (whey predominant). These formulas meet the minimum requirements for various nutrients per 100 kcal, as required by the FDA and deemed appropriate by the AAP. (See product table "Infants' and Children's Formula Products" in *Nonprescription Products: Formulations & Features.*)

Milk-Based Formulas

A milk-based formula is prepared from nonfat cow milk, vegetable oils, and added carbohydrate (lactose). Vitamins and minerals are added in accordance with FDA guidelines. Milk-based formulas are available as iron-fortified (approximately 1.8 mg/100 kcal) or low-iron (approximately 0.16 mg/100 kcal) formulas. Similac is an example of a milk-based formula. Lactofree contains corn syrup solids rather than lactose as its carbohydrate source and thus can be used in infants with lactose intolerance.

Milk-Based Formulas with Added Whey Protein

When whey is added in proper amounts to nonfat cow milk, the ratio of whey proteins to casein can be altered to approximate that of human milk. The high nutritional quality and relatively low renal solute load of these formulas are assets in the therapeutic management of ill infants. Enfamil is an example of a whey-predominant formula.

Therapeutic Formulas

Therapeutic infant formulas are used for infants being treated by medical specialists for conditions that require dietary adjustment. Table 4 lists indications for using various therapeutic infant formulas.

Soy-Protein Formulas

Soy-protein formulas contain methionine-fortified isolated soy protein. Vegetable oils provide the fat content, and corn syrup solids and/or sucrose supply the carbohydrate in these formulas.

The carbohydrate source is an important factor in product selection. Isomil contains corn syrup solids and sucrose; I-Soyalac contains only sucrose; ProSobee contains only corn syrup solids. Infants who are sensitive to corn and corn products and who cannot tolerate a milk-based formula may benefit from a corn-free soy-protein formula.

Soy-protein formulas are lactose free and therefore can be used for infants with primary lactase deficiency or secondary lactose intolerance. Soy-protein formulas also provide an alternative nutritional source for infants whose parents are vegetarians and do not wish to use animal protein–based formulas.

RCF (Ross Carbohydrate Free) soy-protein formula does not contain a carbohydrate source. This formula may be used in the dietary management of infants unable to tolerate the type or amount of carbohydrates in cow milk or other infant formulas. A physician may select a carbohydrate source (sucrose, dextrose, fructose, or glucose polymers) that can be added before feeding. RCF is for use only under medical supervision.

Some infants with gastroenteritis develop intolerance to lactose and sucrose because of secondary lactase and sucrase deficiency. Isomil SF and ProSobee contain corn syrup solids (hydrolyzed corn starch, a glucose polymer) as the carbohydrate source and can thus be used in this situation.

Isomil DF is a specific formula for the management of diarrhea. It contains added dietary fiber from soy.

Soy-protein formulas are promoted for use in the management of allergy to milk or for infants suspected of having milk allergy. However, the AAP recommends that protein hydrolysate formulas rather than soy-protein formulas be used for infants with documented clinical allergy to cow milk and/or soy protein. However, most infants suspected of having adverse reactions to milk-based formulas have not experienced life-threatening manifestations and appear to tolerate soy-protein formulas.

TABLE 4 Indication for the use of therapeutic infant formulas

Problem	Suggested formula	Comments
Allergy or sensitivity to cow milk protein or soy protein	Protein hydrolysate formula (e.g., Alimentum, Nutramigen, or Pregestimil)	Protein allergy or sensitivity
Biliary atresia	Portagen	Impaired digestion and absorption of long-chain fats
Carbohydrate intolerance	RCF, 3232A	Formulas are carbohydrate free; a source of carbohydrate that the patient can tolerate can be added
Cardiac disease	Enfamil, Similac PM 60/40	Whey predominant, low electrolyte content
Celiac disease	Pregestimil or Nutramigen, followed by a soy formula and then a cow milk formula	Advance to more complete formulas as intestinal epithelium returns to normal
Constipation	Routine formula, increase sugar	Mild laxative effect
Cystic fibrosis	Portagen, Pregestimil	Impaired digestion and absorption of long-chain fats
Diarrhea		
Chronic nonspecific	Routine formula or soy formula	Appropriate distribution of calories; impaired digestion of intact protein, long-chain fats, and disaccharides
Intractable	Pregestimil, Alimentum	
Failure to thrive (e.g., when intestinal damage is suspected)	Pregestimil, Alimentum	Advance to more complete formulas as intestinal epithelium returns to normal
Gastroesophageal reflux	Routine formula	Thicken with cereal (1 tbsp/oz of formula); also try small, frequent feedings
Hepatitis		
Without liver failure	Routine formula	Impaired digestion and absorption of long-chain fats
With liver failure	Portagen	
Homocystinuria	Low methionine, Analog XMET	Low content of methionine
Lactose intolerance	Soy formula	Impaired digestion and use of lactose
Maple syrup urine disease	MSUD Diet Powder, Analog MSUD	Low content of leucine, isoleucine, and valine
Necrotizing enterocolitis (with resection)	Pregestimil (when oral feeding is resumed)	Impaired digestion
Phenylketonuria	Lofenalac, Analog XP	Low content of phenylalanine
Prematurity	Preterm infant formulas	Whey predominant, easily digestible sources of carbohydrate and fat; appropriate vitamin and mineral content
Renal insufficiency	Similac PM 60/40	Low phosphate content, low renal solute load

Supplemental information extracted from:
Walker WA, Hendricks KM. *Manual of Pediatric Nutrition.* 2nd ed. Philadelphia: BC Decker; 1990: 79.

Casein Hydrolysate–Based Formulas

Casein hydrolysate–based formulas are effective in the nutritional management of infants with a variety of severe GI abnormalities. These formulas are also indicated during a transition from parenteral feeding to a normal diet.

Use of these formulas for allergy prophylaxis remains controversial. Infants with documented clinical allergic symptoms to cow milk may benefit from a protein hydrolysate formula because approximately 15%–50% of these infants also react to soy protein. Currently, no evidence exists to support the use of hydrolysate formulas for treating colic, restlessness, or irritability. These are common symptoms in infants but they rarely occur as a result of an immune-mediated reaction to cow milk protein.

Extensively hydrolyzed casein protein makes formulas less palatable. However, infants usually accept the feedings satisfactorily. If the formula is rejected when first offered, it may be tried again after a few hours. These products are designed to provide a sole source of nutrition for infants up to 4–6 months of age and to provide a primary source of nutrition through 12 months of age when indicated. Extended use requires physician monitoring on a case-by-case basis.

Pregestimil, Nutramigen, Alimentum, and 3232A are formulas with enzymatic hydrolysates of casein as the protein source. The carbohydrate sources in these formulas vary.

Amino Acid–Based Formula

Occasionally, infants are intolerant to even hydrolyzed casein and require an amino acid–containing formula. Neocate Powder contains 100% free amino acids, as well as 35% medium-chain and 65% long-chain triglycerides. Neocate Powder contains 1 kcal/mL.

Sodium Caseinate Formula

Portagen is a sodium caseinate formula. It has been effective in feeding infants with pancreatic insufficiency (e.g., that caused by cystic fibrosis), bile acid deficiency, intestinal resection, lymphatic anomalies, and celiac disease. It can be used on a physician's recommendation as the sole dietary source for both infants and older children, or as a beverage to be consumed with each meal.

Whey Hydrolysate–Based Formulas

Casein hydrolysate formulas have been used for many years for infants with defects in protein digestion and adverse reactions to intact cow milk protein. Anaphylactic-type reactions have been reported in patients with severe milk allergy who received hydrolysate formulas. Therefore, they should not be used in infants with documented IgE-mediated allergy to cow milk protein. The effectiveness of whey hydrolysate formula in infants who have GI intolerance to cow milk but are not allergic to it suggests that whey hydrolysate formula may be an acceptable alternative to milk-based and soy-protein formulas. This product may be better accepted than casein-hydrolysate formulas, which mothers and infants find noticeably different from milk-based and soy-protein formulas in appearance and taste.

Metabolic Formulas

Infants with inherited metabolic disorders require specific formulas.

Low Birthweight and Preterm Formulas

No commercially available formula is completely satisfactory for LBW or very-low-birthweight (VLBW) infants; however, improvements in special formulas (e.g., Enfamil Premature Formula, Similac Special Care, Similac PM 60/40, Similac Neocare) permit individualization of dietary regimens for these infants.

Preterm and LBW infants are especially susceptible to iron deficiency anemia. Therefore, daily supplementation of elemental iron at 2 mg/kg of iron is recommended by the AAP for infants older than 2 months. Iron supplementation before 2 months of age must be accompanied by ample vitamin E and PUFA additions to the diet to reduce the possibility of hemolytic anemia from vitamin E deficiency. A formula without iron is preferable for VLBW infants in the first 2–4 postnatal weeks to prevent decreased vitamin E serum concentrations.

Human Milk Fortifiers

Whether human milk provides optimal nutrition for VLBW infants is a controversial issue. Mothers who deliver preterm produce milk that is higher in protein, sodium, potassium, and possibly other nutrients than the milk of mothers who deliver at term.

However, human milk, preterm or mature, cannot supply the amount of calcium and phosphorus needed to prevent osteopenia of prematurity. Enfamil Human Milk Fortifier and Similac Natural Care enhance the nutrient content of human milk.

Follow-up Formulas

"Follow-up" or "follow-on" formulas such as Enfamil Next Step and Carnation Follow-Up are designed for infants 6–12 months of age. The AAP has stated that these formulas offer no nutritional advantage over standard formulas.

Formula for Children Aged 1–10 Years

PediaSure, PediaSure with fiber, and Kindercal are nutritionally complete, isotonic, lactose-free enteral formulas designed for young children who cannot tolerate a normal diet or eat solid food. They have a pleasant taste and can be used as supplements to increase caloric intake.

Several therapeutic formulas have also been developed for this age group. Peptamen Junior, a peptide-based elemental formula, and Vivonex Pediatric and Neocate One+, both amino acid–based elemental formulas, are now available.

Potential Problems with Infant Formulas

Diarrhea

The pharmacist should ascertain the severity and duration of the diarrhea, frequency of stools, and method of preparing the infant formula. If the diarrhea is serious (many more stools per day than normal) or has continued for 48 hours, or if the infant is clinically ill (with fever, lethargy, anorexia, irritability, dry mucous membranes, decreased urine output, or weight loss), the infant should be referred to a physician.

A common cause of diarrhea is the improper dilution of a concentrated liquid or powdered formula.

Mild diarrhea of short duration may resolve without medical measures, but the infant should be observed closely. Twenty-four hour discontinuation of usual dietary intake may be helpful. Oral electrolyte replacement solutions (e.g., Pedialyte, Infalyte) may be used cautiously for short-term management of fluid and electrolyte loss. However, these solutions should not be used when parenteral rehydration is required, nor should they be used to provide adequate nutrition. A nutritionally adequate formula should be resumed under a physician's direction.

Formula may be resumed at half strength for 24 hours and then increased to full strength over a 48-hour period. If diarrhea resumes, a lactose-free formula may be used at half strength for 24 hours; then full strength for 1–3 weeks (depending on the severity of the diarrhea). Finally, a milk-based formula may be resumed.

Other Gastrointestinal Problems

Adverse effects of formula on an infant's GI tract range from mechanical obstruction, diarrhea, and dehydration from a hyperosmolar formula to hypersensitivity from specific milk protein.

Hyperosmolar formulas may adversely affect LBW infants during the early neonatal period and may be a potential cause of necrotizing enterocolitis. Appropriately prepared formulas for LBW infants (20–24 kcal/oz) are isotonic, with osmolalities less than or equal to 300 mOsm/kg.

Tooth Decay

Tooth decay can occur in children who bottle-feed beyond the typical weaning period and is especially prevalent in children who sleep with their bottles after 1 year of age.

Formula Preparation

For a discussion of formula preparations, see Chapter 20 of the *Handbook*.

Frequency of Feedings

The frequency of feeding for a newborn infant will vary from every 2 hours to every 4 hours. Smaller infants usually require more frequent feedings. Breast-fed infants desire more frequent feedings than do bottle-fed infants. Infants usually lengthen the interval between feedings to 4 hours by the time they are 3–4 weeks old. Typically, infants begin to stop nighttime feedings by the age of 3–6 weeks.

The amount of formula offered to a bottle-fed infant should be consistent with the RDA for energy based on age and weight. The infant should be fed on demand and not be forced to take more formula than is desired. If the infant finishes a bottle and still seems hungry, another bottle should be offered.

Product Selection Guidelines

When recommending a type of formula, the pharmacist should consider the method of preparation, the parents' ability to follow directions, the parents' attitudes and preferences, and the sanitary conditions and refrigeration facilities available.

Cost may be a critical factor in selecting an infant formula. Convenience is also a consideration. The formula selected should be one that is well tolerated by the infant, convenient to prepare, and priced to fit the family's budget.

CHAPTER 21

Weight Control Products

Questions to ask in patient assessment and counseling

- What is your age, height, and weight?
- Why are you trying to lose weight?
- How long have you had a weight problem?
- How many pounds overweight do you think you are?
- Do you have a family history of obesity? Do either of your parents have a weight problem?
- Do you eat a nutritionally sound diet? How much do you know about nutrition?
- Have you consulted a physician about your desire to lose weight?
- Are you now or have ever you been on a diet to help you lose weight?
- Have you used any weight loss preparations previously? How did they work?
- Do you exercise regularly? Does your physician recommend that you exercise?
- Are you being treated for any chronic disease such as hypertension, angina, diabetes, or a thyroid condition?
- Are you taking any prescription and nonprescription medications?

Body Fat and Obesity

Obesity can be defined as an excessive accumulation of body fat to the extent that it is thought to impair health. When the percentage of body fat equals or exceeds 30% of total weight in women or 25% in men, an individual is considered obese.

Methods of Determining Obesity

Because of the difficulties in measuring body fat, relative weight has become the most popular and convenient indicator of obesity. It is calculated by dividing a person's actual weight by the ideal weight for his or her height and sex. A relative weight of 1.20 or greater (i.e., 20% or more over ideal weight) is used as an operational definition of obesity.

Using relative weight or percentage overweight as an indicator of obesity can be problematic. First, a person may be overweight without being obese because the increased weight reflects muscle mass rather than fat. Second, the point at which increased risk for disease occurs is not clear; the cutoff point of 20% overweight is arbitrary. Third, the concept of ideal weight is based on information from samples that are not representative of the U.S. population. These weights, which are based on data from the Metropolitan Life Insurance Company, may be too liberal for young adults and too restrictive for older persons.

Editor's Note: This chapter is adapted from Paul L. Doering, "Weight Control Products," in Covington, T.R., ed., *Handbook of Nonprescription Drugs,* 11th edition, which is based, in part, on the chapter with the same title that appeared in the 10th edition but was written by Glenn D. Appelt. For a more extensive discussion of obesity, weight loss methods, dietary food supplements, and weight loss products and programs, readers are encouraged to consult Chapter 21 of the *Handbook.*

The 1985 National Institutes of Health Consensus Development Conference on Obesity recommended that body mass index (BMI) be used as an appropriate measure of the tendency toward obesity. It is derived by dividing weight in kilograms by the square of height in meters. For persons of average height, one BMI unit is equivalent to approximately 3.1 kg (6.8 lb) in men and 2.6 kg (5.8 lb) in women. Table 1 presents body weight by height and in correspondence with selected BMI values. The table can be used to approximate an individual's BMI.

Etiology of Obesity

Most obesity is associated with overeating, particularly of carbohydrates or fats. Daily caloric allowances for persons with moderate physical activity may vary with age and sex. As a general rule, an intake of 3500 Cal (kcal) over expenditure will produce a weight gain of approximately 0.454 kg (1 lb) whereas an expenditure of 3500 Cal over intake will result in a 0.454-kg (1-lb) loss of body fat. Daily caloric allowances for average men (weight = 70 kg or 154 lb; height = 1.78 m or 5 feet 10 inches) in a temperate climate range from 3200 Cal at 25 years of age to 2550 Cal at 65 years of age. Corresponding figures for average women (weight = 58 kg or 128 lb; height = 1.63 m or 5 feet 4 inches) are 2300 and 1800 Cal at ages 25 and 65, respectively. The daily caloric requirement for women increases slightly during pregnancy (by 300 Cal) and significantly during lactation (by 500 Cal for one child and 1000 Cal for twins).

Consequences of Obesity

Studies have shown a significant association between morbidity, early mortality, and obesity. Among the more serious and widespread consequences of obesity are cardiovascular disease, diabetes mellitus, skin disorders, cancer, hyperlipidemia, and respiratory problems.

Weight Loss Methods

A variety of methods, alone or in combination, are used to accomplish weight loss. Different approaches are successful for different people.

Dietary Change

Dietary change is the most commonly used weight loss strategy. Methods range from caloric restriction to changes in dietary proportions of fat, protein, and carbohydrate or use of macronutrient substitutes.

Caloric Restriction

The low-calorie diet (LCD) of about 1000–1500 Cal per day may involve a structured commercial program with formulated and calorically defined food products or with guidelines for selecting conventional foods. The very-low-calorie diet (VLCD) at 800 or fewer calories per day is conducted under physician supervision and should be restricted to severely overweight persons. VLCDs are associated with a variety of short-term adverse effects (e.g., fatigue, hair loss, dizziness). The increased risk for gallstones and acute gallbladder disease during severe caloric restriction is more serious.

If total fasting is used to treat obesity, hospitalization and intensive medical supervision are recommended.

TABLE 1 Body weights corresponding to height and body mass index[a]

Height (in.)	Body mass index (kg/m^2)													
	19	20	21	22	23	24	25	26	27	28	29	30	35	40
	Body weight (lb)													
58	91	96	100	105	110	115	119	124	129	134	138	143	167	191
59	94	99	104	109	114	119	124	128	133	138	143	148	173	198
60	97	102	107	112	118	123	128	133	138	143	148	153	179	204
61	100	106	111	116	122	127	132	137	143	148	153	158	185	211
62	104	109	115	120	126	131	136	142	147	153	158	164	191	218
63	107	113	118	124	130	135	141	146	152	158	163	169	197	225
64	110	116	122	128	134	140	145	151	157	163	169	174	204	232
65	114	120	126	132	138	144	150	156	162	168	174	180	210	240
66	118	124	130	136	142	148	155	161	167	173	179	186	216	247
67	121	127	134	140	146	153	159	166	172	178	185	191	223	255
68	125	131	138	144	151	158	164	171	177	184	190	197	230	262
69	128	135	142	149	155	162	169	176	182	189	196	203	236	270
70	132	139	146	153	160	167	174	181	188	195	202	207	243	278
71	136	143	150	157	165	172	179	186	193	200	208	215	250	286
72	140	147	154	162	169	177	184	191	199	206	213	221	258	294
73	144	151	159	166	174	182	189	197	204	212	219	227	265	302
74	148	155	163	171	179	186	194	202	210	218	225	233	272	311
75	152	160	168	176	184	192	200	208	216	224	232	240	279	319
76	156	164	172	180	189	197	205	213	221	230	238	246	287	328

[a]To use the table, find the appropriate height in the left-hand column; then move across the row to a given weight. The number at the top of the column is the body mass index for the height and weight.

Reprinted with permission from NIH Technology Assessment Conference Panel. Methods for voluntary weight loss and control. *Ann Intern Med.* 1993; 119(7 pt 2): 764–70.

Altered Proportions of Food Groups

High-protein, low-carbohydrate diets of 800–1000 Cal per day are often used in weight reduction programs. These and other diets consisting of unbalanced proportions of food groups have been associated with a variety of adverse effects. A low-calorie, balanced diet containing no less than 12%–14% protein, no more than 30% fat (preferably unsaturated), and the remainder composed of complex carbohydrates (low sucrose) is recommended.

Contraindications to Unsupervised Dieting

Unsupervised weight loss is contraindicated for severely overweight persons, pregnant or lactating women, children, persons over age 65, and those with medical conditions that make such an undertaking dangerous.

Exercise

The amount of weight loss that can be achieved by exercise programs alone is more limited than the amount that can be obtained by caloric restriction. Nonetheless, exercise is a key component of a weight control program.

Behavioral Modification

Behavioral modification involves (1) identifying eating or related lifestyle behaviors to be modified, (2) setting specific behavioral goals, (3) modifying determinants of the behavior to be changed, and (4) reinforcing the desired behavior. Behavioral modification can be undertaken through group or individual sessions, under the guidance of professional or lay personnel, and alone or in conjunction with other approaches.

Drug Therapy

Drug treatment of obesity is of limited value. The only satisfactory means of long-term weight control is lifestyle change incorporating caloric reduction and increased physical activity. Drug therapy combined with some degree of caloric restriction can produce weight loss that is equivalent to that obtained with VLCDs alone over comparable periods. Renewed research interest in appetite suppressant drugs has led to some promising discoveries; however, the available drugs are far from ideal.

Dextroamphetamine

Although amphetamines are still labeled for short-term use as appetite suppressants, their use in weight loss programs has diminished greatly. Some states prohibit the prescribing of amphetamines and other related agents for diet purposes. Amphetamines appear to lose effectiveness after a few weeks of therapy and have a substantial abuse potential.

Fenfluramine

Fenfluramine is believed to reduce food intake by partially inhibiting the reuptake of serotonin and releasing serotonin from nerve endings. The D-isomer of fenfluramine, dexfenfluramine (Redux), was recently approved for use in the United States.

Fenfluramine-Phentermine

This combination is being prescribed by large numbers of practitioners around the country, owing in part to media attention. Research indicates that phentermine inhibits reuptake of norepinephrine; the combined mechanism of the two agents seems to prevent the development of tolerance seen with phentermine alone. Although short-term losses have occurred in clinical trials, the losses have often not been sustained at long-term follow-up.

Fluoxetine

Several studies of 5- to 6-months' duration have shown significantly greater weight loss with fluoxetine than with placebo. Long-term studies are needed to determine weight loss continues beyond this period. Fluoxetine is marketed as an antidepressant and is not currently indicated for weight loss.

Phenylpropanolamine

The Food and Drug Administration (FDA) final monograph on OTC weight control products includes only phenylpropanolamine (PPA) and benzocaine as Category I drugs. The FDA has termed PPA to be generally safe and effective for short-term weight control.

Dosage. The FDA permits a PPA dose of up to 37.5 mg in immediate-release products and of up to 75 mg in sustained-release products. The maximum daily dose is 75 mg.

Adverse Effects. Side effects such as nervousness, restlessness, insomnia, dizziness, perspiration, anxiety, headache, nausea, and an excessive increase in blood pressure may occur with PPA, especially if the recommended dose is exceeded. Potentially serious cardiovascular and central nervous system (CNS) adverse effects have been reported following both excessive and recommended doses of products containing PPA. Pharmacists should advise patients of the possible CNS adverse effects of PPA.

However, controlled clinical trials have demonstrated an absence of significant side effects on hypertensive activity with PPA in obese and in healthy, nonobese patients. An FDA advisory panel concluded that the incidence of side effects with oral PPA is low at recommended doses.

Because PPA is an adrenergic substance, it may elevate blood glucose levels and produce cardiac stimulation. The labels on products containing PPA warn that individuals with diabetes mellitus, heart disease, hypertension, or thyroid disease should seek medical advice before taking this drug.

Drug Interactions. Reports of adverse reactions with PPA and PPA-containing combinations should be interpreted within the total context of use. Many involve only one case or a report of multiple drug ingestion. Factors such as hypersensitivity, dosage, product form, concurrent pathology, and the presence of other drugs should be established before the use of PPA is discouraged.

Benzocaine

Recently, citing serious design flaws in clinical trials, the FDA has warned manufacturers of its intent to classify benzocaine as an ineffective weight loss product. Most manufacturers have already removed it from their products.

Dietary Food Supplements

Low-Calorie Balanced Foods

The "canned diet" products are considered substitutes for the usual diet. Any diet of 900 Cal that supplies adequate protein and lowers carbohydrate and fat intake should enable an obese patient to lose weight. When used properly, these products can serve an important function for the person trying to lose weight. Powder, granule, and liquid forms are available; these products are also formulated as cookies and soups.

Artificial Sweeteners

Saccharin

After bladder tumors were discovered in rats fed very large doses of saccharin in utero and throughout life, the FDA removed saccharin from the list of food additives generally recognized as safe. Epidemiologic studies have not revealed a clear-cut relationship between saccharin and urinary bladder carcinoma in humans. Saccharin is permitted in products labeled as diet foods or beverages. Saccharin may accumulate in fetal tissues and should not be used during pregnancy.

Aspartame

The FDA has determined that aspartame is safe as a food additive. Individuals with phenylketonuria or patients who should avoid protein foods must be alerted to the fact that it contains phenylalanine.

Other Sweeteners

Fructose, sorbitol, and xylitol may be used as alternatives to saccharin, but these sweeteners contain calories and should not be viewed as "sugar-free" diet items. Apparently, neither sorbitol nor xylitol causes tooth decay. Some evidence implicates xylitol in the development of urinary tract abnormalities, kidney stones, and tumors in laboratory animals. Ingestion of sufficient amounts of dietetic candies containing sorbitol may result in an osmotic diarrhea in young children.

Fat Substitutes

These substitutes mimic the "mouth-feel" of fat but contain fewer calories. They are used in desserts and baked goods, to replace fat in cheeses and meats, and in cooking and frying.

Nutrient Supplements

If a dieting patient is not receiving adequate quantities of vitamins and minerals in the diet regimen chosen, the administration of vitamins and minerals is warranted. The pharmacist might want to recommend a once-daily vitamin tablet to guard against inadequate intake.

Dosage Forms

Nonprescription products for obesity control are available as liquids, powders, granules, tablets, capsules, sustained-release capsules, wafers, cookies, soups, chewing gum, and candy preparations. If wafers, chewing gum, or candy cubes are substituted for high-calorie desserts or snacks, the candylike nature of the dosage form may offer patients a psychologic aid that is not found when a standard tablet or capsule is used.

Commercial Weight Loss Programs and Products

Weight Loss Programs

People who stay in programs achieve modest weight losses (4.8–15.6 lb during the first 12 weeks and 7–13.2 lb more during the next 12 weeks), but fewer than 20% of participants stay in programs long enough to lose an appreciable amount of weight.

Many weight loss programs include 1000- to 1500-Cal-per-day diets in which projected weight loss averages 1 or 2 lb/wk. The member usually follows a carefully controlled menu plan. In some cases, the participant is required to purchase specially packaged meals available only from the company, and most often these purchases are not reimbursable through health insurance.

Leading weight control programs include TOPS (Take Off Pounds Sensibly), Weight Watchers, Diet Center, Nutri/System, Overeaters Anonymous, and Optifast. Overeaters Anonymous, unlike the others, is a nonprofit program.

Pharmacists are urged to help their patients evaluate the promotional claims of these and all other weight loss plans before paying for them.

Selecting a Weight Loss Method/Program

Pharmacists should advise patients who are evaluating a weight loss method or program to consider the following:

■ The percentage of participants who complete the program;

■ The percentage of those completing the program who achieve various degrees of weight loss;

■ The proportion of weight loss maintained at 1, 3, and 5 years;

■ The percentage of participants who experienced adverse medical or psychologic effects and the kind and severity of those effects;

■ The relative mix of diet, exercise, and behavioral modifications;

■ The amount and kind of counseling (individual sessions and closed groups, in which membership does not change except by attrition, are more successful than open groups, in which members may come and go);

■ The nature of available multidisciplinary expertise (medical, nutritional, psychologic, physiologic, and exercise);

■ The training provided for relapse prevention to deal with high-risk emotional and social situations;

■ The nature and duration of the maintenance phase;

■ The flexibility of food choices and suitability of food types; and

■ The manner in which weight goals are set (unilaterally or cooperatively with the director of the weight loss program).

Weight Loss Products/Diets

A succession of fad diet products has come and gone over the years. Previously popular diets that proved to be ineffective include the Beverly Hills Diet, False Mayo Diet, Twenty-First Century Diet, Immune Power Diet, Fit for Life Diet, Living Healthy Diet, It's Not Your Fault You Are Fat Diet, Atkin's Diet, and Stillman's Diet.

Potentially Dangerous Diet Products

Botanical Products with Stimulant Effects. The FDA is particularly concerned about reports of adverse reactions associated with use of products containing multiple pharmacologically related ingredients, including ma huang (Ephedra sinica or Chinese ephedra, a botanical source of ephedrine, pseudoephedrine, and nor-pseudoephedrine), guarana or kola nut (sources of caffeine), white willow (salicin source), and chromium. These products are often touted for their reported stimulant effects and their ability to enhance metabolism ("fat burners"). Reactions vary from the milder adverse effects known to be associated with sympathomimetic stimulants to chest pain, myocardial infarct, stroke, seizures, psychosis, and death.

Cal-Ban 3000. Cal-Ban's main ingredient is guar gum, a complex sugar that swells when it becomes wet and can create a sense of fullness when ingested. The FDA has ordered that the distribution of Cal-Ban be halted because it may cause esophageal, gastric, and intestinal obstruction.

Weight Loss Teas. Weight loss products, often marketed as "dieter's or slimming teas," contain a variety of strong botanical laxatives (Cassia species [senna], cascara sagrada [botanical name Rhamnus purshiana]) and diuretics. Adverse reactions include severe electrolyte imbalances that may lead to cardiac arrhythmia and death.

The above products are not classified as drugs by the FDA and hence do not undergo premarket review of safety or effectiveness. There is no good dosing information or monitoring advice available, and there are no standards for potency and purity of ingredients. When patients inquire about such products, the pharmacist should review the patient's current prescription and nonprescription drug history. When taking a drug history for any purpose, the pharmacist should ask about the use of botanicals and any other unproven "nutritional" products and should discourage their use by anyone with significant diseases superimposed on obesity.

Products/Diets of Questionable Safety/Efficacy

Among the widely publicized products or systems of unproven efficacy are the Protein-Sparing Modified Fast Diet (PSMF); lipotrophic substances; citrin; the Cleanse, Build, and Burn Pack; the USAI Diet; spirulina; starch blockers; glucomannan; and chromium.

The Pharmacist's Role in Weight Counseling

Patients who request a nonprescription weight loss product may not be well informed about weight-related issues, including physiology and human nutrition. Many have incorrect notions, reinforced by the media, about methods of weight loss and their effectiveness. They often have inflated expectations about the latest diet method. The pharmacist can offer the following assistance:

■ Answer questions about weight loss methods and products;

■ Help the patient set realistic weight loss goals;

■ Counsel the patient on the proper use of drugs and supplements;

■ Refer the patient to a dietitian for evaluation and diet management; and

■ Help monitor the patient for adverse events that may occur during therapy.

The pharmacist should emphasize that even though a caloric deficit must be achieved, the diet must provide all essential nutrients. A regular exercise regimen, which could be as simple as walking, is essential to better health and to maintenance of long-term weight loss. Methods whose primary goal is short-term rapid or unsupervised weight loss and those that rely solely on diet aids such as drinks, prepackaged foods, or pharmacologic agents have never been shown to lead to long-term success.

More particularly, the pharmacist can also help patients spot fraudulent weight loss schemes and recommend legitimate alternatives. The pharmacist should advise patients to be wary of products that:

■ Make exaggerated health claims for particular nutrients or nutrient combinations;

■ Invent their own "physiology" to impress the consumer;

■ Promise quick results for little effort by using "breakthrough formulas";

■ Use anecdotal data, testimonials, radio/television talk show propaganda and info-mercials, or unpublished or unscientific data; or

■ Preach their version of good nutrition and blame a "conspiracy" involving organized medicine for criticizing their "discovery."

Finally, by monitoring the purchase of nonprescription weight loss products, the pharmacist can spot the beginnings of an eating disorder and take steps to get help for the patient.

Product Selection Guidelines

In recommending a nonprescription product for weight control, the pharmacist should:

■ Stress that weight cannot be reduced without a concerted effort to change one's eating and exercise lifestyles and to maintain the new behavior long term;

■ Make the patient aware of the caloric value of various food types;

■ Inquire about diet regimens the patient has attempted so that other nonprescription diet management adjuncts may be considered;

■ Determine if vitamins have been added to a particular weight control product and consider the appropriateness of vitamin supplementation for the individual patient;

■ Consider monitoring the patient's weight reduction efforts.

CHAPTER 22

Ophthalmic Products

Questions to ask in patient assessment and counseling

- Is your vision blurred?
- Do your eyes hurt? Is the pain sharp or dull? Is it constant or intermittent?
- Do your eyes itch or sting?
- Do you have any other eye problems (double vision, redness, scratchy feeling, discharge, or twitch)?
- How long have these symptoms been present? What were you doing when you noticed them? Have you had a similar problem before?
- Have you recently used a nonprescription eye product? Which one(s) did you use? For what symptoms?
- Have you recently been in an accident or injured your head in any way?
- What is the nature of your work?
- Have you been working outside or in an environment that would cause your eyes to water, itch, or burn?
- Have your eyes been exposed recently to irritants such as smog, chemicals, or sun glare? Have you recently applied any pesticides or fertilizers?
- Do you have a chronic disease such as diabetes, glaucoma, or hypertension?
- Have you recently had a head cold or sinus problem?
- Are you taking any prescription or nonprescription medications?
- Do you have any allergies? If so, to what are you allergic?
- Do you wear contact lenses? Are they hard or soft lenses?
- What contact lens products do you use?
- Do you use eye cosmetics? Have you changed brands of eye makeup or used a friend's eye makeup?
- Do you use hair spray or spray deodorants?

Common Ocular Disorders

Ocular inflammation and irritation can be caused by many conditions, some of which can be treated safely and effectively with nonprescription ophthalmic products. These products are used primarily to relieve minor symptoms of burning, stinging, itching, and watering. The Food and Drug Administration (FDA) has suggested that self-medication may be indicated for tear insufficiency, corneal edema, and external inflammation or irritation.

Editor's Note: This chapter is adapted from Mark W. Swanson and Jimmy D. Bartlett, "Ophthalmic Products," in Covington, T.R., ed., *Handbook of Nonprescription Drugs,* 11th edition, which is based, in part, on the chapter with the same title that appeared in the 10th edition but was written by Jimmy D. Bartlett and Mark W. Swanson. For a more extensive discussion of eye anatomy and physiology, ocular disorders, and ophthalmic products, readers are encouraged to consult Chapter 22 of the *Handbook.*

Self-medication also may be effective in managing hordeolum (stye), blepharitis, and conjunctivitis. Referral for medical care is mandatory for embedded foreign bodies, uveitis, flash burns, chemical burns, tear duct infection, and corneal ulcers.

The FDA has recommended that consumers not self-treat ophthalmic conditions for longer than 72 hours without consulting a doctor. The pharmacist should advise patients of this rule when recommending nonprescription ophthalmic products. Figures 1 and 2 provide algorithms that may be used in the decision-making process when managing eyelid irritation and red eye, respectively. If the etiology is not simple external irritation, referral to an optometrist or ophthalmologist is strongly encouraged.

Eyelid Disorders

Blunt Trauma

Under most circumstances, blunt trauma does not result in internal damage and treatment is largely supportive, entailing cold compresses and oral nonprescription analgesics as needed. Nonetheless, all individuals with blunt trauma should be evaluated by an ophthalmologist or optometrist as soon as possible, because internal eye bleeding, secondary glaucoma, and retinal detachment are possible complications.

Blepharitis

Blepharitis is an extremely common inflammatory condition of the eyelid margins. Red, scaly, thickened eyelids, often with loss of the eyelashes, are typical. Itching and burning are the most common complaints. Treatment may include topical antibiotics or nonprescription lid hygiene preparations.

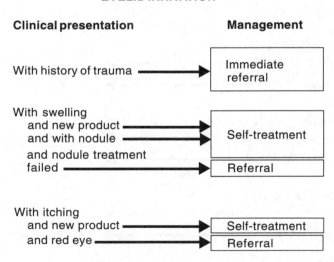

EYELID IRRITATION

FIGURE 1   Decision-making algorithm for management of patients with eyelid irritation.

Lice Infestation

Infestation of the eyelids with the crab louse or head louse may cause symptoms similar to blepharitis. Pediculicides (e.g., RID, NIX, A-200) should not be used around the eye because of potential severe hypersensitivity reactions. A bland ophthalmic ointment (e.g., petrolatum) used for 10 days is effective. A 0.25% physostigmine ointment is effective, but the side effects are not well tolerated. Pharmacists should instruct patients about the need to take hygienic measures, such as washing clothing and bedding.

Contact Dermatitis

Swelling, scaling, or redness of the eyelid, along with profuse itching, are common with contact dermatitis. A change in makeup or soap, or exposure to a foreign substance is usually the cause. The equal involvement of each eyelid suggests allergy. Removal of the offending substance is the best treatment. Nonprescription oral antihistamines, along with cold compresses, help reduce inflammation and itching.

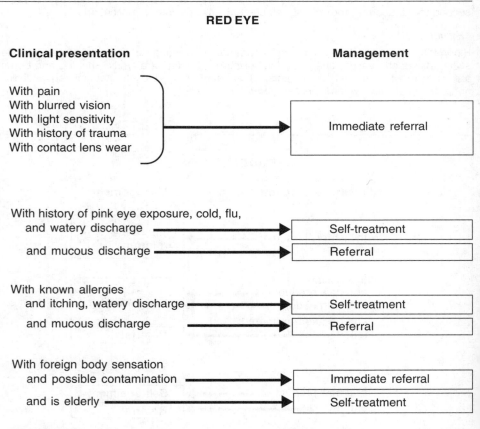

FIGURE 2   Decision-making algorithm for management of patients with red eye(s).

Hordeolum

Hordeolum (stye) is an inflammation of glands in the eyelid. It is generally caused by one of the staphylococcal species associated with blepharitis. A nodule is always present. Swelling of the eyelid, almost to the point of closure, can occur. Hordeola typically respond well to hot compresses applied three to four times daily for 5–10 minutes at each session. Clearing usually occurs within 1 week. Internal hordeola are best treated with oral antibiotics; external hordeola may be treated with a topical antibiotic.

Ocular Surface Disorders

Foreign Substance Contact

Foreign substances often contact the ocular surface. If reflex tearing does not remove the foreign substance, the eye may need to be flushed with sterile saline or specific eyewash preparations (irrigants). Metallic foreign bodies are often not removed by irrigation and can cause abrasion, scarring, and chronic red eye if not removed. Immediate medical referral is indicated.

Abrasions

Contact with foreign matter can also cause abrasions of the cornea and conjunctiva. Self-treatment is not recommended owing to the risk of bacteria or fungi contaminating and infecting the eye.

Chemical Exposure

Chemical exposure by splash injury, a solid chemical, or fumes is a medical emergency. The initial treatment should include flushing the eye with sterile saline for at least 10 minutes. If saline is not available, water may be used. This type of injury should be referred immediately to an emergency facility.

Thermal Damage

One minor form of thermal damage occurs from exposure to UV radiation during snow skiing without protective goggles. It usually responds well to artificial tear solutions or ointments. If such treatment does not provide relief within 24 hours, medical referral is indicated. More severe forms of thermal injury may require a visit to the optometrist or ophthalmologist.

Conjunctivitis

Conjunctivitis is the term given to inflammation of the bulbar conjunctiva. Four general types of conjunctivitis are commonly seen: viral, allergic, bacterial, and chlamydial.

Viral Conjunctivitis. Patients with this condition usually have a "pink eye" with copious watery discharge, ocular discomfort, and a mild sensation that a foreign body is in the eye. Viral conjunctivitis is usually self-limiting; symptoms resolve over 1–3 weeks. Treatment is aimed at relief of the major symptoms using artificial tear preparations and ocular decongestants. Because certain forms of viral conjunctivitis can be extremely contagious, counseling should include warnings about washing hands, not sharing towels, and properly disposing of tissues used to blot the eye.

Allergic Conjunctivitis. The hallmark symptom of ocular allergy is itching, usually accompanied by a red eye with a watery discharge. The most common allergens include pollen, animal dander, and topical eye preparations. Questioning the patient about

271

exposure to an allergen may help identify the offending substance. Removal or avoidance of the cause is the best treatment, but ocular decongestants, ocular decongestant antihistamine preparations, nonprescription oral antihistamines, and cold compresses help relieve symptoms.

Bacterial Conjunctivitis. Bacterial conjunctivitis is characterized by a red eye with purulent discharge and general eye discomfort. The eyelids are often stuck together on awakening. The condition is typically self-limiting within 2 weeks, but topical antibiotics can clear the infection more quickly.

Chlamydial Conjunctivitis. Chlamydial conjunctivitis may have many signs and symptoms in common with both viral and bacterial conjunctivitis, and it is often initially misdiagnosed. Misdiagnosis can be a serious problem because afflicted individuals often harbor other sexually transmitted diseases. Self-treatment should be discouraged if symptoms and signs are vague.

Keratitis

Keratitis is the inflammation of the cornea. It is potentially a vision-threatening problem. Individuals with red eye and signs of keratitis (i.e., blurred vision, photophobia, pain) need to be evaluated as soon as possible by an optometrist or ophthalmologist. This is especially true for patients who wear contact lenses, because ulceration and loss of the eye are more likely among this population.

Corneal Edema

Halos or "star bursts" around lights, with or without reduced vision, are a hallmark symptom of corneal edema. Once the diagnosis is established, hypertonic saline in solution or ointment form, usually in 2% and 5% concentrations, can be used to dehydrate the cornea. Pharmacists should warn individuals using a 5% solution that profound stinging may occur on instillation.

Dry Eye

This condition is characterized by a white or mildly red eye; a sandy, gritty feeling or complaint of something in the eye is common, as is excessive tearing. Antihistamines, anticholinergics or drugs with anticholinergic properties (e.g., antihistamines and anti-depressants), diuretics, and beta-blockers are common pharmacologic causes of dry eye. Dry eye can also be associated with aging or a number of diseases. Treatment entails the instillation of nonprescription artificial tears and lubricants. Preparations without preservatives have been shown to have a greater beneficial effect. Vitamin A preparations may be of greatest benefit in treating severe dry eye associated with glandular tissue destruction.

Internal Eye Conditions

Uveitis

Uveitis is the term for inflammation of the uveal tract (iris, ciliary body, or choroid). Pain, blurred vision, and photophobia are common. The eye is usually mildly to markedly red with reflex tearing. Treatment involves topical, depot, or systemic oral steroids, depending on the cause. Because of the severe consequences of untreated or improperly treated uveitis (i.e., secondary glaucoma, blindness), care must be taken in recommending self-treatment.

Angle-Closure Glaucoma

Angle-closure (narrow-angle) glaucoma may present as a red, painful eye. The most common symptoms are brow-ache or headache, often accompanied by nausea and vomiting. Individuals complaining about headache or eye pain after an eye examination that involved pupillary dilation should be referred immediately to their eye doctor.

Ophthalmic Drug Formulations

Ophthalmic medications available without a prescription are formulated to reduce the stinging and other side effects common with many prescribed ophthalmic drugs. Among the inactive ingredients of these products, the drug vehicle and preservative systems are the most important.

Vehicles

An ophthalmic vehicle is an agent other than the active drug that is added to a formulation to enhance drug action by providing increased viscosity that retards drainage of the active ingredient from the eye. Among the most commonly used vehicles for ophthalmic solutions are povidone, polyvinyl alcohol (PVA), hydroxypropyl methylcellulose (HPMC), and poloxamer 407. Ointments that consist of a mixture of white petrolatum and mineral oil, with or without a water-miscible agent, are also used as vehicles. Patients should be informed that using these agents coat the eye and may temporarily cause blurred vision.

Preservatives

Preservatives are incorporated into ophthalmic products designed for multidose use. They are intended to destroy or limit multiplication of microorganisms inadvertently introduced into the product. Commonly used preservatives include the quaternary surfactants benzalkonium chloride and benzethonium chloride, chlorhexidine, thimerosal, chloro-butanol, methylparaben and propylparaben, and ethylenediaminetetraacetic acid. Thimerosal may produce allergic reactions with prolonged use; ethylenediaminetetraacetic acid may also induce contact allergies.

Major Categories of Nonprescription Ophthalmic Products

Numerous nonprescription ophthalmic products for treating minor ocular irritations are available for self-administration under minimal or no supervision. Such products are also adequate for treating certain clinical conditions that have been diagnosed by health practitioners. The pharmacist must assist patients in selecting the appropriate product that will enhance compliance, minimize or avoid side effects, and reduce the attendant costs of therapy.

Lubricants

Artificial Tear Solutions (Demulcents)

These solutions are usually administered three to four times daily but may be given more or less frequently, depending on patient need. Products commonly used in these preparations include cellulose ethers, PVA, and povidone.

In recent years, artificial tear preparations have been introduced in preservative-free formulations. This is beneficial for patients who are sensitive to certain preservatives. In general, nonpreserved formulations have the disadvantage of increased cost, and they can become easily contaminated by the patient during use. Unused solution should be discarded after 12 hours. No single formulation of artificial tears will universally improve clinical signs and symptoms of dry eyes while maintaining patient comfort and acceptance.

A sterile, buffered isotonic solution is available specifically for cleaning and lubricating artificial eyes.

Table 1 summarizes guidelines for self-administration of eyedrops.

Nonmedicated Ointments (Emollients)

The principal advantage of nonmedicated (bland) ointments is their enhanced retention time in the eye.

Ointment formulations are usually administered twice daily but may be administered as often as every few hours or only occasionally as needed.

Blurred vision is a common problem during ointment therapy. It can usually be resolved by decreasing the amount of ointment instilled or by administering it at bedtime. As a rule, it is better to recommend nonmedicated ointments without preservatives for the treatment of dry eye to overcome potential problems that might occur with the use of products with preservatives.

Table 2 summarizes guidelines for self-administration of eye ointments.

Decongestants

Phenylephrine

Only the 0.12% and 0.125% concentrations are available without a prescription.

Even the low concentrations of phenylephrine used in nonprescription topical decongestants may dilate the pupil. This is not uncommon in persons who wear contact lenses, who may instill the medication following lens wear. Patients should be cautioned against instilling this and other ophthalmic decongestants too often. They should be encouraged to seek professional eye care if offending ophthalmic signs or symptoms do not resolve within 72 hours.

TABLE 1 Procedure for self-administration of eyedrops

1. Wash hands thoroughly.

2. Tilt head backward.

3. Gently grasp lower outer eyelid below lashes and pull eyelid away from eye to create a pouch.

4. Place dropper over eye by looking directly at it.

5. Just before applying a single drop, look upward.

6. After applying the drop, look downward for several seconds.

7. Release the eyelid slowly.

8. Close eyes gently for 1–2 minutes. Minimize blinking or squeezing the eyelid.

9. With a finger, put gentle pressure over the opening of the tear duct at the inner corner of the eye.

10. Blot excessive solution from around the eye.

TABLE 2   Procedure for self-administration of eye ointments

1. Wash hands thoroughly.
2. Tilt head backward.
3. Gently grasp lower outer eyelid below lashes and pull eyelid away from eye.
4. Place ointment tube over eye by looking directly at it.
5. With a sweeping motion, place 1/4- to 1/2-inch of ointment inside the lower eyelid by gently squeezing the tube.
6. Release the eyelid slowly.
7. Close eyes gently for 1–2 minutes.
8. Blot excessive ointment from around the eye.
9. Vision may be temporarily blurred. Avoid activities requiring good visual ability until vision clears.

The most important and common side effect following chronic use of phenylephrine for ocular decongestion is rebound congestion of the conjunctiva. Such patients should be referred for professional eye care.

Systemic adverse effects are extremely rare following the topical instillation of nonprescription phenylephrine. The drug should be used cautiously, however, by patients with cardiovascular disease or diabetes and by patients taking atropine, tricylic antidepressants, monamine oxidase inhibitors, reserpine, guanethidine, or methyldopa.

Imidazoles

The imidazoles include naphazoline, tetrahydrozoline, and oxymetazoline. They are clinically useful in constricting conjunctival vessels. These drugs have only minimal effect on underlying vessels of the episclera and sclera.

The imidazoles generally do not induce ocular or systemic side effects. However, patients should be cautioned that their liberal or indiscriminate use can lead to excessive systemic absorption and the possibility of cardiovascular side effects. Some patients may experience abnormal dryness with prolonged use. Because rebound congestion appears to be less likely following use of naphazoline or tetrahydrozoline, these agents should generally be recommended over phenylephrine or oxymetazoline. Naphazoline 0.02% can be recommended with confidence as an ocular decongestant of choice.

Antihistamines

Two nonprescription antihistamines are available for topical ophthalmic use: pheniramine maleate and antazoline phosphate. They are indicated for the rapid relief of symptoms associated with seasonal or atopic conjunctivitis. All nonprescription preparations contain the decongestant agent naphazoline because the combination has been shown to be more effective than either agent alone. The FDA has classified the topical antihistamines in the less than effective category primarily because clinical trial data on effectiveness are lacking.

The recommended dosage is one or two drops applied to each eye three or four times daily. Burning, stinging, and discomfort on instillation are the most common side effects. Pheniramine may be somewhat more comfortable. Antihistamines are contraindicated in persons with a known risk of angle-closure glaucoma.

Irrigants

Irrigants are used on a short-term basis to cleanse ocular tissues and maintain their moisture. They are also used for ocular lavage following chemical injury to the eye. Although physiologic saline is the ideal irrigant for this purpose, water is acceptable if nothing else is available. Alkali or acid burns warrant immediate evaluation and treatment by an ophthalmologist or optometrist. Continuous eye pain, changes in vision, continued redness or irritation of the eye, or worsening of an ocular condition also merit referral.

Ocular irrigants should not be used in conjunction with eye care products containing PVA. Commercial products that use an eyecup should be avoided because of difficulties in cleaning the eyecup and the risk of contamination.

Hyperosmotics

Hyperosmotic formulations are intended to increase the tonicity of the tear film, thereby promoting movement of fluid from the cornea. They may provide subjective relief of discomfort and improve vision for patients with mild-to-moderate corneal epithelial edema. Sodium chloride, in solution and ointment formulations, is the only ophthalmic hyperosmotic agent available without a prescription. Application of 5% sodium chloride tends to produce stinging and burning, and patients often prefer the 2% concentration.

One or two drops of the solution are usually instilled every 3–4 hours. The ointment requires less frequent instillation. Because vision associated with an edematous cornea is often worse on arising, several instillations of the solution during the first few waking hours may be helpful. Topical hyperosmotic sodium chloride is contraindicated in patients with clear, edematous corneas with a traumatized epithelium. Such patients should be referred for immediate professional eye care.

Antiseptics

Silver Protein

For mild ocular infections, several drops of silver protein are generally instilled every 3–4 hours for several days. Frequent application for prolonged periods should be avoided to prevent permanent discoloration of the eyelid skin or conjunctiva. This agent is incompatible with topically applied sodium sulfacetamide.

Boric Acid

Boric acid is indicated for the treatment of irritated or inflamed eyelids. It should be applied in a small quantity to the inner surface of the lower eyelid once or twice daily. If ocular irritation persists or increases, the patient should receive medical attention.

Zinc Sulfate

Zinc sulfate is a mild astringent for temporary relief of minor ocular irritation. It is generally used in a dosage of one to two drops up to four times daily.

Eyelid Scrubs

The mainstay of blepharitis therapy is careful eyelid hygiene. The patient can accomplish this by applying hot compresses for 15–20 minutes, two to four times daily. Each application should be followed by lid scrubs using a mild detergent cleanser compatible with ocular tissues (Table 3).

Although baby shampoo is often used for this purpose, other commercially available cleansers produce less stinging, burning, and toxicity. Lid scrub products are intended for the removal of oils, debris, or desquamated skin associated with the inflamed eyelid. They can also be used for hygienic eyelid cleansing in people who wear contact lenses. These products are designed to be used full strength on eyelid tissues and must not be instilled directly into the eye. If signs or symptoms fail to improve, the patient should be referred for a professional ocular examination and treatment with antibacterial agents.

Patient Counseling

The safety and effectiveness of ophthalmic products can be enhanced by paying strict attention to drug selection, contraindications, dosage schedules, and administration technique. Careful consideration of the patient's medical history, including concomitant medication use, can minimize the risk of adverse reactions. Appropriate dosing procedures are important.

Patient History

A careful history, focusing particularly on concomitant medications, can alert the pharmacist to possible adverse drug reactions and assist in selecting the most appropriate product.

Drug Interactions/Allergies

Drug interactions can potentiate or impair drug effects and exacerbate any potential adverse reaction. For example, topically applied phenylephrine may heighten the pressor effects of certain prescription drugs.

Inquiry regarding a history of drug allergies is essential. Hypersensitivity to thimerosal and other mercurial compounds is not uncommon among those who wear contact lenses, and topically applied ophthalmic medications containing mercurial preservatives, especially when used long term, can lead to allergic reactions.

TABLE 3 Procedure for eyelid scrubs

1. Wash hands thoroughly.

2. Apply three to four drops of baby shampoo or eyelid cleanser to cotton-tipped applicator or gauze pad.

3. Close one eye and clean the upper eyelid and eyelashes using side-to-side strokes, being careful not to touch eyeball with applicator or fingers.

4. Open eye, look up, and clean lower eyelid and eyelashes using side-to-side strokes.

5. Repeat the procedures on other eye using a clean applicator or gauze pad.

6. Rinse eyelids and eyelashes with clean, warm water.

Coexisting Medical Conditions

Patients with systemic hypertension, arteriosclerosis, and other cardiovascular diseases may be at risk if they use topically applied ocular decongestants.

It is prudent to limit topical ophthalmic dosing in pregnant women. Artificial tears can be used without limit.

Medical Referral

Patients who fail to respond to nonprescription therapy within 72 hours should generally be referred for medical evaluation, especially if they are not currently under the care of an ophthalmic practitioner. It is important for patients with acute ocular disease to receive a prompt diagnosis, including baseline visual acuity, before the appropriateness of nonprescription therapy is considered.

Many patients with chronic ocular conditions, especially dry eye, may fail to respond to initial nonprescription therapy with artificial tears or other lubricants. In many cases, the most appropriate strategy is to switch to a different lubricant, especially one with a different polymer or preservative system. If there is still no response, the patient should be encouraged to seek care from an ophthalmic practitioner.

Self-Administration of Ophthalmic Medications

The following guidelines should help promote the safe and effective use of nonprescription ophthalmic products:

- Nonprescription ophthalmic products should be used only in situations in which vision is not threatened, and they should generally not be used for longer than 72 hours without medical referral if the condition being treated persists or worsens.
- Nonprescription ocular medications should not be recommended to patients who have demonstrated an allergy to any of the active ingredients, preservatives, or excipients in the product.
- Patients who are already using a prescription ophthalmic product should use nonprescription products only after consulting an ophthalmic practitioner or pharmacist.
- Patients with a history of narrow anterior chamber angles or narrow-angle glaucoma should not use topical ocular decongestants.
- The lowest concentration and conservative dosage frequencies should be used.
- Drug application should be conservative in patients with hyperemic conjunctiva.
- Patients should be reminded to use all medications only as directed. There is generally no additional benefit from using more than the intended amount of the drug.
- If multiple drop therapy is indicated, the best interval between drops is at least 5 minutes.
- If both drop and ointment therapy are indicated, the drop should be applied at least 10 minutes before the ointment.
- Patients should wipe excessive solution or ointment from the eyelids and lashes after instillation.
- Because ointments may blur the patient's vision during the waking hours, they should be used with caution if visual acuity is critical; otherwise, bedtime instillation is most appropriate.
- Use of eyecups should be discouraged because of potential bacterial, fungal, or viral contamination.
- Ophthalmic medications should not be used beyond their expiration dates. Eyedrop bottles should be replaced or discarded 30 days after the sterility safety seal is opened.
- Patients should store all medications out of children's reach.

CHAPTER 23

Contact Lens Products

Questions to ask in patient assessment and counseling

- What types of lenses do you wear? Hard, soft, or rigid gas-permeable (RGP)? Are your lenses disposable or for extended wear?
- How long have you been wearing lenses? When did you start wearing this particular pair?
- What problems are you having with your lenses? Are they related to eye irritation or to changes in vision? When did the problems start?
- How many hours a day do you wear your lenses before problems start? Do you remove your lenses during the day?
- When did you last see your optometrist or ophthalmologist?
- How do you take care of your lenses?
- Have you recently changed brands of any of your solutions?
- How often do you change your storage solutions?
- How often do you clean or replace your storage container? Does it need to be replaced?
- Have you become pregnant or begun using oral contraceptives since you were prescribed lenses?
- What nonprescription and prescription medications are you now taking?
- Do you have any allergies?

Types of Contact Lenses

Contact lenses can be classified as hard, rigid gas-permeable (RGP), or soft. The majority of contact lens-wearing patients (85%) are fitted with soft (hydrophilic) lenses. About 74% of patients wearing contacts wear some type of disposable or planned replacement lenses. When used with a fastidious care and cleaning program, daily-wear soft lenses can have an average life of 12–14 months; similarly used RGP lenses last between 18 and 36 months.

Hard Lenses

Hard contact lenses were the first lenses to be used in the United States. They are made of esters of polymerized plastics. In rigid lenses, a small colored dot marker or an etch mark on one lens identifies it as being for the right eye. The hardness of these lenses is less than that of glass but more than that of RGP or soft lenses. Thus, reasonable care must be exercised to avoid scratching or chipping them. Inadequate care or neglect of hard lenses may lead to corneal problems or wearer discomfort, but the lens will still maintain its optical qualities.

One phenomenon associated with hard lenses is spectacle blur. A hard lens alters the topography of the eye and creates hypoxic edema. As a result, the patient may not see well with glasses immediately after removing the lens.

Editor's Note: This chapter is adapted from Janet P. Engle, "Contact Lens Products," in Covington, T.R., ed., *Handbook of Nonprescription Drugs,* 11th edition. For a more extensive discussion of contact lenses and lens care products and procedures, readers are encouraged to consult Chapter 23 of the *Handbook.*

RGP Lenses

RGP lenses, which are made of several different gas-permeable materials, combine the optical qualities of hard lenses with the oxygen permeability of soft lenses. To maintain rigidity (important for the correction of astigmatism and the fit of the lenses), RGP lenses are generally thicker than soft lenses. Some RGP lenses have been approved for 1–7 days of extended wear. The use of extended-wear lenses is somewhat controversial because they have been implicated in causing corneal ulcers (eruptions on the corneal surface), which in rare instances can lead to partial or complete blindness.

Soft Lenses

The difference between rigid lenses and soft lenses is that the latter will absorb and hold water. Soft lenses are easier to remove and more comfortable than rigid lenses, an effect most apparent during the initial break-in period. Photophobia is not likely with soft lenses. Soft lenses are also less likely than rigid lenses to trap dust particles, eyelashes, or other foreign material.

Because soft lenses cannot be as precisely tailored to the cornea, the fitting process is less exact than it is with rigid lenses. As a result, the quality of vision with soft contact lenses does not usually equal that of a properly fitted pair of rigid lenses.

Soft lenses can absorb chemical compounds from topically administered ophthalmic products. Ocular irritation may result, and the lens may be damaged. With the exception of a few specifically formulated rewetting solutions, no solution should be instilled into the eye with a soft lens in place. If a drug solution has been instilled into the eye, the wearer must wait until the solution has cleared the precorneal (conjunctival) pocket before inserting the lens. This takes about five minutes. If no instructions accompany an ophthalmic prescription for a soft lens wearer, the prescribing practitioner should be contacted. This is also true for a nonprescription ophthalmic product not specifically designed for use with contact lenses.

Use of Contact Lenses

Indications

The decision to wear contact lenses rather than eyeglasses is sometimes based on therapeutic necessity. For example, with keratoconus, a gradual protrusion of the central cornea, satisfactory vision is usually unattainable with ordinary eyeglasses but can be obtained with rigid contact lenses.

Other indications for the use of contacts include refractive errors such as myopia (nearsightedness), hyperopia (farsightedness), astigmatism, and presbyopia.

Contraindications

Some individuals who require vision correction cannot or should not wear contact lenses. Contraindications are often based on lifestyle, including occupational conditions, as well as on medical history. Contact lenses should not be used for cosmetic reasons if a patient has active pathologic intraocular or corneal conditions. Medical reasons that contraindicate contact lens wear include chronic conjunctivitis; blepharitis; recurrent viral, bacterial, or fungal infections; and poor blink rate or incomplete blink. Chronic common colds or allergic conditions such as hay fever and asthma may make lens wear extremely uncomfortable or impossible. Contact lenses should be used with caution by patients with epilepsy or severe arthritis. The corneal topography may be altered by pregnancy or oral contraceptives. Contact lenses can be used with care by elderly persons.

During the period needed for adapting to rigid contact lenses, the eyelids may become hyperemic; this condition may lead to blepharitis. Short pseudoblinks, by new wearers of hard lenses, may irritate the conjunctiva of the upper eyelid. Chin elevation and squinting may result from the patient's efforts to minimize the irritation.

Precautions

Some patients wearing contact lenses with high water content may experience hazy vision around the edge of objects. In some cases, patients wearing hard lenses experience night-time "ghosting," which occurs when the pupils dilate to such an extent that the patient can see the edges of the lens. Other patients complain of spider web vision, also usually at night. This can be due to crazing (i.e., the developing of fine cracks) and it is most common in RGP lenses.

Adverse Effects of Drugs

Topical Drugs

Many undesired effects have been reported when a patient who wears contact lenses topically applies certain drugs (Table 1). Patients should be counseled not to place any ophthalmic solution, suspension, gel, or ointment into the eye when contact lenses are in place. The only exceptions to this rule are products specifically formulated to be used with contact lenses or products that an eye care practitioner has recommended for use with contact lenses.

Airborne Drugs

Some drugs that are present in indoor air (e.g., ribavirin, nicotine) may damage lenses.

Systemic Drugs

Some systemic medications are secreted into tears and may interact with (primarily soft) contact lenses.

Cosmetics

Patients who wear contact lenses should choose cosmetics with care. They should insert their lenses before applying makeup and avoid touching the lens with eyeliner or mascara. Cosmetics, moisturizers, and makeup removers should have an aqueous base. Mascara should be applied only to the tips of the lashes. Eyeliner should never be applied inside the eyelid margin. Any aerosol product must be used with caution. Nail polish, hand creams, and perfumes should be applied only after the lenses have been inserted.

Patients often contaminate their lenses with hair preparations and spray deodorants; they should take care to clean their hands thoroughly before handling their contacts. Soaps containing cold cream or deodorants should be avoided. If the lens comes in contact with residual petrolatum-based lotion on the patient's fingers, its surface can be modified. This modification cannot be detected by inspection; it will be noted, however, once the lens is worn.

Corneal Hypoxia and Edema

Even when properly fitted, rigid and soft lenses can produce a progressive hypoxia of the cornea while the lenses are in place. One major effect of this hypoxia is corneal edema. Symptoms include photophobia; rainbows around a light; sensations of hotness, grittiness and itchiness; fogging of vision; and blurred vision. A patient experiencing corneal edema

TABLE 1 Drug–contact lens interactions

Changes in tear film and/or production

Tear volume decreased

Anticholinergic agents
Antihistamines
Diuretics

Timolol (topical)
Tricyclic antidepressants

Tear volume increased

Cholinergic agents

Reserpine

Changes in lens color (primarily soft lenses)

Diagnostic dyes
(i.e., fluorescein)
Epinephrine (topical)
Fluorescein (topical)
Nicotine

Nitrofurantoin
Phenazopyridine
Phenolphthalein
Phenothiazines
Phenylephrine

Rifampin
Sulfasalazine
Tetracycline
Tetrahydrozoline
(topical)

Changes in tonicity

Pilocarpine (8%)

Sodium sulfacetamide (10%)

Lid/corneal edema

Chlorthalidone
Clomiphene

Oral contraceptives
Primidone

Ocular inflammation/irritation

Gold salts
Isotretinoin

Salicylates

Changes in refractivity (i.e., induction of myopia)

Acetazolamide
Sulfadiazine
Sulfamethizole

Sulfamethoxazole
Sulfisoxazole

Miscellaneous

Digoxin (increased glare)
Ribavirin (cloudy lenses)
Topical ciprofloxacin/Prednisolone acetate
(precipitate)
Hypnotics/Sedatives/Muscle relaxants
(decreased blink rate)

Adapted with permission from Engle JP. Contact lens care. *Am Druggist*. 1990 Jan; 201: 54–65.

from overuse of contact lenses can be treated with one to two drops of sodium chloride (2% or 5%) every 3–4 hours after the lenses have been removed. Transient stinging or burning may occur upon instillation of the drops. The patient should be counseled not to overuse the lenses.

Corneal Abrasions

Corneal abrasions are surface defects in the epithelial layer of the cornea. The pain associated with corneal abrasion is usually of greater magnitude than the damage. The epithelium regenerates quickly. The lens should not be worn for 2–7 days. Extensive abrasions require the attention of an eye care specialist.

Symptoms of Lens Problems

The following list provides perspective for counseling a lens wearer. Most of this information is particularly applicable to rigid lens wear.

- *Deep aching of eye:* This pain persists even after the lens is removed, and it may be caused by poorly fitted lenses. An eye care practitioner must be consulted.

- *Blurred vision:* This effect may be produced by improper refractive power, wearing lenses in the wrong eye or inside out, tear film buildup, cosmetic film buildup, corneal edema, or oral contraceptives.

- *Excessive tearing:* Tearing is normal when lenses are first worn; however, tearing may also be caused by poorly fitted lenses or rough edges on the lenses.

- *Fogging:* Misty vision can be caused by corneal edema, overwearing of contact lenses, deposits on lens surfaces, or poor wetting of the lens while on the eye.

- *Flare:* Point sources of light having a sunburst or streaming quality can be caused by inadequate optic zone size or decentration of a poorly fitting lens.

- *Lens falling out of eye:* Poorly fitted lenses could be the cause; however, properly fitted rigid lenses may also occasionally slide off the cornea.

- *Inability to wear lenses in the morning:* This may be caused by corneal edema or mild conjunctivitis. Most likely, however, the patient's eyes dry out overnight owing to incomplete eyelid closure.

- *Pain after removal of lens:* This effect is usually caused by corneal abrasion. The lens anesthetizes the cornea by producing hypoxia. When sensation returns 4–6 hours after the lens has been removed, pain develops.

- *Sudden pain in the eye:* Sudden pain may be caused by a foreign body or chipped or folded lens.

- *Squinting:* This effect is caused by excessive lens movement or a poorly fitted lens.

Lens Care Products and Procedures

Contact Lens Solutions

Formulation Considerations

The manufacturing and marketing of contact lenses are regulated by the ophthalmic devices division of the Food and Drug Administration (FDA).

The basic considerations for a well-formulated contact lens solution include pH, viscosity, isotonicity with tears, stability, sterility, and provision for maintenance of sterility (bactericidal action).

Routine daily use of any contact lens solution allows the potential for bacterial contamination. The solution must, therefore, contain a bactericidal agent that is both effective over the long term and nonirritating with daily use in the eye. Few preservatives fulfill these criteria. Commonly used agents are benzalkonium chloride, thimerosal, and sorbic acid products, all of which can cause irritation, depending on concentration and patient sensitivity.

Preservatives

Benzalkonium Chloride. Some persons using a solution preserved with benzalkonium chloride develop ocular irritation. Switching to a solution with a lower benzalkonium chloride concentration may alleviate this, but change to a solution with a different agent may be required. Benzalkonium chloride should not be used with soft contact lenses because it is adsorbed onto the lens.

Thimerosal. Thimerosal does not pose a significant problem when used with hard contact lenses; however, most practitioners have discouraged its use in soft lens care products because of the high incidence of sensitivity.

Sorbic Acid or Potassium Sorbate. Less irritating than mercurials, sorbic acid or potassium sorbate is the preservative ingredient often included in products labeled "thimerosal-free" or "for sensitive eyes." Sorbic acid's maximum antimicrobial activity is at a pH that is too low to be of optimum value for use on the eye.

Chlorhexidine. At the concentration in which it is used in soft lens solutions, chlorhexidine is less effective against several yeasts and fungi than is optimal. Chlorhexidine-containing solutions that appear greenish should not be used because the color change indicates decomposition of the product.

Sodium Salts of EDTA. Sodium salts of ethylenediaminetetraacetic acid (EDTA) disrupt the integrity of bacterial cell walls and enhance the action of other preservatives. Addition of EDTA to nonpreserved saline solutions will increase their shelf life after opening.

Polyquaternium-1. Few toxicity or sensitivity problems have been noted with this preservative.

Polyaminopropyl Biguanide. No significant adverse effects to polyaminopropyl biguanide have been reported. The higher concentrations used with hard lenses do not seem to cause toxicity to the wearer because RGP lenses do not adsorb the preservatives to the degree that soft lenses do.

Solutions from different manufacturers should not be mixed because a precipitate may result.

Care of Hard Lenses

Hard lens care involves important steps: cleaning, soaking, and wetting (Figure 1). All three steps should be performed each time the lenses are removed from the eye.

Cleaning Solutions

Cleaning solutions generally contain surfactants that emulsify oils and aid in solubilizing other debris. Proteins and lipids are soluble in highly alkaline media, but a high pH can cause lens decomposition. Weak alkaline solutions, in conjunction with the surface tension-lowering properties of the surfactants, may help dislodge deposits from the lens.

Lenses should be thoroughly rinsed after cleaning. Lenses should never be wiped dry with tissue because this can cause surface scratches. Homemade cleaning solutions, such as mixtures of baking soda with distilled water or cleaning solution, should not be used; they may scratch the lens and may not be easily rinsed off. Dishwashing detergent, lighter fluid, toothpaste, or other cleaners not formulated for contact lens use may accumulate and cause ocular irritation or damage.

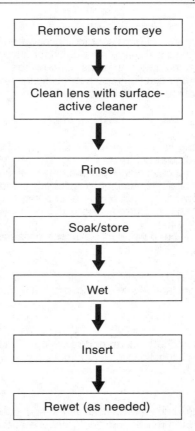

FIGURE 1 Hard contact lens care.

There are four techniques for cleaning rigid lenses.

Friction Rubbing. A contact lens cleaning solution or gel is applied to both surfaces of the lens. The lens is rubbed between the thumb and forefinger or between the forefinger and palm of the opposite hand for about 20 seconds.

Spray Cleaning. The lenses are placed into a perforated holder and held under a stream of tap water. The pressure of the water dislodges debris that has been loosened by overnight soaking in the storage case.

Hydraulic Cleaning. The lenses are placed into separate baskets in a plastic container that has a rotating cap. The unit is filled with a special cleaning solution to assist in the removal of deposits.

Ultrasonic Cleaning. The lenses are placed in a water bath through which ultrasound waves are passed. These high-priced units have not been shown to be superior in cleaning contact lenses.

Soaking Solutions

A soaking solution is used to store hard contact lenses whenever they are removed from the eyes. The solution maintains the lens in a constant state of hydration. It also aids in removing deposits that accumulate on the lens during wear.

To maintain sterility, storage solutions use essentially the same preservatives as wetting solutions. The main difference is that the concentration of a soaking solution can be somewhat higher.

Wetting Solutions

Not all patients need wetting solutions. If the lens is thoroughly cleaned before insertion, lacrimal fluid can adequately wet the lens.

The concentration of the cushioning polymer in wetting solutions affects both eye comfort and the quality of vision immediately following insertion. In some individuals, a concentration that is too low causes discomfort after a short time. In other wearers, a high polymer concentration results in blurred vision. If the solution spills onto the lids and eyelashes, it may cause crusting.

Saliva should never be used to wet contact lenses because it can lead to infection.

Multifunctional Products

The major problem with an all-purpose solution is that ingredients required in its formulation perform different and somewhat incompatible functions. Such solutions are marginally effective.

Rewetting Solutions

Rewetting solutions are intended to clean and rewet the contact lens while the it is in the eye. Although these products function well to recondition the lens, the cornea benefits more if the lens is actually removed, cleaned, and rewetted.

Other Products

Other ophthalmic products, such as artificial tears and ocular decongestants, are not recommended for use with the lenses in place. Because of their emollient and lubricating effect, artificial tears can be used to soothe the eye. Topical decongestants can induce conjunctival hypoxia and routine use should be avoided. If symptoms requiring their use persist, a visit to a vision specialist is advised.

Product Selection Guidelines

Selecting hard lens care products can be difficult because of the large number of products available and the availability of single- and multiple-function products within the same product line. Thus, product selection is an area in which the pharmacist can perform a much-needed consulting role. Usually a surfactant cleaner, soaking solution, wetting solution, and rewetting solution should be recommended. Unfortunately, information at hand is not always sufficient to provide a complete foundation for patient consultation. Product labeling is often inadequate.

Insertion and Removal

Instructions for inserting and removing hard lenses appear in Table 2.

TABLE 2 Insertion and removal of hard lenses

Insertion

- After washing hands, remove the lens from the lens storage case, rinse it with fresh conditioning/soaking solution, and inspect it for cleanliness and signs of damage (cracks or chips).
- If a wetting or conditioning solution is being used, place a few drops on the lens.
- Place the lens on the top of the index finger. Place the middle finger of the same hand on the lower lid and pull it down. With the other hand, use a finger to lift the upper lid. Then place the lens on the eye. Release the lids and blink.
- Check vision immediately to ascertain that the lens is in the proper position. If the lens is not placed correctly after three to four blinks (blurry vision), it may be off center, on the wrong eye, or dirty. Instill one to three drops of rewetting or reconditioning drops into the eye.
- If there is no improvement, remove the lens, place several drops of wetting/conditioning solution onto both surfaces, and reinsert. Repeat this procedure with the other lens.

Removal

- Before removing the lens, fill the storage cases with soaking/conditioning solution. Remove the top from the cleaning solution. Place a hand (or a towel) under the eye. Two methods are appropriate for removing the lens from the eye:
  - *Two-finger method:* Place the tip of the forefinger of one hand on the middle of the eyelid by the lashes. Place the forefinger of the other hand on the middle lower lid margin. Push the lids inward and then together. The lens should pop out. If it only becomes decentered onto the white part of the eye, recenter and try again.
  - *Pull/blink method:* Place an index finger on the outer edge of the lower and upper lids. Widen the eyelids a little, initially. Stretch the skin outward and slightly upward without allowing the lid to slide over the lens. Blink briskly. The lens will pop out because of the pressure of the eyelids at the top and bottom of the lens. Blinking facilitates removal after the lids have been tightened around the lens.

Care of RGP Lenses

Procedures

The diversity and variation in materials used in RGP lenses preclude generalizations. Lens wearers should be advised by their eye care professional about the products and regimens recommended for their particular lenses.

The care of an RGP lens is similar to that of a hard contact lens. The major difference is the need to clean the lens with an enzymatic cleaner once a week. Failure to comply with this cleaning step may result in the need for professional polishing or replacement of the lens.

It is important to counsel the patient to rinse the lens carefully and not to apply too much pressure when cleaning. Care should be taken to clean both surfaces of the lens. The lenses should be cleaned in the palm of the hand to decrease the risk of chipping an edge.

Products containing chlorhexidine gluconate should not be used with silicone or styrene lenses. Fluorosilicone acrylate lenses should not be disinfected with hydrogen peroxide or cleaned more than one time with MiraFlow. Cracking, changes in parameters, and brittleness have been noted when this type of lens is cleaned repeatedly with MiraFlow.

Product Selection Guidelines

Lens wearers should be advised against substituting other products for those specifically recommended by their eye care professional.

Insertion and Removal

Wearers of RGP lenses should be counseled to follow the insertion and removal procedures for hard lenses (Table 2).

Care of Soft Lenses

Conventional hard lens solutions should never be used with soft lenses. Lens disinfection is crucial to prevent ocular infection and damage to the lens material by bacteria and fungi. Wearers of soft hydrophilic contact lenses should also be cautious in exposing their lenses to chemicals.

The regimen of care for soft lenses is different from that for hard lenses (Figure 2). The only exception is with daily-wear disposable soft contact lenses. Because they are disposed of within 2 weeks, enzymatic cleaners are usually not necessary. Disposable lenses should, however, be cleaned and disinfected after each wearing until disposal. Products such as Opti-One are multipurpose solutions (for cleaning and disinfecting) formulated specifically for contact lenses that have a replacement schedule of 2 weeks or less.

Cleaning Products

A troublesome aspect of soft lens wear is the accumulation of deposits on the lens. Soft contact lenses require two cleaning steps to rid them of debris. Cleaning with a surface-active cleaner must be done daily or, in the case of extended-wear lenses, each time they are removed from the eyes. Cleaning with an enzymatic cleaner should be done weekly or more often if necessary.

Surface-Active Cleaners. A common method of cleaning soft lenses uses surface-active materials and friction rubbing. With both methods, care must be used to avoid cutting the soft lens with a fingernail or scratching the lens surfaces with grit or dirt on the hands. Rinsing is essential; it should be carried out using a sterile isotonic buffered solution. Tap water should never be used.

Enzymatic Cleaners. Although the surface-active cleaners generally are effective in removing lipid deposits, they are less successful in removing protein debris. Enzymatic cleaners can help solve this problem. For the enzyme solution to work properly, the lens must be first cleaned with a surface-active cleaner.

Enzymatic cleaners are used in the following manner. The enzyme tablet (papain, pancreatin, or subtilisin) is placed in a solution recommended by the manufacturer, and the lens is soaked from 15 minutes (high-water lenses) to as long as overnight (low-water lenses). The enzymatic cleaner is thoroughly rinsed from the lens. With most enzymatic products (certain subtilisin products are the exception), the lens then must be disinfected. It is usually sufficient to use enzyme cleaning as a once-a-week supplement to daily cleaning with surface-active chemicals. Some enzymatic regimens have been developed to be used simultaneously with thermal and chemical disinfection.

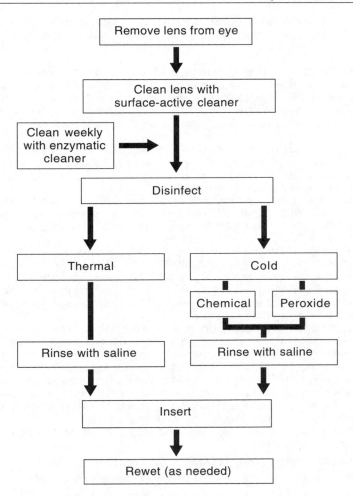

FIGURE 2 Soft contact lens care.

Disinfecting Methods

The FDA recommends disinfecting soft contact lenses before each reinsertion. Disinfection occurs after cleaning the lens. Two methods of disinfection are currently approved: thermal and chemical. Both are reliable for most ocular pathogens.

Thermal Disinfection. Thermal disinfection involves placing the cleaned lenses into separate compartments of a storage case filled with saline. The case is then placed into a heating unit, and the temperature is increased to a specific level for a prescribed time.

In situations where it is not possible to use a heat disinfection unit, the patient may place the tightly closed lens case containing the lenses and saline in a pot of boiling water for at least 10 minutes (15 minutes if at an altitude above 7,000 feet). The water must not boil away. The pot with the water and lenses should then be removed from the heat and allowed to cool for 30 minutes. The patient should resume use of the heat disinfection unit as soon as possible.

Chemical Disinfection. Two basic chemical disinfection methods are available in the United States. The first is based on the original chemical disinfecting solutions, which consisted of antimicrobial preservatives of sufficient concentration in storage solutions primarily composed of saline. The second uses hydrogen peroxide as the antimicrobial agent.

Patients should soak their lenses in the chemical disinfecting solution for a minimum of 4 hours.

When contact lenses are disinfected with hydrogen peroxide, a second step must be taken to neutralize the peroxide to trace levels. This can be accomplished by the catalytic action of a platinum disc; by soaking the lenses in a solution containing catalase, sodium pyruvate, or sodium thiosulfate; or by dilution techniques.

Most hydrogen peroxide systems that require two steps for disinfection and neutralization work in only 20–30 minutes. Patients who use the platinum disc (i.e., AO Sept) for neutralization should be counseled to replace the disc after 100 uses or 3 months, whichever comes first.

One potential disadvantage of hydrogen peroxide disinfection is that patients may insert the lens directly from the peroxide solution without neutralization. A peroxide-soaked lens placed on the eye will cause great pain, and, perhaps, corneal epithelial damage. If this occurs, the patient should immediately remove the lens from the eye and flush the eye with sterile saline solution. The pain should subside within a few hours. If it does not, the patient should consult an eye or vision care specialist.

Two hydrogen peroxide products, UltraCare and AO Sept, can help the patient avoid the possibility of forgetting to do the neutralization step. With one product, UltraCare, the user adds a delayed-release neutralizing tablet at the beginning of the disinfection cycle. This tablet contains cyanocobalamin, which turns the solution pink, thus reminding the user that the tablet has been added. There are no additional steps to remember as disinfection and neutralization will occur at the appropriate time intervals. Another advantage of UltraCare is that the lenses are exposed to the disinfecting effects of hydrogen peroxide for 2 hours, the time necessary for optimal activity against *Acanthamoeba.*

The following points should be discussed with patients who are using hydrogen peroxide disinfecting systems:

■ Neutralizers from different peroxide systems should never be mixed.

■ A neutralizing solution should never be placed in a case with a catalytic disc.

■ Lenses should not be soaked in the peroxide solution for longer than the recommended time; otherwise, it may take longer to neutralize the peroxide.

■ Household hydrogen peroxide solutions should not be used to disinfect soft lenses.

■ The lens cup that comes with a product should be used. Lens cases/cups should not be switched between products.

■ Product expiration dates should be observed.

Saline Solutions

Soft contact lenses must be maintained in a constant state of hydration. Isotonic normal saline is the basic solution used for rinsing, disinfecting, and storing soft contact lenses.

Prepared saline is available in preserved or preservative-free forms. Because thimerosal and chlorhexidine can cause sensitivity reactions or irritation, sorbic acid–preserved products are commonly promoted for sensitive eyes and appear to be acceptable to most wearers.

Several preservative-free salines are also available. Some nonpreserved saline products contain EDTA. EDTA, although not a preservative, will inhibit the growth of certain bacteria, thus extending the shelf life of the product.

Patients should avoid using other forms of saline such as intravenous normal saline or saline squirts because these products are usually too acidic.

Some persons prepare their own preservative-free saline using salt tablets and USP purified water. The clear superiority of commercial salines argues strongly against it.

Rewetting Solutions

Accessory solutions for use with soft lenses permit lubricating and rewetting of the lens in the eye. These solutions are particularly useful to patients with highly hydrated lenses, such as the extended-wear type. To minimize contaminations, the tip of the applicator bottle should not touch the eye or any other surface. The pharmacist should be aware of the preservative content of these products. Some are available without thimerosal and may be less sensitizing to patients with preservative allergies.

Product Selection Guidelines

Many problems associated with soft lens wear arise from the way people handle their lenses. Specific questions about the care and maintenance regimen used by a wearer may bring these problems to light.

Surface-Active Cleaners. Some surface-active cleaners have a lower viscosity and may be easier to rinse off the lens (e.g., Bausch & Lomb Sensitive Eyes Daily Cleaner). These products are good choices for patients who have difficulty completely rinsing the cleaner off their lens.

Some products (e.g., Opti-Clean II) contain mild abrasives. These products should be shaken before use. Care should be taken to be sure that no residue from the cleaning solution remains on the lens prior to insertion.

One surfactant cleaner (MiraFlow) contains isopropyl alcohol. This product is useful for patients who discover heavy lipid deposits on their lenses.

Enzymatic Cleaners. Enzymatic cleaners can be recommended based on the disinfection system the patient uses. If the patient uses thermal disinfection, ReNu Thermal is a good choice because it eliminates the need to perform the enzymatic cleaning and disinfection steps separately. If the patient uses a hydrogen peroxide cleaning system, Ultrazyme is a good choice. This product can be placed in the peroxide solution, thus cleaning and disinfecting at the same time. If the patient uses Opti-Free disinfecting solution, Opti-Free Enzymatic Cleaner would be a good choice as it can be placed directly in the Opti-Free solution during the disinfection cycle. If the patient uses another chemical disinfection system, the comparisons between products become very idiosyncratic unless the patient has an allergy to one of the components.

Disinfecting Methods. When counseling a patient about the best disinfection method to use, the pharmacist should ask what type of lenses the patient wears. If the patient wears low-water lenses, heat disinfection or UltraCare is best. If a patient wears high-water lenses or is not sure what type of lenses he or she has, a hydrogen peroxide system or a second-generation chemical system (i.e., Opti-Free or ReNu) can be recommended.

Soft lens wearers may switch from thermal to chemical disinfection methods, but the switch from chemical to thermal may present problems. Prolonged soaking in several changes of saline is recommended to clean the lenses before using a heating unit.

Product Incompatibility. Several incompatibilities may occur when mixing soft lens products.

Insertion and Removal

Steps for inserting and removing soft lenses are summarized in Table 3.

Patient Counseling

General Instructions

Pharmacists should ask patients wearing contact lenses the questions at the beginning of this chapter. The pharmacist should then ask specific questions related to the type of lens the patient is currently wearing. Only then can the pharmacist give appropriate counseling information.

Specific Instructions

Hard Lenses

- Do you soak your lenses when they are not in use?
- How often do you clean your lenses?
- What lens care products do you use? Do you use a combination-type solution, which may not provide optimal lens care?
- Do you inspect your lenses regularly for chips and scratches?

TABLE 3 Insertion and removal of soft lenses

Insertion

- Wash the hands with noncosmetic soap and rinse thoroughly; dry the hands with a lint-free towel.
- Remove the lens for the right eye from its storage container. Rinse it with saline solution to dilute any preservatives left from disinfection.
- Place the lens on the top of a finger and examine it to be sure it is not inside out. This can be done by using the "taco test." Gently fold the lens at the apex (not the edges) between the thumb and forefinger. The edges should look like a taco shell, with the edges pointed inward. If the edges roll out, the lens is inverted and must be reversed.
- Examine the lens for cleanliness. If necessary, clean it and rinse again with saline.
- Insert the lens on the right eye.
- Repeat the process for the left eye.

Removal

- Before removing the lenses, wash hands with a noncosmetic soap; rinse the hands thoroughly and dry them with a lint-free towel.
- Using the right middle finger, pull down the lower lid of the right eye. Touch the right index finger to the lens and slide the lens off the cornea.
- Using the index finger and thumb, grasp the lens and remove it.
- Repeat the procedure for the left eye.

The following special instructions will help ensure successful hard contact lens wear.

- The eyes should not be rubbed while lenses are in place.

- Contact lenses should not be rinsed with very hot or very cold water because temperature extremes may warp the lenses.

- Lenses should be cleaned before storage.

- Wearers should not get oils or lanolin on the lens.

RGP Lenses

- What brand of RGP lenses do you wear?

- Do you routinely use enzymatic cleaners? How often? What do you use to dissolve the enzymatic tablet?

- Do you clean your lenses immediately upon removal from the eye?

- Do you routinely use a soaking/conditioning solution formulated for your type of RGP lenses?

Soft Lenses

- What type of soft lenses do you wear (i.e., brand, high- or low-water content, ionic or nonionic)?

- Do you clean your lenses before disinfection?

- What method of disinfection do you use?

- How often do you disinfect your lenses?

- Do you use commercial saline solutions or do you mix your own? How often do you replace your solution?

- Do you use any cosmetics that are applied to the eye area? How do you apply these products?

- Do you routinely use enzymatic cleaners? How often? How do you dilute the enzymatic tablet?

- Are your lenses extended-wear lenses? How long do you wear them?

Extended-Wear Lenses

Extended-wear lenses can be either RGP or soft. The following instructions should be given to patients wearing extended-wear lenses:

- Each morning, look carefully at your eyes. Is there unusual, persistent redness? (Some redness is normal upon wakening; it should abate within 45 minutes.) Is there any unusual discharge? Pain? If any of the above are present, remove the lens and call your lens care practitioner.

- Can you see well with your lenses? (Some hazy vision is normal upon awakening.) Application of a few drops of rewetting agent may improve the hydration of the lens and help resolve the hypoxia. If it does not, remove the lenses, clean them, and reinsert. If your vision still has not improved within an hour, remove your lenses and call your lens care practitioner.

- Female patients should remove eye makeup before sleeping.

- If your lenses appear to be lost upon awakening, check your eyes to see if the lenses were displaced. Soft lenses can fold over on themselves and get lodged underneath the top or bottom eyelid.

Storage Case

Choice of a lens case is important. The case should have left and right clearly identified on the caps and in the lens wells. There should be ridges or flutes in the lens wells so that the RGP lens does not adhere to the case.

As important as lens care is the proper care and cleaning of the contact lens storage case. A storage case should be able to hold at least 2.5 mL of the storage solution. The lens case should be cleaned thoroughly and replaced at least every 3 months. Routine cleaning entails air drying the case between periods of use and scrubbing it weekly. Air drying should be done daily. If the case can withstand boiling (such as those cases made of polycarbonate or noryl plastic), it can be boiled in a pot of water for 10 minutes weekly. It should be examined for cracks and replaced periodically.

CHAPTER 24

Otic Products

Questions to ask in patient assessment and counseling

Earache

- Do you have an earache? How long have you had it?
- Is the pain sharp and localized or dull and generalized?
- Is the pain constant? It is made worse by pulling on the ears or chewing?
- Do you have or have you recently had a cold or the flu?
- Do you have a fever?
- Have you been swimming during the past few days?
- Have you attempted to clear your ears recently to remove earwax? If so, what method did you use?
- Are your ear canals dry and flaky or wet and sticky?
- Have you had similar symptoms in the past? If so, how long ago?
- What, if anything, have you already done to treat your earache?
- Do you wear dentures or have any dental problems?
- What is your occupation?

Hearing Loss

- When did you notice that your hearing is not as good as it used to be?
- Do you have a cold or the flu?
- Have you been swimming during the past few days?
- Are your eardrums damaged from a prior illness or injury?
- Have you been traveling in an airplane recently or been in any places where the air pressure has changed suddenly (e.g., fast elevators)?
- Does anyone in your family have a hearing loss?
- Do any of your relatives wear a hearing aid?
- Are you taking any prescription medications?
- Have you been hospitalized recently? If so, why?
- Would you be interested in taking a 5-minute hearing test for your own information only?

Tinnitus

- Are the abnormal sounds you are sensing continuous or intermittent?
- Are you taking aspirin or any prescription or nonprescription medications? If so, in what doses?

Editor's Note: This chapter is adapted from Keith O. Miller, "Otic Products," in Covington, T.R., ed., *Handbook of Nonprescription Drugs,* 11th edition. For a more extensive discussion of the anatomy and physiology of the ear, common ear problems, and treatment of ear disorders, readers are encouraged to consult Chapter 24 of the *Handbook.*

Discharge

- *Could you describe the appearance and the amount of discharge from your ear(s)?*
- *Was your ear itchy before the discharge appeared?*
- *Did you have any ear pain after the discharge appeared? Before the discharge started?*
- *Have you taken oral analgesics (e.g., aspirin) or pain-relieving eardrops, or have you tried to rinse out the ear?*
- *Do you have diabetes or any other medical condition?*
- *Do you have dandruff?*

Patients often complain of earache, impacted ear, running ear, cold in the ear, itching in the ear, or a combination of these symptoms. Home remedies and nonprescription drugs may be effective for self-limited, minor disorders of the external ear. Before recommending any nonprescription product to persons with ear disorders, the pharmacist should recognize the symptoms of the various disorders and their corresponding pathophysiology.

Common Problems of the Ear

Many disorders of the external ear are minor and easily resolved. However, the pharmacist should keep in mind that pain associated with minor disorders can be significant. Some untreated ear problems can result in hearing loss. The pharmacist can assist the patient by assessing the symptoms (Table 1), discussing the proper course of action, and recommending a nonprescription product when appropriate.

Self-treatment of ear disorders is inappropriate whenever drainage, pain, or dizziness are present; whenever an infection is suspected; whenever there is known injury in or perforation of the eardrum; or within 6 weeks following otic surgery.

Disorders of the Auricle

Disorders associated with the auricle, the external part of the ear, are generally minor and self-limiting. They often involve lacerations, boils, and dermatitis, as described below.

Trauma

Scrapes and cuts involving only the skin of the auricle usually heal spontaneously. Wounds that do not heal normally should be checked by a physician, as should deep wounds. A hematoma may require aspiration or incision by a physician because it may obliterate normal auricular contours.

Boils

Boils (furuncles) are usually localized infections of the hair follicles. A boil often involves the anterior portion of the external auditory canal. It usually begins as a red papule and develops into a pustule. The lesion gradually enlarges, becomes firm, and then generally softens and opens within 2 weeks. Even minimal swelling may cause severe pain.

Perichondritis

Perichondritis is an inflammation involving the perichondrium (the fibrous connective tissue surrounding the auricular cartilage) usually following a poorly treated or untreated burn, injury, hematoma, or local infection. Its onset is characterized by a sensation of heat, stiffness of the auricle, and pain. The auricle becomes dark red, swollen, and shiny. Some patients may experience fever and malaise. Patients suspected of having perichondritis should be referred to a physician.

TABLE 1 Symptoms of selected otic disorders

	Boil	Otomycosis	Bacterial external otitis	Nonsuppurative otitis media	Impacted cerumen	Suppurative otitis media
Pain[a]	Often	Possibly	Often	Rarely	Rarely	Usually
Hearing deficit	Rarely	Possibly	Possibly	Possibly	Often	Usually
Purulent discharge	Rarely	Rarely	Often	Rarely	Rarely	Occasionally and indicative of perforation
Bilateral symptoms	Rarely	Rarely	Possibly	Often	Rarely	Occasionally
Appropriateness of self-medication	Auricle only	Never	Never	Never	Never	Never

[a]Pain is increased with chewing, traction on the auricle, and pressure on the tragus except in otitis media, where pain may be knifelike and steady.

297

Dermatitis of the Ear

Dermatitis may result from an abrasion of the auricle; if untreated, a dermal infection may develop. Inflammatory conditions such as seborrhea, psoriasis, and contact dermatitis (e.g., poison ivy, poison oak) may also affect the skin of the auricle and the external ear canal. Contact dermatitis may be caused by an allergic response to jewelry, cosmetics, detergents, or topical applications of antihistamines or antibiotics (dermatitis medicamentosa). Dermatitis lesions may spread from ear molds.

Symptoms include itching and local redness followed by vesication, weeping, and erythema. The lesions form scales and yellow crusts. Excessive scratching may cause the lesions to become infected. Topical drugs should be used cautiously because of their potential allergenicity. Because seborrheic dermatitis of the ear is usually associated with dandruff, treatment of the scalp with a dandruff-control shampoo is recommended. Cases that are difficult to control should be referred to a physician.

Itching

Itching commonly begins as an itch-scratch cycle that results in trauma, infection, epidermal barrier destruction, and inflammation of the affected areas following repeated scratching. Ear scratching may be a compulsive habit. Careful observation to determine the cause of itching is often helpful before any attempt is made to provide symptomatic relief.

An itchy ear canal may mask the preinflammatory stages of acute external otitis. Itching can be related to dryness. It may also be caused by infections, allergic seborrheic dermatitis, eczema of the skin around the ears, psoriasis, contact dermatitis, superficial fungal infection, or neurodermatitis.

Aural Drainage

Excess fluids in the external auditory canal may cause a feeling of fullness. Fluid can be removed by having the patient tilt the head to one side with the affected ear down. Any patient with a discharge or drainage from the ear should be referred to a physician.

Disorders of the External Auditory Canal

Boils

Symptoms induced by boils include pain at the infected site, which is usually exacerbated by chewing. The ear canal may be partially occluded. Edema and pain over the mastoid bone may occur. Traction of the auricle or the tragus is very painful. Patients should be referred to a physician.

Otomycosis

Otomycosis, a fungal infection of the ear, is most common in warm, tropical, or semitropical climates. Antibiotic treatment of a bacterial ear infection with resultant suppression of normal bacterial flora, immunosuppression (drugs, disease), and diabetes mellitus may predispose an individual to a fungal infection. Intense itching is the primary complaint.

Keratosis Obturans

Keratosis obturans is a rare condition with an unclear etiology. Wax accumulates in the deeper parts of the external auditory canal and, with adjacent epithelial cells, leads to an obstruction that exerts pressure on the surrounding tissue.

Pain in the ear and decreased hearing are common symptoms. A discharge and tinnitus may also occur. Mechanical removal of the obstruction is necessary and should be performed by a physician—preferably an otolaryngologist.

Impacted Cerumen

The accumulation of cerumen in the external auditory canal may be caused by overactive ceruminous glands, a small canal or an abnormal narrowing of the canal, or secretion of abnormal cerumen that may interfere with the normal epithelial migration process. Individuals who get water in their ears while swimming or showering sometimes experience a sudden loss of hearing in one ear. This may be caused by the increased bulk of the earwax or by water trapped behind the wax. Cerumen is often packed deeper into the external auditory canal by repeated attempts to remove it. Ordinarily there is no pain unless the ear is secondarily infected.

Foreign Objects in the Ear

An object lodged in the ear canal usually causes a hearing deficiency, pain, or pressure in the ear during chewing. An exudate may form because of secondary bacterial infection. Olive oil (sweet oil) drops or mineral oil may be used to suffocate insects in the canal.

Foreign objects lodged in the ear canal may not always cause symptoms and may be found only during a routine physical examination. Mechanical removal should be performed only by a physician.

External Otitis

External otitis (inflammation of the skin lining the external auditory canal, often due to infection) is one of the most common diseases of the ear. A bacterial infection of the external auditory canal may progress through the fibrous layer of the tympanic membrane, perforate the membrane, and spread infection into the middle ear; this results in intense pain and discomfort. External otitis is particularly difficult to control in individuals who have diabetes.

Symptoms often develop following attempts to clean the ear with cotton swabs, hairpins, matchsticks, pencils, fingers, or other objects. Symptoms may also be caused by foreign debris or scratching of the ear. This may traumatize and damage the horny skin layer, forming an opening that allows invasion by microorganisms.

Swimmer's Ear. Heat, humidity, and moisture cause the stratum corneum of the skin to swell and block the follicular glands. Introduction of extraneous moisture or water during swimming or bathing increases the maceration of the skin lining the ear canal and sets up a condition favorable for bacterial growth. Within a day following exposure to excess moisture, symptoms of itching, pain, and possible draining from the ear may occur, with swelling causing partial occlusion.

Acute External Otitis. Symptoms of acute external otitis are related to the severity of the pathologic condition. There is usually mild or moderate pain. A discharge may be present. Hearing loss may occur if the ear canal is obstructed.

Allergic External Otitis/Dermatitis of the External Auditory Canal. In allergic external otitis and dermatitis of the external auditory canal caused by seborrhea, a common symptom is itching, burning, or stinging of the lesions.

Chronic External Otitis. Chronic external otitis is usually caused by the persistence of predisposing factors. Many cases are of fungal origin and occur in individuals whose ear canals are exposed to excessive moisture. The most common symptom is itching. Tender lymph nodes may be felt anterior to the tragus, behind the ear, or in the upper neck. Chronic or progressive cases should be referred to a physician.

Malignant External Otitis. Malignant external otitis is the most progressive form of otitis. It occurs in persons who are elderly, cancer patients, patients with granulocytopenia, and persons with poorly controlled diabetes. The most common complaints are severe, persistent pain and swelling.

Disorders of the Middle Ear

All bacterial infections of the middle ear should be promptly evaluated and treated by a physician. The usual treatment is systemic antibiotic therapy.

Otitis Media

Otitis media is an inflammatory condition of the middle ear that occurs most often during childhood. Upper respiratory tract infection, allergy, adenoid lymphadenopathy, and cleft palate predispose individuals to otitis media. Symptoms are mild intermittent pain, mild hearing loss, and fullness in the ear.

Nose blowing and sneezing against occluded nostrils may worsen the condition and should be avoided. nonprescription otic drugs should never be used to treat otitis media.

Purulent (Suppurative) Otitis Media. The most common symptoms in the acute phase of purulent otitis media are pain, hearing loss, and fever. Pain is described as sharp, knifelike, and steady. Excessive nose blowing may worsen the condition. Nonprescription eardrops or prescription antibiotic drops do not help resolve acute otitis media.

Chronic Otitis Media

Chronic serous otitis media occurs most often in small children. The most common symptom is impaired hearing. The onset may be insidious. Children may have acute symptoms. Frequently, parents may note that the child has become inattentive and disobedient, and the child's school performance may decline. The condition requires referral to a physician.

Tympanic Membrane Perforation

The most common causes of traumatic perforation of the tympanic membrane are water sports. Other causes include blows to the head with a cupped hand, foreign objects entering the ear canal with excessive force, and introduction of a caustic agent into the ear. At the moment of injury the pain is severe, but it decreases rapidly. Hearing acuity usually diminishes quickly. Any patient suspected of having an acute perforated tympanic membrane should be referred to a physician.

Barotrauma

Barotrauma occurs during a quick descent from high altitude. It may occur in individuals who fly with an upper respiratory tract infection or with any condition associated with impaired eustachian tube ventilation. Pretreatment with antihistamines or decongestants may help avoid symptoms during air travel. Treatment of acute episodes consists of oral decongestants, antihistamines, and autoinflation of the eustachian tube. Swallowing or blowing against pressure may help equalize the pressure.

Hearing Disorders

Tinnitus

Tinnitus is alien noise in the ear that is audible only to the patient. It is described as sounding like steam escaping from a small pipe, ringing, roaring, pulsating, chirping, or humming. Tinnitus may be constant or intermittent.

Patients with tinnitus caused by such drugs as salicylates, quinidine, or quinine usually notice a decrease in the intensity of the tinnitus following discontinuation of the offending medication. Any patient who experiences tinnitus should receive a medical examination and evaluation. Nonprescription eardrops are not effective.

Patient Assessment

To choose appropriately between patient self-treatment and physician referral, as well as to make the proper product selection and to instruct the patient appropriately, the pharmacist must be able to assess the nature and severity of the patient's otic condition by evaluating overt signs and symptoms (Table 1).

The pharmacist should have the patient describe the symptoms and should ask whether the patient has experienced similar symptoms previously and, if so, when and how they were treated. Evaluation of the patient's present health status must also be based on information in the medical and drug history records, as well as on information concerning predisposing factors or conditions that may influence the patient's response to self-treatment (e.g., seborrheic dermatitis, psoriasis, eczema, allergies, contact dermatitis, and chronic diseases that may impair healing, such as diabetes mellitus).

The patient should always be referred to a physician if the symptoms include severe pain, lymphadenopathy, discharge from ear, possible hearing deficit, or fever. Appropriately selected nonprescription drug products can be relied upon to provide a suitable therapeutic response in certain conditions.

Hearing loss should be evaluated and diagnosed by a physician or audiologist. A 5-minute hearing test (available from the American Academy of Otolaryngology—Head and Neck Surgery, Inc., 1 Prince St., Alexandria, VA 22314-3357, 703–836–4444) is sometimes useful to assess some patients with a suspected hearing deficit. Acute hearing loss without pain may be experienced and identified during an examination of the ear canal.

Patients with impacted cerumen without secondary complications may be treated safely with nonprescription cerumen-softening agents. Patients with hearing loss without pain, and whose tympanic membrane is visible and not obstructed, should be evaluated and treated by a physician. Such decreased hearing may be due to a perforated tympanic membrane. Usually the patient with this injury has experienced a sharp pain of short duration at the time of the injury.

Treatment

External Ear Disorders

Boils

Small boils may be treated by good hygiene combined with topical compresses. Self-treatment may be instituted by applying hot compresses of saline solution to the affected area, followed by an antibiotic ointment. A soft cotton applicator is useful for applying a topical drug over and around the boil. An antibiotic ointment may be used in the absence of known or suspected sensitivity. The lesion usually clears after several days of frequent applications of heat and ointment. Boils that do not respond rapidly to topical therapy should be examined by a physician.

External Otitis

Treatment of external otitis typically includes antibiotic and hydrocortisone drops applied in the ear canal. When cellulitis and lymphadenopathy are present, oral antibiotics are effective. The ear canal should be kept clean and dry at all times.

A 5% aluminum acetate solution (Burow's solution) may be used to obtain rapid resolution of eczematous or weeping skin. Soaking with warm water, saline, or aluminum acetate solution is often useful in the treatment of crusting and edema.

Cleansing repeatedly with saline or water at body temperature helps clear debris from the ear canal. The irrigation solution should be at body temperature. A bulb ear syringe may be appropriate for cleansing. Proper technique is important. The water column should be superior against the canal wall so that the returning stream can push the cerumen from behind. The use of a forced water spray should be reserved for health professionals trained in aural hygiene.

Cleansing the ear may be uncomfortable but should never be painful. Severe, knifelike pain occurs if the tympanic membrane is ruptured, and it may be followed by intense vertigo. If this occurs, irrigation must be stopped at once.

Pharmacologic Agents

Because most bacteria or fungi do not thrive in acidic environments, any otic solution should have an acidic pH.

All nonprescription otic preparations may be contraindicated in individuals who are susceptible to local irritation and hypersensitivity. Patients should be advised to discontinue using the medication if rash, local redness, or other adverse symptoms occur.

Acetic Acid Solutions

Acetic acid solution in the form of household vinegar has been used for years to treat mild forms of external otitis. It is recommended for treatment of swimmer's ear. Acetic acid is well tolerated and nonsensitizing, and it does not induce resistant organisms.

A suitable concentration of acetic acid can be made in the pharmacy from white distilled household vinegar, which is usually 5% acetic acid. A 50:50 mixture of distilled household vinegar with either water, propylene glycol, glycerin, or rubbing alcohol (70% isopropyl or 70% ethyl alcohol) provide a 2.5% acetic acid solution.

Patients can be treated at home with dilute acetic acid solution using eight drops of white vinegar diluted to 10 mL with 10% isopropyl alcohol or aluminum acetate solution. The solution should be applied as two to four drops into the ear using the following technique:

■ Tilt head downward, affected ear up.

■ If there is possibility that there is a hole in the eardrum, carefully squeeze a medicine dropper full of the solution into the ear canal.

■ With one hand, move the ear back and forth to move the solution all the way into the ear.

■ Tilt the head to the other, affected side to let the solution out, gently tapping the unaffected side.

■ Repeat the procedure in the opposite ear.

Aluminum Acetate Solution (Burow's Solution)

External otitis or local itching of the external ear caused by external ear dermatitis may be treated with an astringent such as 1:10 or 1:40 aluminum acetate solution. One tablet or one packet dissolved in 500 mL of water yields a concentration of 1:40. Aluminum acetate solution is used widely for conditions involving the external ear. Its major value is its acidity.

When the ear canal is swollen, weeping, and inflamed, an aluminum acetate solution is helpful. Aluminum acetate solution may also be used to treat the edema and crusting associated with acute moist ear canals, for which the abundant desquamative debris that forms requires special cleansing.

A wet compress may be used with a gauze dressing on the auricle. Drops may be instilled into the canal. The usual dosage of aluminum acetate solution is four to six drops every 4–6 hours until itching or burning subsides. Aluminum acetate solution is suitable for children and adults. It is nonsensitizing and well tolerated. Adverse reactions are rare.

Boric Acid

Boric acid is a weak, local anti-infective and is nonirritating to intact skin in a dilute solution of 1%–5%. Because of its toxicity, boric acid should be used with caution, particularly in children and on open wounds.

Cerumen-Softening Agents

Cerumen-softening and cerumenolytic agents soften and loosen, but do not remove, cerumen. Patients can remove minor amounts of excessive ear wax by rinsing the ear canal with an ear syringe. Hardened earwax should be removed by a physician.

Carbamide Peroxide. Carbamide peroxide 6.5% formulated in an anhydrous glycerin vehicle is safe and effective for occasional nonprescription use as an aid to soften and remove excessive earwax. The FDA recommends usage twice each day for up to 4 days if needed, or as directed by a physician. Five drops of the solution should be instilled into the affected ear and allowed to remain at least 15 minutes. Failure to obtain relief after 4 days of treatment could indicate a more serious condition, and a physician should be consulted. This process is not recommended for children under 12 years of age.

Unless it is under physician supervision, carbamide peroxide should not be used if there is ear drainage, pain, or dizziness; if there is known injury or perforation of the eardrum; or if ear surgery has been performed within the past 6 weeks. This treatment should be discontinued whenever irritation or rash appears. It is not recommended for treating pain of raw inflamed tissue, swimmer's ear, or itching of the ear canal.

Other Cerumen-Softening Products. The occasional instillation of olive oil, mineral oil, glycerin, diluted hydrogen peroxide solution, or propylene glycol in the ear can soften the cerumen and promote its removal. The patient may rinse the ear canal every few days with a mixture of 20%–30% alcohol and water or aluminum acetate solution to prevent cerumen buildup. Patients can be instructed to use cerumen-softening agents for 3–4 days, at which time the cerumen should be softened enough to be easily removed by rinsing with an ear syringe.

Glycerin

Glycerin may be used as a solvent, an emollient, or a humectant. It is widely used as a vehicle in many otic preparations to open wounds or abraded skin.

Olive Oil (Sweet Oil)

Olive oil is used as an emollient and topical lubricant. It may be instilled into the ear canal to alleviate itching and burning and to soften earwax. If an insect becomes trapped in the ear canal, olive oil can be instilled to smother the insect.

Propylene Glycol

Propylene glycol is a solvent that has preservative and humectant properties. It is hygroscopic and its viscosity increases contact time with tissues of the external auditory canal.

Other Medications

Agents whose safety and effectiveness in the treatment of otic disorders have not been established include antipyrine, benzocaine, camphor, chloroform, ichthammol, menthol, phenol in glycerin, and thymol.

Patient Counseling

Cleansing procedures and self-treatment for ear disorders should not be performed by patients unless they understand proper techniques. Patients must be evaluated for their ability to understand the hazards of inappropriate self-treatment.

Patients should be instructed on the use of nonprescription drugs for the ear. They should understand the proper use of medicine droppers for administering eardrops and of ear syringes for irrigating the ear. Water that is to be used to irrigate the ear canal should be sterile or sterilized by boiling. Eardrops should be warmed to body temperature by holding the medication container in the palm of the hand or placing it into a vessel of warm water for a few minutes before administration. Heated eardrops should never be applied to the ear. Eardrops may be applied as often as four times daily. The involved ear should be tilted up for at least 2 minutes following the placement of two to four eardrops to permit effective contact of the medication.

A cotton wick may be inserted gently into the ear canal to help the medication maintain contact with the affected area in the ear canal. Gently pulling the auricle backward may allow medication to reach a greater depth in the ear canal. Cotton wicks, however, usually require insertion with appropriate instruments and should be used only by trained personnel.

Patients should be advised that symptoms usually begin to subside within 1–2 days if self-treatment is appropriate. If symptoms persist or if an adverse reaction to the medication occurs, the patient should consult a physician immediately.

CHAPTER 25

Oral Health Products

Questions to ask in patient assessment and counseling

General Assessment

- What are your symptoms?
- How long have you had this dental problem?
- Have you seen a dentist about the problem? When?
- What remedies have you tried? How long did you use them? Did they work?
- Have you had this problem before?

Mouth Pain

- Where is the pain?
- Is the pain severe? Is there swelling in the area?
- Is the pain continuous and throbbing, or does it come and go?
- Is the pain triggered or made worse by hot or cold substances or by chewing?
- Does anything make the pain go away? If so, what?
- Do you feel ill?
- Do you have a cold, sinus infection, or ear infection?
- Do you have a fever?
- Are there any prior events such as trauma associated with the pain?
- Are there any other symptoms associated with the pain?

Mouth Irritation or Discomfort

- Where is the area of irritation or lesion? Is it visible? What color is it?
- Is the discomfort continuous?
- Is the discomfort aggravated by eating or drinking?
- Is there a discharge from the lesion?
- Do your gums bleed when you brush your teeth?
- Do you have a bad taste in your mouth?
- Do you have bad breath continuously?
- Are any of your teeth loose?
- Do you wear dentures? Are they loose?
- Do your dentures cause sore spots?

Editor's Note: This chapter is adapted from Arlene A. Flynn, "Oral Health Products," in Covington, T.R., ed., *Handbook of Nonprescription Drugs*, 11th edition. For a more extensive discussion of dental anatomy and physiology, common oral problems, and therapeutic considerations in special populations, readers are encouraged to consult Chapter 25 of the *Handbook*.

General State of Oral Health

- *How do you brush your teeth or clean your dentures? How often?*
- *Do you use dental floss? How often?*
- *How often do you see your dentist for checkups?*
- *Do you use supplemental fluoride (e.g., rinse, tablet)?*

Patient-Specific Factors

- *Do you suffer from any chronic illness (e.g., diabetes mellitus, rheumatic heart disease, asthma, seizure disorder, high blood pressure)?*
- *Are you taking any prescription or nonprescription medications? If so, what are they?*
- *Do you have a pacemaker?*
- *Have you had joint replacement surgery?*
- *Do you smoke or use any tobacco product (including smokeless tobacco products)?*
- *Do you have any food or drug allergies? If so, what are they?*

Patient Assessment and Counseling

On the basis of thorough patient assessment, the pharmacist can advise the patient regarding self-care or the need for professional referral for oral health. Questions the pharmacist should ask the patient presenting with a dental problem are presented at the beginning of this chapter.

It is important for the pharmacist to assess each complaint to determine whether the problem is recurrent, is likely to resolve with self-treatment using nonprescription products, could lead to serious consequences, or presents a dental emergency. It is also important for the pharmacist to determine if the patient is currently under a dentist's care and is experiencing a problem related to a recent dental procedure. A recurrent problem (e.g., swelling, drainage, chronic pain) may signal a condition that warrants referral to a dentist. Previous self-treatment with nonprescription oral products needs to be evaluated for possible misuse, abuse, or inappropriate response.

Clinical Manifestations

Pain

Pain can accompany many common oral problems. Tooth pain triggered or worsened by heat, cold, or pressure upon biting often indicates a pulpal response to deep carious lesions or a cracked or broken tooth. Continuous tooth pain may indicate pulpal infection and necrosis, an abscess, or serious periodontal disease. Fever, malaise, and swelling may indicate an oral abscess. A patient who exhibits these symptoms should be referred to a dentist for immediate professional care.

Mouth Irritation or Discomfort

Continuous irritation, soreness, or pain that is associated with the soft tissues of the mouth and is more severe upon eating or drinking is a common symptom of canker sores and acute atrophic candidiasis. Pain along the gingival ridge under a denture prosthesis suggests ill-fitting dentures, denture stomatitis, or candidiasis. Examples of pathologic color changes include the white plaques of candidiasis, the erythema on the margins of cold sores or canker sores, and the gingival erythema associated with periodontitis. Halitosis may result from poor oral hygiene, acute necrotizing ulcerative gingivitis (trench mouth), periodontal disease, or dentopyogenic infections and merits inquiry and possible referral.

Patient-Specific Factors

The patient's medication profile should be reviewed. This history may suggest potentially serious dental or medical complications, such as endocarditis secondary to an oral abscess in a patient with rheumatic heart disease. Patients who have undergone surgery for placement of a pacemaker or prosthetic joint may be at high risk for bacterial endocarditis. Signs and symptoms of oral candidiasis (e.g., white plaques with a milk curd appearance, erythematous tissue, angular cheilitis) might be observed in the presence of a disease (e.g., leukemia, autoimmunodeficiency syndrome, cancer) or with some treatment regimens. Patients treated with an antihistamine with high anticholinergic activity that dries the mouth, an orally inhaled steroid that decreases the immune response in the mouth, a broad-spectrum antibiotic that results in overgrowth of nonsusceptible organisms, or therapy (e.g., cancer chemotherapy) that produces an immune deficiency disorder may be at risk.

General Oral Health

Poor oral hygiene or infrequent dental care can greatly increase the likelihood of dental caries, infection, periodontal disease, ill-fitting or broken dentures, and other oral health problems. Patients sometimes notice bleeding gingiva, plaque and calculus on teeth, and loose teeth during brushing and flossing. Such symptoms should prompt the pharmacist to refer the patient to a dentist for evaluation. Lifestyle risk factors that may impair dental health include alcohol consumption, use of tobacco products, and chewing ice cubes.

Common Oral Problems

Plaque and Calculus

Plaque is the source of microbes that cause caries and periodontal disease; thus, plaque buildup is related to the incidence of oral disease. If not removed within 24 hours, dental plaque begins to calcify by precipitating calcium salt from the saliva and forms calculus or tartar. This hardened deposit is removable only by professional dental cleaning.

The best way to ensure healthy teeth and gingival tissues is to remove plaque buildup by brushing at least twice daily and flossing at least once a day. Eating fibrous foods such as celery, apples, or carrots does not prevent plaque accumulation or aid in its removal. Chemical management of plaque and calculus can enhance mechanical removal. Chemical agents may be particularly appropriate for patients are unable to brush and floss effectively.

Plaque Removal

Two classes of products have made antiplaque claims. One class includes products that rely on the mechanical action of abrasives to remove plaque. The other includes products that claim to reduce or remove plaque by chemical or antimicrobial activity. These products are available in multiple forms (e.g., dentifrices, gargles, mouthwashes).

Products for plaque removal may have cosmetic and/or therapeutic activity. The American Dental Association (ADA) seal program is the consumer's guide to dental product safety and efficacy. ADA evaluates dental products on the basis of data regarding their safety and effectiveness for their intended use. Products that carry ADA seals or statements have scientifically earned their recognition.

Toothbrushes and Similar Devices

The toothbrush is the most universally accepted device for removing dental plaque. Dentists recommend toothbrushes based on the individual patient's manual dexterity, oral anatomy, and periodontal health. The toothbrush should be of a size and shape to allow the patient to reach every tooth.

Characteristics considered desirable in selecting a toothbrush include a relatively small brush head for easy access; a multitufted, dense, straight-trimmed brushing surface; and soft, resilient, nylon filaments with rounded ends.

The proper frequency and method of brushing varies from patient to patient. Thoroughness of plaque removal without gingival trauma is more important than method. Patients should brush thoroughly at least twice a day. A gentle scrubbing motion with the bristle tips at a 45-degree angle against the gumline is indicated. Excessive force should be avoided. Gentle brushing of the upper surface of the tongue is recommended to reduce debris, plaque, and bacteria.

Although 3 months has been suggested as a guide for toothbrush life expectancy, patients should replace them at the first sign of bristle wear. Toothbrushes have been found to be a receptacle for bacteria. Patients with infectious diseases of the oral tissue should change brushes every 2 weeks. Patients should be advised to replace a toothbrush following a respiratory infection to prevent reinfection. Toothbrushes should be rinsed thoroughly after each use.

Standard electric toothbrushes have not consistently proven superior to properly manipulated manual toothbrushes; however, they may benefit patients who are handicapped, who lack manual dexterity, who require someone else to clean their teeth, or who wear orthodontic appliances. Positive results (i.e., significant reductions in dental plaque accumulation) depend to some extent on proper use of the device.

Oral Irrigating Devices

Oral irrigators direct a high-pressure stream of water through a nozzle to the tooth surfaces. These devices can remove only a minimal amount of plaque from tooth surfaces. Oral irrigators cannot be viewed as substitutes for a toothbrush, dental floss, or other plaque-removal devices but should be considered as adjuncts in maintaining oral hygiene.

Dental Floss

Plaque accumulation in the interdental spaces contributes to proximal caries and periodontal pocketing. Interdental plaque removal reduces gingival inflammation and prevents periodontal disease and dental caries. Dental flossing is the most widely recommended method of removing dental plaque from tooth surfaces not adequately cleaned by toothbrushing alone.

Proper flossing requires practice. Patients should be instructed to use approximately 18 in. of floss and wrap most of it around a middle finger. The remaining floss should be wound around the same finger of the opposite hand. About an inch of floss should be held between the thumbs and forefingers. The patient should use a gentle, sawing motion to guide the floss to the gumline. When the gumline is reached, the floss should be curved into a C-shape against one tooth and gently slid into the space between the gum and tooth until there is resistance. The patient should hold the floss tightly against the tooth and gently scrape the side of the tooth while moving the floss away from the gums. Next, the patient should curve the floss around the adjoining tooth and repeat the procedure. Waxed floss may pass between teeth more easily than unwaxed floss. If contacts at the crowns of teeth are too tight to force floss interdentally, floss threaders can be used to pass floss between the teeth and around fixed bridges.

Specialty Aids

Cleaning devices that adapt to irregular tooth surfaces better than dental floss does are recommended for interproximal cleaning of teeth with large interdental spaces, such as is found in patients with periodontal disease. Specialty brushes and aids are available to remove plaque from hard-to-clean areas and dentures. The most common aids are tapered triangular wooden toothpicks (Stim-U-Dent), holders for round toothpicks (Perio-aid), miniature bottle brushes (Py-Co-Prox or Proxabrush), rubber stimulator tips, denture brushes, and denture clasp brushes.

Disclosing Agents

Disclosing agents are available for home use as either a solution or a chewable tablet. These agents should be used intermittently as a plaque indicator to monitor cleaning technique. Disclosing products should be expectorated completely. The mouth should be rinsed with water and the water should also be expectorated.

Dentifrices

Dentifrices are used with a toothbrush for cleaning accessible tooth surfaces. Use of a dentifrice enhances removal of dental plaque and stain, resulting in a decreased incidence of dental caries and gum disease, reduced mouth odors, and enhanced personal appearance. Dentifrices are available as powders, pastes, or gels. The ideal dentifrice abrasive would maximally aid in cleaning and minimally cause damage to tooth surfaces. Such a product does not exist.

Unless advised otherwise by their dentists, patients—especially those with periodontal disease, significant gum recession, and exposed root surfaces—should choose the least abrasive dentifrice that effectively removes stained pellicle. Low-abrasive dentifrices usually have 10%–25% concentration of silica abrasives. Baking soda, a mild abrasive, is found in a number of dentifrices. Toothpastes with baking soda have not been shown to be better at cleaning teeth than toothpastes without it.

The most common therapeutic agent added to dentifrices is fluoride for its anticaries activity. Other therapeutic agents (e.g., potassium nitrate) are added to treat hypersensitive dentin.

Chemical agents to control plaque and help prevent or reduce calculus formation have received much attention as additives to dentifrices and mouthrinses. No dentifrice is currently accepted by the ADA as efficacious in the antiplaque/antigingivitis therapeutic category, and patients should not forgo the benefits of fluoride in favor of chemical antiplaque ingredients. Certain fluoride dentifrices for which antiplaque claims are made bear the ADA seal of approval for their anticaries effect only.

A number of fluoride dentifrices containing anticalculus or tartar-control compounds are marketed. Although plaque, not calculus, is the primary etiologic factor in marginal periodontal disease, the reduction of calculus formation is still a goal of oral hygiene. Patients who form heavy calculus between dental visits may consider using a fluoride dentifrice with added tartar-control ingredients instead of a plain fluoride dentifrice. The ADA regards inhibition of supragingival calculus as a nontherapeutic use and therefore does not evaluate anticalculus claims.

Use of tartar-control toothpastes has been related to a type of contact dermatitis in the perioral region. Patients experiencing such a reaction should be advised to switch to a non–tartar-control fluoride product.

Cosmetic dentifrices are usually chosen by patients because of taste, whitening ability, or antistain properties. Some dentifrices claiming to remove stubborn coffee or tobacco stains may contain high concentrations of abrasives. They are not advised for long-term use or for use by patients with exposed root surfaces. Plain baking soda or toothpastes containing baking soda have limited polishing and stain removal capacity. Other products may contain a pigment (e.g., titanium dioxide) that produces a temporary brightening effect.

Mouthrinses (Mouthwashes)

Mouthrinse and dentifrice formulations are very similar. A mouthrinse approximates a diluted liquid dentifrice containing ethanol and no abrasive. Mouthrinses can be classified by appearance, alcohol content, and active ingredients. Patients who request a mouth-wash to eliminate halitosis should be reassured that some degree of oral malodor (e.g., morning breath) is normal in a healthy individual.

The alcohol content in mouthrinses ranges from zero to 27%. Ingestion of alcohol-containing products poses a danger for children, who may be attracted by bright colors and pleasant flavors. There is a potential association between the use of mouthrinses containing alcohol and an increased risk of oral cancer. Alcohol-free formulations in the various mouthrinse categories are entering the market.

The quaternary ammonium compounds and sanguinarine compounds have some merit, but studies of their efficacy in plaque and gingivitis reduction are mixed.

Clinical trials with mouthrinses containing cetylpyridinium chloride alone or in combination with domiphen bromide have reported reductions in plaque accumulation. The potential for oral toxicity with these agents is low, and the potential for a gingival health benefit exists. However, studies consistent with ADA guidelines have not been evaluated, and further study is needed.

Another approach to plaque control is based on principles of surfactant action to loosen plaque. Advanced Formula Plax was shown to effect statistically significant reductions in subjects' plaque levels compared with placebo.

Mouthrinses claiming anticalculus or tartar-control activity contain the same active ingredients as anticalculus dentifrices.

Mouthrinses are intended for use twice daily after brushing, with the exception of Advanced Formula Plax, which should be used prior to brushing. In general, an amount equal to 1–2 tbsp of rinse should be swished vigorously in the mouth and between the teeth for about 30 seconds and then expectorated; the rinses should not be swallowed. Patients should be advised to refrain from smoking, eating, or drinking for 30 minutes following use. These products are generally safe when used as directed, but occasional burning sensation and irritation have been reported. Overuse should be discouraged. Consultation with a health professional is indicated if irritation occurs and persists after use of the product is discontinued. Unsupervised use is contraindicated in patients with mouth irritation or ulceration.

Patients should be cautioned that use of a mouthrinse with plaque or calculus control properties does not substitute for normal oral hygiene.

Tooth Whiteners

Tooth whiteners, which claim to bleach teeth, contain oxidizing ingredients such as hydrogen peroxide, carbamide peroxide, or perhydrol urea. The ADA accepts none of the available nonprescription products for unsupervised consumer use as a tooth-whitening agent.

Patients should be strongly discouraged from attempting tooth bleaching without a dentist's direct supervision. Serious adverse effects (i.e., loss of surface enamel) resulting from misuse or overuse of such products have been reported.

Periodontal Disease

Etiology and Pathophysiology

The primary etiologic cause of periodontal disease is accumulated bacterial plaque. The basic pathologic process is inflammatory. The more common forms of periodontal disease are gingivitis, acute necrotizing ulcerative gingivitis (ANUG), and periodontitis.

Gingivitis. The etiology of gingivitis is thought to be associated with the accumulation of supragingival plaque. The inflamed gingiva generally bleeds readily when probed or during toothbrushing. In the early stage of gingivitis, it is possible to reverse the inflammatory process with effective oral hygiene. Disease progression is usually slow and often painless. Left untreated, gingivitis is a common precursor to the more advanced inflammatory condition of chronic destructive periodontal disease, or periodontitis.

Acute Necrotizing Ulcerative Gingivitis. ANUG, also referred to as Vincent's stomatitis and trench mouth, is an acute bacterial infection characterized by necrosis and ulceration of the gingival surface with underlying inflammation. The disease most commonly starts in the gingiva between teeth. It may involve a single tooth, a group of teeth, or the entire oral cavity. Symptoms include severe pain, bleeding gingival tissue, halitosis, foul taste, and increased salivation. Lymphadenopathy, fever, and malaise may accompany localized symptoms. ANUG is seen most frequently in the United States in teenagers and young adults. Professional dental treatment is indicated.

Periodontitis. Whereas gingivitis is the inflammation of the gingiva without loss or migration of epithelial attachment to the tooth, periodontitis occurs when the periodontal ligament attachment and alveolar bone support of the tooth have been compromised or lost.

Adult periodontitis, especially slight or moderate, is very common. Periodontitis in juveniles is relatively rare.

Preventive Measures

Adequate removal and control of supragingival plaque is the single most important factor in reversing gingivitis and preventing and controlling periodontal disease.

Dental Caries

Etiology and Pathophysiology

Dental caries is a destructive microbial disease that affects the calcified tissues of the teeth. A carious lesion starts slowly on the enamel surface and initially produces no clinical symptoms. Once the demineralization progresses through the enamel to the softer dentin, the destruction is much more rapid and becomes clinically evident as a carious lesion. At this point, the patient can become aware of the process by visualization or by symptoms of sensitivity to stimuli, such as heat, cold, or chewing. If untreated, the carious lesion can result in damage to the dental pulp itself (with continuous pain as a common symptom) and, eventually, in necrosis of vital pulp tissue.

Preventive Measures

Because a combination of diet (carbohydrate substrate), oral bacteria, and host resistance is involved in the process, intervention to prevent dental caries should be aimed at modifying these factors. Frequency of refined carbohydrate intake should be reduced; plaque, which supports cariogenic bacterial growth, should be removed; and host resistance should be increased through appropriate exposure to fluoride ion.

The Role of Fluoride. Nonprescription topical fluoride-containing products such as dentifrices, mouthrinses, and self-applied gels provide a means of increasing contact of fluoride with the tooth surfaces. Patient groups with high caries activity or risk may especially benefit from multiple sources of fluoride application.

Fluoride Dentifrices. Use of fluoride-containing dentifrices is the one method of caries prevention common to all countries that shows a reduction in caries. Fluoride-containing toothpaste and gel dentifrice formulations with abrasive systems compatible with delivery of the fluoride compound are accepted by the ADA as being safe and effective in caries prevention.

Included among the ADA-accepted dentifrices are the standard 1000-ppm and 1100-ppm fluoride ion concentrations as well as a more recent 1500-ppm fluoride ion product. This extra-strength product is clinically and statistically superior to its regular-strength counterpart. It should not be used by children under 2 years of age, and children under 6 should be supervised while using it.

Fluoride Mouthrinses and Gels. Many fluoride mouthrinses contain 0.05% sodium fluoride. Fluoride gel formulations contain 1.1% sodium fluoride or 0.4% stannous fluoride. For a complete list of products, consult "Oral Hygiene Products" in *Nonprescription Products: Formulations and Features.*

Studies of fluoride mouthrinsing have given consistently positive results. Orthodontic patients may benefit because they are at risk of developing decalcified areas while under treatment and their ability to clean interdental spaces thoroughly may be inhibited.

Fluoride rinses provide a therapeutic fluoride treatment; they should not be confused with a mouthrinse, and package directions should be followed closely. When recommending a nonprescription sodium fluoride mouthrinse, the pharmacist should stress that:

■ The fluoride rinse should be used after brushing the teeth with toothpaste and should be expectorated;

■ A measured dose of the rinse (most commonly 10 mL) should be vigorously swished between the teeth for 1 minute;

■ Nothing should be taken by mouth for 30 minutes after use;

■ The mouthrinse can benefit the patient for as long as the patient has natural dentition; and

■ The fluoride is preventive in action and will not cure carious teeth.

The self-applied fluoride gels are used once daily after the teeth are brushed with a fluoride dentifrice. The gel is brushed on the teeth, left for 1 minute, and then expectorated.

Orofacial Pain

Toothache

Toothache usually indicates dental pathology involving tooth substance, dental pulp, or the supporting periodontium. Pain may also be referred to the teeth from the sinuses, eyes, or ears. Pain may be intermittent, often indicating viable pulp with reversible damage. If pain is continuous and throbbing, this usually indicates irreversible pulp damage.

Topical oral mucosal anesthetics/analgesics classified as Category I for relief of pain associated with minor irritation or injury to soft tissue are not considered effective for relieving toothache from a cavity. The patient with toothache should be advised to seek professional dental assistance. If the patient wears a removable prosthesis that attaches to the painful tooth, removing the appliance may help temporarily. Nonprescription analgesics such as ibuprofen, aspirin, or acetaminophen may be taken internally for short-term pain relief; however, none of these products, and particularly not aspirin, should ever be placed on gingival tissue or in a cavity.

Hypersensitive Teeth

Hypersensitive teeth result from exposed areas of the root at the cementoenamel junction. Pain may be intense and may condition patients to limit oral hygiene, which in turn will contribute to plaque accumulation and the progression of disease. A patient who has self-diagnosed sensitive teeth should be referred to a dentist. Once the dentist diagnoses the pain as dentinal hypersensitivity, this condition can be treated with a desensitizing dentifrice.

Patients should be advised to apply at least a 1-in. strip of dentifrice to a soft bristle brush and to use the product twice daily. Brushing thoroughly for at least 1 minute will apply the desensitizing agent to all sensitive surfaces. Onset of effect may take up to 2 weeks. These dentifrices should be used until the sensitivity subsides or as long as a dentist recommends. The patient should then switch to a low-abrasion dentifrice.

The FDA has proposed a Category I classification for the combination of a Category I fluoride ingredient with 5% potassium nitrate for use in relieving dentinal hypersensitivity and preventing dental caries. Such a product (e.g., Sensodyne for Sensitive Teeth and Cavity Prevention, Crest Sensitivity Protection Mild Mint Paste) would be a good recommendation. Dentifrices containing 5% potassium nitrate are not recommended for children under 12 years of age.

Oral Mucosal Lesions

Oral Malignancies

Oral carcinomas can appear as red or white lesions, ulcerations, or tumors. It is important that the pharmacist question patients who seek product recommendations for treatment of persistent oral lesions and refer such individuals to a physician or dentist.

Canker Sores and Cold Sores

Two of the most common oral problems for which patients seek nonprescription treatment are canker sores and cold sores (fever blisters). Both conditions yield to symptomatic self-treatment, and the conditions should be self-limiting unless a secondary infection occurs. Although many nonprescription products are available for symptomatic treatment of cold sores and canker sores, none has been shown conclusively to decrease the recurrence rate of lesions or to be curative.

Canker Sores. Canker sores appear as an epithelial ulceration on nonkeratinized mucosal surfaces of movable mouth parts, such as the tongue, the floor of the mouth, the soft palate, or the inside lining of the lips and cheeks. Patients may develop single or multiple lesions. The color is usually gray to grayish-yellow with an erythematous halo of inflamed tissue. The lesions can be painful and may inhibit eating, drinking, swallowing, and talking, as well as oral hygiene. Most lesions persist for 7–14 days and heal spontaneously without scarring. Canker sores are neither viral in origin nor contagious.

The main goal in treating canker sores is to control discomfort and protect the sores from irritating stimuli. Coating the ulcers with topical oral protectants such as Orabase, denture adhesives, or benzoin tincture can be effective. These products can be applied as needed. The ADA accepts both Orabase Plain and benzoin tincture as topical oral mucosal protectants.

Topical application of local anesthetic/analgesic pastes or gels affords temporary pain relief. Benzocaine and butacaine are the most commonly used local anesthetics in

313

nonprescription products. Benzocaine should not be used by patients with a history of hypersensitivity to other benzocaine-containing products.

Pharmacists should discourage the sustained use of potentially inflammatory products containing substantial amounts of menthol, phenol, camphor, and eugenol as anesthetic, counterirritant, or antiseptic treatments for canker sores. None of these ingredients has been accepted as safe and effective by the ADA for treating canker sores.

Products that release nascent oxygen (e.g., 10%–15% carbamide peroxide, 3% hydrogen peroxide, perborates) can be used as debriding and cleansing agents. Such products can be used up to four times daily (after meals) but should be used for no more than 7 days. It is important that the patient follow specific package directions. The solution should never be swallowed. If no improvement is seen in a week or if the condition worsens, professional consultation is indicated.

Systemic nonprescription analgesics (e.g., aspirin, ibuprofen, acetaminophen) afford additional relief of discomfort.

Saline rinses (1–3 tsp of table salt in 4–8 oz of warm tap water) may be soothing and can be used prior to topical application of a medication.

Cold Sores.   Cold sores or fever blisters are lesions that are generally caused by the herpes simplex type 1 virus (HSV-1). They commonly occur on the lip or on areas bordering the lips; the usual site is at the junction of mucous membrane and skin of the lips or nose. The lesions are recurrent, painful, and cosmetically objectionable. The primary infection is reported most often in childhood. HSV-1 is contagious and thought to be transmittable by direct contact.

Cold sores are often preceded by burning, itching, tingling, or numbness in the area of the forthcoming lesion. The lesion becomes visible as small, red papules of fluid-containing vesicles. Often, many lesions coalesce. A mature lesion often has a crust over the top of many coalesced, burst vesicles; its base is erythematous. The presence of pustules or pus under the crust of a cold sore may indicate a secondary bacterial infection and should be evaluated promptly and treated with an appropriate antibiotic.

Cold sores heal without scarring, usually within 10–14 days. Patients often associate predisposing factors such as sun or wind exposure, fever, systemic infectious diseases (colds and flu), menstruation, extreme physical stress and fatigue, or local trauma with the onset of cold sores. Those who identify sun exposure as a precipitating event should be advised to use a lip sunscreen product.

The primary goals in treating cold sores are to control discomfort, allow healing, and prevent complications. The cold sore should be kept moist. Skin protectant ingredients (e.g., allantoin, petrolatum, cocoa butter) can relieve dryness. Topical local anesthetics (e.g., benzocaine, dibucaine) in emollient vehicles aid in relieving itching and pain. If there is evidence of secondary bacterial infection, topical application of a thin layer of triple antibiotic ointment (e.g., Mycitracin, Neosporin) three to four times daily is recommended, along with systemic antibiotics if indicated. Systemic nonprescription analgesics may provide pain relief.

The FDA review of over-the-counter (OTC) products for fever blisters and cold sores classified external analgesics, alcohols, ketones, and amine and caine-type local anesthetics as Category I. A partial listing of Category I ingredients includes benzocaine 5%–20%, dibucaine 0.25%–1%, dyclonine hydrochloride 0.5%–1%, benzyl alcohol 10%–33%, camphor 0.1%–3%, and menthol 0.1%–1%. The FDA has proposed topically applied nonprescription skin protectants or externally applied analgesic/anesthetic drug products as the only currently effective nonprescription treatment for relieving the discomfort of fever blisters. Products that are highly astringent should be avoided.

Lesions should be kept clean by gently washing with mild soap solutions. Hand washing is important in preventing lesion contamination and minimizing autoinoculation of

HSV. Factors that delay healing (e.g., stress, local trauma, wind, sunlight, fatigue) should be avoided.

Minor Oral Mucosal Injury or Irritation

Minor wounds or inflammation resulting from dentures, orthodontic appliances, minor dental procedures, accidental injury (e.g., biting the cheek or suffering an abrasion from sharp, crisp foods), or other irritations of the mouth or gums may be treated with various drugs. Combination preparations to treat minor oral mucosal injury may contain a single anesthetic/analgesic with either a single astringent, an oral mucosal protectant, or a denture adhesive; or benzocaine combined with menthol or phenol preparations. Labeling advises that these products must not be used for more than 7 days unless directed by a physician or dentist.

The FDA has determined that no ingredient is generally recognized as safe and effective for use as a nonprescription oral wound-healing agent. Four active ingredients— carbamide peroxide in anhydrous glycerin, hydrogen peroxide, sodium perborate monohydrate (1.2 g), and sodium bicarbonate—are generally recognized as safe and effective for use as nonprescription oral health care debriding agents/oral wound cleansers.

Prolonged rinsing with oxidizing products could lead to soft-tissue irritation, decalcified tooth surfaces, and black hairy tongue. Alternatives are a sodium bicarbonate rinse (1/2 to 1 tsp in 4 oz of water) or a salt water rinse (1–3 tsp of salt in 4–8 oz of warm tap water). A saline rinse can be used safely for cleansing and soothing.

Oral Infections

Dentopyogenic Infections

Dentopyogenic infections are pus-producing infections that are associated with a tooth or its supporting structures. Symptoms range from minor generalized pain, throbbing, and sensitivity, to fever, malaise, swelling, localized pain, erythema, warmth at the infection site, and septic shock. Persons with minimal symptoms may unwisely attempt self-treatment.

Candidiasis

Candidiasis appears in debilitated patients, immunocompromised patients, and patients taking a variety of drugs. The acute pseudomembranous form of candidiasis (thrush) is characterized by white plaques with a milk curd appearance.

Patients with suspected candidiasis should be referred for medical or dental evaluation. Listerine has exhibited anti-*Candida* properties when used as an antifungal rinse for treatment of patients wearing removable dentures. It may also be useful for the prevention of oral candidiasis in immunocompromised patients.

Halitosis

Halitosis may be symptomatic of oral or nonoral pathology. Any patient who complains of severe or lingering halitosis without a readily identifiable cause should be advised to see a dentist. Masking foul taste and odor with cosmetic mouthrinses may delay necessary treatment.

Therapeutic Considerations in Special Populations

Geriatric Patients

Edentulism (toothlessness) is decreasing; more than half of older Americans have retained natural dentition. Topical fluoride application in the form of dentifrice, rinse, or gel is indicated for the prevention of coronal and root caries as long as there is natural dentition. In counseling geriatric patients on oral health care, it is important to consider medication profiles. Because the elderly are likely to be taking multiple medications, the likelihood of drug-induced or disease-related changes in oral physiology increases.

Xerostomia

About 20% of the elderly are affected with xerostomia, a condition in which salivary flow is limited or arrested. Pharmacists should review medication profiles (prescription and nonprescription) for patients complaining of dry mouth to determine if the condition is drug induced.

Xerostomia can produce difficulty in talking and swallowing, stomatitis and burning tongue, increased caries, or periodontal disease. Treatment should be directed toward the control of dental decay and the relief of soft-tissue distress. The commercially available artificial salivas relieve soft-tissue discomfort and are more effective and longer lasting than rinses and lozenges. Because they do not stimulate natural salivary gland production, however, they must be considered as replacement therapy, not as a cure for xerostomia.

Artificial salivas can be used on an as-needed basis. Xerostomic patients with a history of caries susceptibility should use a professionally designed topical fluoride program in addition to artificial saliva products. These patients should also use very soft toothbrushes and avoid mouthrinses with high alcoholic content, given that alcohol contributes to xerostomia.

Denture Problems

Denture stomatitis (an inflammation of the oral tissue in contact with a removable denture), inflammatory papillary hyperplasia, and chronic candidiasis can be caused by ill-fitting dentures, trauma, and poor denture hygiene. Poor denture hygiene contributes to fungal and bacterial growth. It not only affects the patient aesthetically (unpleasant odors and staining) but also seriously affects oral health. Refitting, relining, or repairing dentures requires professional dental treatment.

Denture Cleansers. Patients should be instructed to clean dentures thoroughly at least once daily. Only products specifically formulated for denture cleansing should be used. Whitening toothpastes meant for natural dentition should be discouraged because their abrasivity is too high. More than one product may be required to meet patient needs.

A combination regimen of brushing and soaking is recommended. Abrasive products should be used with care. Plaque removal is enhanced by brushing the denture after it has soaked. The denture should be thoroughly rinsed before reinsertion.

Denture cleansers are either chemical or abrasive in their action. The three types of chemical cleansers are alkaline peroxides, alkaline hypochlorites, and dilute acids.

Alkaline peroxide cleaners are the most commonly used chemical denture cleansers. These products are most effective on new plaque and stains that are soaked for 4–8 hours. Alkaline peroxides have few serious disadvantages and do not damage the surface of acrylic resins.

Denture-cleansing products should be completely rinsed off the denture before insertion. They should be kept out of the reach of children. Patients should not soak or clean dentures in hot water or hot soaking solutions because distortion or warping may occur. Stains that are resistant to proper denture brushing and soaking in available solutions should be evaluated by a dentist.

Denture Adhesives. Denture adhesives may be the most overused dental products purchased by patients. Pathologic changes in soft tissue under the denture have been reported with the inappropriate use of denture adhesives and ill-fitting dentures. Excessive application of adhesives could cause denture repositioning with resultant malocclusion.

Patients who believe that daily use of denture adhesives is necessary should be referred to their dentist.

The ADA has accepted some denture adhesive products provided that the labeling indicates that they are to be used only temporarily or upon the recommendation of a dentist.

Denture Reliners and Cushions. Extended use of reliners or cushions for dentures harms the patient and damages the denture. The ADA does not accept any of these products as safe and effective and discourages their use.

Patients with dentures need periodic professional dental evaluations. As time passes, it is normal to expect the original fit to need adjustment.

Denture Repair Kits

Broken dentures can be evaluated and repaired only by a dentist. Pharmacists should discourage the use of denture repair kits. They should advise patients to save all pieces of the denture or appliance to take to the dentist and to seek professional treatment without delay. Prolonged periods without wearing a partial denture can result in position changes among the remaining teeth and a loss of fit.

Pediatric Patients

It is important to start oral hygiene early in life. A wet gauze pad may be used to wipe the baby's gums after each feeding. Deciduous teeth usually start to erupt at about 6 months of age. Decay is a possibility at any time. "Baby bottle caries" results when an infant is allowed to nurse from a bottle of juice, milk, or sugar water when put to bed. When the teeth have erupted, a soft child-size toothbrush can be used. Parents must do the brushing and should take care to use only a very small amount of fluoride toothpaste or none at all.

Teething Discomfort

If teething causes sleep disturbances or irritability, symptomatic treatment may be considered. Topical local anesthetics such as benzocaine or phenol and frozen teething rings may provide symptomatic relief. Systemic nonprescription analgesics (e.g., acetaminophen) may be used. When teething is accompanied by fever, nasal congestion, or malaise, a dentist or physician should be contacted.

Pediatric Toothbrushes

Soft bristles are recommended for children's toothbrushes. Toothbrush size and shape should be individualized according to the size of the child's mouth. Children are usually unable to brush by themselves until they are 4 or 5 years old, and they may require supervision until 8 or 9 years of age.

Dental Fluorosis

Fluoride dentifrices contribute to the amount of fluoride ingested by children. Other sources are dietary, recommended systemic supplements, and any other topical fluoride preparations. Children who live in a community with an optimally fluoridated water supply may exceed optimal daily amounts. This places them at risk for mild forms of dental fluorosis, a mottled appearance of surface enamel.

Limiting ingestion of fluoride dentifrice is advised. Parents should apply the toothpaste (a pea-sized amount) to a child-size toothbrush and should brush the teeth of preschoolers until the children can manage it properly themselves. Children should be taught to rinse thoroughly and expectorate after brushing. Only regular-strength fluoride toothpaste is recommended for use by children under 6 years of age.

Swallowing should also be avoided when fluoride rinses are used. Ethanol content of most nonprescription fluoride rinses ranges from 6% to 8% and may pose a hazard for very young children. Fluoride rinses should be used only by children 6 years of age and older who have mastered the swallowing reflex. Fluoride gels are not recommended for children under 6, and children under 12 should use these products only under supervision.

Orthodontia

Fixed orthodontic appliances require careful attention to oral hygiene. Patients with these appliances need a combination of toothbrush types to clean all surfaces effectively. Powered toothbrushes or oral irrigating devices may help remove plaque and debris. It may be advisable for orthodontic patients to use a nonprescription fluoride mouthrinse while undergoing treatment.

Patients with removable orthodontic appliances should consult their orthodontist about using a denture cleanser.

Pregnancy Gingivitis

Pregnant patients are more susceptible to dental caries and gingivitis. Pregnancy gingivitis can be prevented or resolved with thorough plaque control. The severity of the inflammatory response and resulting gingivitis will decrease postpartum.

CHAPTER 26

Dermatologic Products

Questions to ask in patient assessment and counseling

Dermatitis and Scaly Dermatoses

- How long have you had this condition?
- What skin areas, including mucous membranes, hair, and nails, are involved?
- How does the affected area feel (e.g., itchy, painful)? Is it dry or oozing?
- Do you scratch the affected area? If so, how often? At what time of day is it worse?
- Has your condition changed in appearance?
- Have you had this condition before? Does it seem to come and go?
- Have you ever had other skin conditions?
- Do others in your family have a similar condition?
- Do you or any family members have allergies, asthma, or hay fever?
- Do you notice a seasonal change in your condition?
- What is your occupation?
- Is there anything that seems to make the condition worse (e.g., engaging in work activities or hobbies; cleaning house; changing soaps, deodorants, or shampoos; wearing jewelry; taking medications)?
- Have you consulted a physician about your condition? If so, what treatment was suggested? Did you follow, or are you currently following, any treatment? How effective have previous treatments been for this condition?
- Are you using any prescription or nonprescription medications? If so, what are they?
- What is your age?

Skin Infections

- What area of the skin is affected? How extensive is the area involved?
- Is the skin broken? Is there pus? Is it painful?
- How long have you had this condition? Have you ever had it before?
- Did the condition develop as the result of a previous rash or skin condition?

Editor's Note: This chapter is adapted from Dennis P. West and Phillip A. Nowakowski, "Dermatologic Products," in Covington, T.R., ed., *Handbook of Nonprescription Drugs,* 11th edition, which is based, in part, on the 8th edition chapter "Dermatitis, Dry Skin, Dandruff, Seborrheic Dermatitis, and Psoriasis Products," written by Joseph R. Robinson and Laura J. Gauger, and the 10th edition chapter "Dermatologic Products," written by Joye Ann Billow. The 11th edition chapter has also been updated and expanded to include discussions of viral and fungal skin infections and skin hyperpigmentation, the core material of which appeared in the 10th edition chapters "Topical Anti-Infective Products," written by Dennis P. West and Susan V. Maddux, and "Personal Care Products," written by Donald R. Miller and Mary Kuzel. For a more extensive discussion of the anatomy and physiology of the skin, percutaneous absorption of drugs, specific skin conditions, and skin products, readers are encouraged to consult Chapter 26 of the *Handbook.*

- *Has the condition worsened?*
- *Are any other members of your family affected?*
- *Do you have a fever or any flulike symptoms?*
- *Do you have diabetes? Any other medical conditions?*
- *Do you have any allergies to topical medications?*
- *What treatments have you tried for this condition? Were they effective?*
- *What oral or topical medications are you using? Have they been effective?*

Skin Hyperpigmentation Products

- *Have you been using a hyperpigmentation product? If so, for how long?*
- *For what type of "skin spot" do you use it?*
- *How long have you had that mole?*
- *Has the mole changed color or enlarged?*
- *Do you have any medical problems?*
- *Is there any possibility that you are pregnant?*
- *Are you taking any medications, including birth control pills?*

Hair Loss

- *How long ago did you begin to lose your hair? What areas of the scalp are involved? How extensive is the hair loss?*
- *Do others in your family suffer from hair loss?*
- *Have you tried any treatments for hair loss? Did you see any improvement in the condition?*
- *Have you been diagnosed as having an autoimmune disorder, a nutritional deficiency, or an endocrine disorder?*
- *Have you undergone chemotherapy or used a hormonal medication?*
- *(If female) Have you recently given birth?*
- *Have you suffered any trauma to the scalp?*

Dermatitis

Dermatitis is a nonspecific term that describes a number of dermatologic conditions that are inflammatory and generally characterized by erythema. The terms eczema and dermatitis are often used interchangeably. Known causes of dermatitis include allergens, irritants, and infections.

Dermatitis may be acute or chronic. Initial signs and symptoms include pruritus, erythema, and edema. Edema may be accompanied by vesicles, which often break and ooze. Over time, the weeping may diminish, giving way to a dry, scaly condition. If the dermatitis is chronic, the skin is dry and scaly, and fissures may appear. If itching results in excessive scratching, the epidermis may appear thick and ridged. Infections may occur as sequelae to pruritus-induced scratching. Pigment production may be altered, and hyper- or hypopigmentation may occur. Table 1 describes the dermatologic terms used in assessing skin lesions.

TABLE 1 Selected dermatologic terms used in the assessment of skin lesions

Term	Type of lesion[a]	Definition
Crust (scab)	Secondary	Dried exudate containing proteinaceous and cellular debris from erosion or ulceration of primary lesions
Erythema	Primary	Reddened skin
Fissure	Secondary	A split in the epidermis extending into the dermis
Lichenification	Secondary	Thickening and hardening of the skin into an irregular plaque due to excessive rubbing or scratching
Macule	Primary	Flat, nonpalpable, discolored lesion less than 1 cm in diameter. Lesions larger than 1 cm are termed *patches*
Necrosis	Secondary	Dead cells or groups of cells caused by severe trauma or an infectious process
Papule	Primary	A solid, circumscribed, elevated lesion less than 1 cm in diameter
Plaque	Primary	A palpable, papular, relatively flat lesion more than 1 cm in diameter
Pustule	Primary	A circumscribed, elevated lesion less than 1 cm in diameter containing pus. A larger lesion is termed an *abscess* or *furuncle*
Scale	Secondary	Accumulation of loose, desquamated, hyperkeratitic epidermal cells
Ulcer	Secondary	An erosion of the epidermis exposing the dermis. Deep ulcers may result in destruction of the dermis
Vesicle	Primary	A sharply circumscribed, elevated lesion containing fluid. Diameter of a vesicle may be up to 1 cm. A fluid-filled cavity of diameter greater than 1 cm is termed a *blister* or *bulla*

[a]Primary lesions are changes in the skin as a result of the undisturbed disease process. Secondary lesions are the result of external influences on the primary lesion. Primary and secondary lesions frequently coexist.

Adapted from Cahn RL, Longe RL. *The Skin: Assessment*. Palo Alto, Calif: Syntex Laboratories; 1986: 4–5.

Specific Conditions

Atopic Dermatitis

Atopic dermatitis, also called eczema, occurs primarily in infants, children, and young adults. The signs, symptoms, and areas most commonly affected are listed in Table 2.

Etiology and Characteristics. Atopic dermatitis is not contagious but is known to be genetically linked. Atopic dermatitis may be exacerbated by various factors, such as irritants (e.g., solvents, industrial chemicals, fragrances, soaps, fumes, tobacco smoke, paints, bleach, wool, astringents), allergens, extremes of temperature and humidity, dry skin, emotional stress, and cutaneous infections. The patient should be encouraged to identify the role of these factors so that they may be minimized or avoided. The role of food allergies in exacerbating atopic dermatitis is not clear.

Secondary or associated cutaneous infections are often difficult to prevent. Patients should seek medical attention promptly when signs of bacterial or viral skin infection such as pustules, vesicles, crusting, and fever blisters or cold sores are noted.

Assessment and Treatment. The pharmacist should ask questions such as those at the beginning of this chapter. Because atopic dermatitis is primarily a disease of the young, patient age is important in assessment.

If atopic dermatitis is not extreme and the patient is not under 2 years of age, initial treatment may be attempted with nonprescription measures.

The first step is to substitute sponge baths with tepid water for full-body bathing several days per week. Because of the drying effects of most soaps, mild cleansers (e.g., Cetaphil) are recommended.

Treatment of acute weeping or oozing lesions includes applying wet tap-water compresses for 20 minutes, four to six times daily. Bathing with tepid water containing colloidal oatmeal may be soothing. Hydrocortisone in an oil-in-water base may be used. If the condition does not resolve or involves a large area of the body, a physician should be consulted.

Treatment of chronic or dry lesions focuses on measures to maintain skin hydration and decrease itching. Colloidal oatmeal may be used for bathing, or a water-miscible bath oil may be added to the water near the end of the bath. The skin should be patted dry. An emollient should be applied while the skin is still damp. Topical hydrocortisone may be used for inflammation and itching, preferably in an ointment base. If the condition is not relieved, a physician should be consulted.

Adjunctive measures may be used to minimize scratching. Fingernails should be kept short, smooth, and clean. Wearing cotton gloves or socks on the hands at night helps lessen the mechanical damage related to scratching. Antihistamines are of limited value in decreasing the itching, but those with a sedative effect (e.g., diphenhydramine) may be used to promote sleep. A major limitation with the use of classic antihistamines is the undesired drowsiness the following morning.

Contact Dermatitis

Contact dermatitis, one of the most common ailments directed to pharmacists for consultation, refers to a rash that results from an allergen or irritant contacting susceptible skin. Lesions are often asymmetric in distribution and sharply demarcated. See Table 2.

Etiology and Characteristics. Irritant contact dermatitis is a nonallergenic, nonimmunologic irritation. Inflammation may be produced by exposure to many substances if concentration and duration of contact are sufficient. Allergic contact dermatitis is an immunologically mediated and delayed hypersensitivity reaction to contact allergens.

TABLE 2 Characteristics of selected forms of dermatitis and dry skin

Condition	Symptoms	Location	Signs
Atopic dermatitis	Itching, scratching	2 mo: chest, face 2 y: scalp, neck, and extremities 2–4 y: neck, wrist, elbow, knee 12–20 y: flexors, hands	Red, raised vesicles; dry skin; oozing Less acute lesions; edema; erythema Dry, thickened plaques; hyperpigmentation
Contact dermatitis (irritant and allergic)	Acute: itching Chronic: stiffness, dry	Irritant: contact areas Allergic: exposed contact areas (transferable by touch)	Irritant (mild, acute): red, oozing blisters Irritant (mild, chronic): dry, thick, fissured skin Irritant (severe): blisters, ulcers Allergic: unusual pattern of lesions; sharp margins with angles and straight lines
Hand dermatitis	Itching, dry	Sides of fingers, occasionally palms	Red, dry, chapped, fissured skin
Dry skin (chapped)	Often none; moderate to severe itching	Lower legs, backs of hands, forearms, occasionally entire body	Dry, fine scale; patches, diffuse or round; if severe, fissures

Adapted from Ricciatti–Sibbald DJ. In: Clark C, ed. *Self-Medication: A Reference for Health Professionals.* 4th ed. Ottawa: Canadian Pharmaceutical Association; 1992: 65.

The most common contact allergen comes from poison ivy, oak, and sumac (see Chapter 32). Particles in smoke and indirect contact with pets may cause allergic contact dermatitis in very sensitive persons. A number of metals (e.g., cobalt, chromium, nickel) may cause allergic contact dermatitis.

Assessment and Treatment. It is important to identify the offending substance, because its removal will usually result in improvement of the condition. Asking questions about the patient's environment and practices (e.g., home, work, recreation, laundry products, the wearing of unwashed new clothes, and medication use) may allow an irritant or allergen to be identified.

Agents that may act as sensitizers include neomycin, iodine-containing products, sulfonamides, mercury-containing antiseptics, and ethylenediamine. Many topical skin preparations used for medicinal effect, including benzocaine, may also be a source of allergens. Topical antihistamines such as diphenhydramine may also cause sensitization. Once a patient has become sensitized by the topical product, oral administration of diphenhydramine may also produce dermatitis.

A patient may be sensitive to, or irritated by, more than one drug or chemical. Therefore, before recommending any product for the treatment of contact dermatitis, the pharmacist should first encourage the patient to try to identify possible offending substance(s).

Choice of treatment depends on the severity of the condition. Mild to moderate dermatitis is usually amenable to treatment with nonprescription agents. The involved area should be washed gently, but well, to remove traces of the offending agent. If the area is oozing, compresses of cool tap water applied for 20 minutes, four to six times daily, may be recommended to aid in drying the lesions. Application of calamine lotion between compress applications and use of colloidal oatmeal baths may be soothing and help relieve itching. Topical hydrocortisone cream may be added to the regimen to reduce inflammation and itching. If the condition does not improve in a couple of days or if it worsens, a physician should be consulted. A person with a severe reaction or involvement of large areas of the body should also be referred to a physician.

To patients who have experienced topical allergic reactions to cosmetics, fragrances, hair care products, nail polish, hair dyes, deodorants, and soaps, a wide range of hypoallergenic products may be recommended.

Hand Dermatitis

Etiology and Characteristics. Hand dermatitis (hand eczema) often occurs in individuals whose occupation requires frequent hand washing or contact with moisture and mild irritants (e.g., hairdressers, bartenders, food handlers, medical personnel).

Hand dermatitis is marked by erythema, dryness, chapping, and, in severe cases, oozing vesicles and pruritus. In severe, untreated cases, fissures may allow infection that can proceed to tissue necrosis.

Treatment. Acute and subacute hand dermatitis are usually treated in the same manner. Wet dressings may be applied, followed by hydrocortisone ointment. After the acute condition subsides, a nonmedicated emollient or hydrocortisone ointment should continue to be applied at least four times a day until the condition has healed.

Treatment of chronic (i.e., dry, scaling, and fissured) hand dermatitis focuses on maintaining skin hydration by applying water-in-oil emollients often, especially after immersion in water. The emollient can be alternated with hydrocortisone ointment, if necessary. Medical attention should be sought if the condition does not improve within 1–2 weeks.

A number of adjunctive measures, such as wearing vinyl (not rubber) gloves while doing "wet work," can be recommended. Patients should be reminded that wearing a glove with a hole in it will trap irritants and is worse than wearing no glove at all. Thin cotton liners worn under vinyl gloves may be helpful. When washing the hands, the patient should use lukewarm water and a minimal amount of soap. The patient should avoid creams and lotions because they may be too drying and may contain common allergens such as unrefined lanolin or fragrances.

Dry Skin

Etiology and Characteristics. Dry skin is characterized by roughness, scaling, loss of flexibility, fissures, inflammation, and pruritus. It appears most often on lower legs, dorsa of the hands, and forearms. Dry skin is especially prevalent during the winter. It may occur secondary to prolonged detergent use, malnutrition, damage to the stratum corneum, or systemic disorders (e.g., hypothyroidism, dehydration).

Dry skin is caused not by a lack of natural skin oils but by a lack of water in the stratum corneum. Conditions that may cause dry skin include frequent or prolonged bathing or showering with hot water, excessive use of soap, low humidity, and damage to the stratum corneum. Dry skin occurs with an increased incidence among elderly people.

Treatment. The key to treatment is to maintain skin hydration. Full-body bathing may be cut back to every other day or less often, or replaced by sponge baths or quick showers with warm water. Bath products such as colloidal oatmeal, oilated oatmeal, or bath oil added near the end of the bath may enhance skin hydration. Oil-based emollients should be applied immediately after bathing while the skin is damp and should be reapplied frequently. More severe cases of dry skin may require a urea- or lactic acid-containing product. Topical hydrocortisone ointment may be applied on a short-term basis to reduce inflammation and itching. If resolution does not occur within 1 or 2 weeks, a physician should be consulted.

Pharmacologic Agents for Dermatitis and Dry Skin

Nonprescription products for dermatitis and dry skin include bath products, emollients, hydrating agents, keratin-softening agents, astringents, antipruritics, protectants, and hydrocortisone. Keratolytics and agents that reduce the mitotic activity of the epidermis, such as tars, are usually avoided because of their irritant properties.

Bath Products

Bath Oils. Bath oils are minimally effective in improving a dry skin condition. Their effect may be maximized by adding the oil near the end of the bath and patting the skin dry rather than rubbing it. Bath oils may also be applied as wet compresses (1 tsp in 1/4 cup of warm water) to help lubricate dry skin.

Bath oils make the tub and floor slippery, creating a safety hazard. There is no clear superiority of one type of product over another; however, patients with dermatologic disorders should generally avoid products with fragrance.

Oatmeal Products. Colloidal oatmeal bath products are less effective than bath oils; however, oilated oatmeal products combine the effect of oatmeal (i.e, soothing and antipruritic) and a bath oil.

Cleansers. Some authorities recommend special soaps that contain extra oils to minimize the drying effect of washing; however, these soaps usually clean poorly. Unscented Dove is one example of a cleansing agent with minimal drying effect to skin. Although there is little objective proof of their superiority, the glycerin soaps are advertised for and well accepted by people with skin conditions. Mild cleansers such as Cetaphil may be recommended if soap should be avoided.

Emollients/Moisturizers

Emollients are used to prevent or relieve the signs and symptoms of dry skin. They act primarily by leaving an oily film on the skin surface through which moisture cannot readily escape. Commonly used emollients include petrolatum, lanolin, mineral oil, and dimethicone.

Frequency of application depends on the severity of the condition as well as on the hydration efficiency of the occlusive agent. Care should be exercised to avoid excessive hydration, which may lead to tissue maceration. Contact with the eye or with broken or abraded skin should be avoided because formulation ingredients may cause irritation.

Petrolatum is an effective occlusive agent. Mineral oil is not as effective, and silicones are even less effective. Petrolatum should not be applied over puncture wounds, infections, or lacerations because its high occlusive ability may lead to maceration and further inflammation. Application to intertriginous areas, mucous membranes, and acne-prone areas should also be avoided. Similar precautions should be taken with dimethicone.

Patients with a history of allergic reactions to lanolin should avoid lanolin-containing products. Refined lanolin-containing products are less likely to be sensitizing.

Humectants

Humectants are hygroscopic materials that may be added to an emollient base. Their function is to draw water into the stratum corneum. Commonly used hydrating agents are glycerin, propylene glycol, and phospholipids.

Keratin-Softening Agents

Chemically altering the keratin layer softens skin and improves its appearance. This treatment approach does not need a substantial addition of water, but all the attendant dry skin symptoms may not be alleviated unless water is added to the keratin layer.

Urea. Urea (carbamide) in concentrations of 10%–30% is mildly keratolytic and increases water uptake in the stratum corneum. It is considered safe and has been recommended for use on crusted necrotic tissue. Concentrations of 10% have been used on simple dry skin; 20%–30% formulations have been used for treating more resistant dry skin conditions. Urea-containing creams can cause stinging, burning, and irritation, particularly on broken skin.

Alpha-Hydroxy Acids. Lactic acid is an alpha-hydroxy acid that has been useful in concentrations of 2%–5% for treating dry skin conditions. Lactic acid may be added to urea preparations.

Allantoin. The Food and Drug Administration (FDA) has recommended that allantoin be considered safe and effective as a skin protectant for adults, children, and infants when applied in concentrations of 0.5%–2.0%. It is less effective than urea.

Astringents

Astringents retard the oozing, discharge, or bleeding of dermatitis. When applied as a wet dressing or compress, they cool and dry the skin through evaporation. They cause vasoconstriction and reduce blood flow in inflammation. They also cleanse the skin of exudates, crust, and debris.

The FDA has identified two astringent solutions as being safe and effective: aluminum acetate (Burow's solution) and witch hazel (hamamelis water). Aluminum acetate solution (USP) must be diluted 1:10 to 1:40 with water before use.

The patient may soak the affected area in the astringent solution two to four times daily for 15–30 minutes or apply a loose compress of washcloths soaked in the solution and then wrung gently. The dressings should be rewetted and reapplied every few minutes for 20–30 minutes, four to six times daily. Isotonic saline solution, tap water, or diluted white vinegar (1/4 cup per pint of water) may also be used.

Antipruritics

The itching associated with dermatitis may be mediated through several different mechanisms, which may explain how three major classes of pharmacologic agents—local anesthetics, antihistamines, and steroids—are useful as antipruritics.

Local anesthetics relieve itching as well as pain. Because local anesthetics may also cause systemic side effects, they should not be used in large quantities or over long periods of time, particularly if the skin is raw or blistered. Nonprescription topical anesthetics that appear to be safe and effective are dyclonine and benzocaine.

Antihistamines are considered safe and effective for use as nonprescription external analgesics. Because of their sensitizing potential, the FDA does not recommend the topical use of these agents for more than 7 consecutive days except under the advice and supervision of a physician. Oral antihistamines have been used to treat the itching of dermatologic disorders with variable results.

Protectants

Skin protectants protect injured or exposed skin surfaces from harmful or annoying stimuli. Zinc oxide (1%–25%) is one of the most widely used. Other protectants include aluminum hydroxide and bismuth subnitrate. Covering the lesions or applying a product with an occlusive barrier may increase the degree of tissue maceration and prevent heat loss, resulting in discomfort.

Topical Hydrocortisone

Hydrocortisone is the only corticosteroid available without a prescription for the topical treatment of dermatitis. It relieves the redness, heat, pain, swelling, and itch associated with various dermatoses.

Concentrations of 0.5%–1% are appropriate for the treatment of localized dermatitis. Hydrocortisone should be applied sparingly by massaging it well, but gently, into the affected area three or four times a day. An ointment formulation is best for chronic, non-oozing dermatoses.

Before recommending a hydrocortisone product, the pharmacist should be certain that the area of application is not infected, because topical hydrocortisone may mask the symptoms of dermatologic infections and allow them to progress. Signs of bacterial infection include redness, heat, pus, and crusting. Fungal infections may be marked by erythema and scaling.

Topical hydrocortisone rarely produces systemic complications. Because response decreases with continued use, intermittent courses of therapy are advised.

Product Selection Guidelines

When deciding on which product to recommend for dermatitis or dry skin, the pharmacist must evaluate the active ingredients, secondary ingredients, and the vehicle. Secondary ingredients added to enhance product elegance and stability include emulsifiers, emulsion stabilizers (thickening agents), and preservatives. Many of these have the potential for producing contact dermatitis.

The type of vehicle (e.g., ointment, cream, lotion, gel, solution, aerosol) may have a significant effect on dermatitis. The following guidelines may be used to choose an appropriate vehicle:

- "If it's wet, dry it." If a drying effect is desired, solutions, gels, and occasionally creams may be recommended.
- If slight lubrication is needed, creams and lotions are preferred.
- "If it's dry, wet it." If the lesion is very dry and fissured, ointments are the vehicle of choice. However, they should be avoided in intertriginous areas. Also, in an acute process, ointments may cause further irritation because of their occlusive effect.
- Aerosols, gels, or lotions may be recommended when the dermatitis affects a hair-covered area of the body.

Efficacy of any skin care product may need to be sacrificed or compromised somewhat to achieve patient acceptance. The most efficacious product that the patient will accept should be recommended.

Table 3 lists the amount of drug needed to cover a given area of the body three times daily over a 1-week period.

Scaly Dermatoses

Dandruff, seborrheic dermatitis (seborrhea), and psoriasis are chronic, scaly dermatoses. They may be placed on a spectrum ranging from dandruff, a minor problem that is primarily cosmetic, to psoriasis, a condition that can have significant physical, psychologic, and economic consequences. Nonprescription products are appropriate for all degrees of dandruff. Many cases of seborrheic dermatitis will respond to the same nonprescription drug regimen used to treat dandruff. Psoriasis that involves mild inflammation may be responsive to nonprescription treatment. Initial diagnosis and management of acute flare-ups require the attention of a physician.

TABLE 3 Amount of topical medication needed for three times daily application for 1 week

Part of the body	Cream/ointment (g)	Lotion/solution/gel (mL)
Face	5–10	100–120
Both hands	25–50	200–240
Scalp	50–100	200–240
Both arms or both legs	100–200	240–360
Trunk	200	360–480
Groin and genitalia	15–25	120–180

Adapted from Bingham EA. Topical dermatologic therapy. In: Rook A, Parish LC, Beare JM, eds. *Practical Management of the Dermatologic Patient*. Philadelphia: JB Lippincott; 1986: 227–8.

Dandruff

Dandruff is a chronic, noninflammatory scalp condition that results in excessive scaling of scalp epidermis. It is characterized by accelerated epidermal cell turnover, an irregular keratin breakup pattern, and the shedding of cells in large scales. The specific cause of accelerated cell growth seen in dandruff is unknown.

Treatment. Dandruff is more of a cosmetic than a medical problem. The patient needs to understand that there is no direct cure for dandruff and that the condition can usually be well controlled. Washing the hair and scalp with a nonmedicated shampoo every other day or daily is often sufficient to control dandruff. If not, medicated nonprescription antidandruff products may be used. The patient should be counseled to allow medicated shampoo to remain on the hair for approximately 1 minute before rinsing and repeating. Thorough rinsing is important.

A cytostatic agent such as pyrithione zinc, selenium sulfide, or coal tar is recommended. Coal tar–containing shampoos may discolor light hair as well as clothing and jewelry and may not appeal to some patients. Next, a keratolytic shampoo containing salicylic acid or sulfur may be used. If dandruff proves resistant to these agents, the patient should be referred to a physician.

Seborrheic Dermatitis

Seborrheic dermatitis is a general term for a group of eruptions that occur predominantly in the areas of greatest sebaceous gland activity (e.g., the scalp, face, trunk). Seborrhea occurs mostly in middle-aged and elderly persons, particularly men.

The distinctive characteristics of the disorder are its occurrence in hairy areas (especially the scalp); the appearance of dull, well-demarcated, yellowish-red lesions; and the presence of oily-appearing, yellowish scales. Pruritus is common. The most common form, seborrhea of the scalp, is characterized by greasy scales on the scalp. When seborrhea of the scalp occurs in newborns and infants, it is referred to as cradle cap and is treated primarily by gentle massaging with baby oil followed by a nonmedicated shampoo.

The cause of seborrhea is unknown. Emotional and physical stress are aggravating factors.

Assessment

Seborrhea fluctuates in severity, often as a result of stress. Lesion distribution is a key factor in distinguishing seborrhea from psoriasis. Seborrhea commonly involves the face, whereas psoriasis is rarely found on the face. The scalp is generally involved in both conditions, but seborrhea is marked by oily, yellow scales, whereas psoriatic scales are dry and silvery. The Auspitz sign (small bleeding points) is indicative of psoriasis.

Fungal infections may be mistaken for seborrhea. Thus, proper assessment is important because fungal infections may be worsened by seborrhea therapy using hydrocortisone. If the lesion is located in the groin, tinea cruris (jock itch) must be considered. Scalp lesions must be evaluated for the possibility of tinea capitis (ringworm of the scalp).

Treatment

The treatment of seborrheic dermatitis is similar to that of dandruff. Seborrhea generally responds to shampoos containing pyrithione zinc, selenium sulfide, salicylic acid, or coal tar.

Topical corticosteroids, while not indicated for dandruff, may be used for seborrheic dermatitis when erythema persists after therapy with medicated shampoos. Hydrocortisone lotions for scalp dermatitis are available without a prescription. The patient should be instructed to apply the hydrocortisone product two to three times a day until symptoms subside and then intermittently to control acute exacerbations. The hair should be parted and the product applied directly to the scalp and massaged in thoroughly. This process should be repeated until desired coverage is achieved. Absorption is enhanced if the lotion is applied after shampooing.

The patient should be encouraged to minimize prolonged use of hydrocortisone because a rebound flare may occur when prolonged therapy is discontinued. If the condition worsens or symptoms persist for more than 7 days, or the seborrhea spreads to the ear canal, eyelashes, or eyelids, a physician should be consulted.

Nonprescription products used to treat seborrhea are to be avoided for children under 2 years of age, except under the advice and supervision of a physician.

Psoriasis

Psoriasis is a papulosquamous erythematous skin disease marked by the presence of silvery scales.

Psoriatic lesions tend to appear on the scalp, elbows, knees, fingernails, lower back, and the genitoanal region. Lesions may develop at sites of trauma and have even been reportedly produced by shock and noise. Itching is a significant manifestation of the disease in 30%–70% of cases.

Psoriasis is primarily manifested in the epidermis; mucous membranes are rarely involved. About 7% of psoriatic patients have a unique form of arthritis, psoriatic arthritis.

Initial onset peaks in the late 20s and declines with advancing age. It is distributed almost equally between men and women.

Psoriasis lesions may last a lifetime or may disappear quickly. The disease is marked by spontaneous exacerbations and remissions. It is not contagious. There seems to be an inherited predisposition to psoriasis. Controlled exposure to sunlight usually improves the condition. Emotional stress often affects psoriasis adversely. Antimalarial agents, beta-blockers, and lithium can exacerbate or precipitate a psoriasis-like eruption. Abrupt withdrawal of corticosteroids may precipitate a severe rebound flare.

Assessment

Assessment usually is straightforward, although the diagnosis and management of acute flare-ups require the attention of a physician. Sites of involvement, the dry silvery appearance of scales, and a small area of bleeding after gentle scale removal are characteristic. Pruritus and joint involvement may be present. Information regarding precipitating factors such as disease, pregnancy, a recent vaccination, emotional stress, or physical trauma is useful.

It is important to differentiate psoriasis from other diseases that may have similar symptoms but call for different treatment. When the scalp or the flexural and intertriginous areas are involved, psoriasis must be differentiated from a fungal infection or seborrhea. A fungal organism may be identified from lesion scrapings; when nails are involved, differentiation requires laboratory analysis. Psoriasis of the scalp may be distinguished from seborrhea by the Auspitz sign and by the difference in scale appearance and color. The psoriatic plaque has a full, rich, red color with a depth of hue and opacity not typically seen in seborrhea or dermatitis. In dark skin, this distinction may be lost.

Treatment

Pruritic dry skin is very common in psoriasis, and emollients and lubricating bath products often provide relief for these symptoms. Gentle rubbing with a soft cloth following the bath helps remove scales. If this is insufficient, self-treatment may progress to the use of keratolytics, coal tar, and topical hydrocortisone. Vigorous rubbing should be avoided.

Acute localized flares call for local therapy with emollients and hydrocortisone. Tars, salicylic acid, and aggressive ultraviolet (UV) radiation therapy must be avoided.

The FDA recommends that only mild cases of psoriasis be self-treated. If a nonprescription product is used, the pharmacist should counsel the patient to consult a physician if the condition does not improve in 1–2 weeks or if it worsens. Individuals with severe cases involving large areas of the body should be under a physician's care.

Psoriasis cannot be cured, but signs and symptoms can usually be controlled with appropriate patient education and treatment. If the pharmacist can help the patient understand and accept the condition, it may reduce the patient's emotional stress and therefore decrease psychogenic exacerbations. Prevention of flares, achieved by minimizing precipitating factors such as emotional stress, skin irritation, and physical trauma, should be emphasized.

Pharmacologic Agents for Scaly Dermatoses

Active ingredients cited as Category I by the FDA include the following:

- *Dandruff:* Coal tar preparations, pyrithione zinc, salicylic acid, selenium sulfide, sulfur, and sulfur in combination with salicylic acid;
- *Seborrheic dermatitis:* Coal tar preparations, pyrithione zinc, salicylic acid, and selenium sulfide;
- *Psoriasis:* Coal tar preparations and salicylic acid. Topical hydrocortisone is useful in the self-treatment of seborrhea and psoriasis.

Cytostatic Agents

Cytostatic agents decrease the rate of epidermal cell replication. They represent a direct approach to controlling dandruff and seborrhea.

Pyrithione Zinc. For pyrithione zinc products intended to be applied and washed off after a brief exposure, the FDA allows concentrations of 0.3%–2% for treating dandruff and 0.95%–2% for treating seborrhea. Concentrations for products intended to be applied and then left on the skin or scalp are 0.1%–0.25% for treating both dandruff and seborrhea. Shampoos and soaps are available in 1% and 2% concentrations.

Before using one of these products, the patient should be advised to shampoo with a nonmedicated, nonresidue shampoo (e.g., Prell, Breck, Johnson and Johnson Baby Shampoo). This may be followed by a pyrithione zinc shampoo worked into the scalp vigorously for at least 5 minutes and then rinsed thoroughly. This treatment should be repeated twice weekly for 2 weeks and then once weekly as needed.

Long-term use of 1%–2% pyrithione zinc products has not been associated with toxicity. Patients should be cautioned against using this agent on broken or abraded skin.

Selenium Sulfide. Selenium sulfide is more effective with longer contact time and thus should be applied in the same manner as pyrithione zinc. The product must be rinsed from the hair thoroughly or discoloration may result. Frequent use of selenium sulfide tends to leave a residual odor and an oily scalp. It is available in a nonprescription strength of 1% and in a higher concentration, by prescription, for use in resistance cases.

Selenium sulfide causes irritation of scalp and adjacent skin areas. Contact with the eyes should be avoided. If such contact does occur, the patient should flush the eyes with copious amounts of water. Selenium sulfide is toxic if ingested.

Coal Tar

Crude coal tar (1%–5%) and UV radiation therapy have been used together in the treatment of psoriasis since 1925 (the Goeckerman treatment). Coal tar is available in creams, ointments, pastes, lotions, bath oils, shampoos, soaps, and gels. Tar gels represent a unique product form that appears to deliver the beneficial elements of crude coal tar in a form both convenient to apply and cosmetically acceptable. They may have a drying effect on the skin, necessitating the use of an emollient. Side effects of coal tar include folliculitis, staining of the skin and hair, photosensitization, and dermatitis.

Known active photosensitizers of coal tar include acridine, anthracene, and pyridine. If the patient is using other photosensitizing drugs such as tetracyclines, phenothiazines, thiazides, or sulfonamides, the pharmacist should give appropriate warnings. Patients should be cautioned that the use of coal tar may increase their tendency to sunburn for up to 24 hours after application. However, physicians sometimes instruct patients to spend time in the sunlight following evening application of coal tar.

The FDA considers the benefits of coal tar to outweigh the risks for use in shampoo formulations and has granted approval for coal tar in concentrations of 0.5%–5% in the self-treatment of dandruff, seborrhea, and psoriasis.

Keratolytic Agents

Keratolytic agents are used in dandruff and seborrhea products to loosen and lyse keratin aggregates, thereby facilitating their removal from the scalp in smaller particles.

These agents have a concentration-dependent irritant effect, particularly on mucous membranes and the conjunctiva of the eye. They also have the potential of acting on hair keratin as well as on skin keratin. Thus, hair appearance may be altered as a result of extended use. The directions and precautions for use of keratolytic shampoo are similar to those for shampoos containing cytostatic agents.

Salicylic Acid. Topical salicylic acid is useful for psoriasis when thick scales are present. A patient should soak the psoriatic lesions in warm water for 10–20 minutes before applying the preparation, which may then be covered by an occlusive dressing. Application over extensive areas should be avoided because of the potential for percutaneous absorption and systemic toxicity. Initially, lower concentrations should be used to minimize the possibility of irritation.

At concentrations of 1.8%–3%, the keratolytic effect typically takes 7–10 days.

Sulfur. Sulfur has been approved in concentrations of 2%–5% for the self-treatment of dandruff. Sulfur is often combined with salicylic acid. This combination has been commonly used for the self-treatment of seborrhea.

Topical Hydrocortisone

Topical hydrocortisone is not indicated in the treatment of dandruff. It may be useful for seborrhea accompanied by inflammation and should be reserved for scalp seborrhea unresponsive to medicated shampoos.

Nonprescription hydrocortisone products play an important role in the management of psoriasis. Efficacy may be enhanced by an occlusive dressing. However, continued use of topical steroids beyond 2 or 3 weeks may render the drug less effective. If the patient does not respond adequately, physician referral is appropriate.

Adverse effects include local atrophy of the skin after prolonged use and the aggravation of certain cutaneous infections. The concentrations of hydrocortisone available in nonprescription preparations are unlikely to cause systemic sequelae.

The patient should be instructed to apply the hydrocortisone as a thin film two to four times a day at the onset of therapy and intermittently thereafter to control exacerbations. The medication should be thoroughly but gently massaged into the skin. Frequent use is discouraged because topical steroids may become less effective with prolonged use, promote local rebound, cause adverse local effects, and, most important, fail to induce remissions of psoriasis. The patient should be instructed to rely primarily on other treatments and to use topical hydrocortisone only when necessary.

The systemic use of corticosteroids is contraindicated in all but the most severe forms of psoriasis.

Patient Counseling Guidelines

Dandruff and Seborrheic Dermatitis

- The patient should shampoo daily at first and then at least every other day. If shampooing every other day does not control the condition, a medicated shampoo should be used.
- The patient should wet the hair first and then lather a generous amount of medicated shampoo into the entire scalp, paying special attention to the hairline and other areas of activity, such as around the ears, nose, and eyebrows. The shampoo should be left on the scalp and skin for about 1 minute and then rinsed off. The process should then be repeated. Adequate contact time is important.
- The patient should be reassured that dandruff and seborrhea are extensions of normal physiologic events and that total control may not be possible. If the patient has tried one medicated shampoo without success, the next alternative should be a product with a different mechanism of action.
- If the erythema or itching persists after a trial period with a medicated shampoo, a hydrocortisone lotion or gel may be added to the regimen. It should be applied sparingly once a day and worked into the scalp thoroughly. Improvement should be seen within the first week.
- Recalcitrant cases and cases in children under 2 years of age should be referred to a physician.

Psoriasis

Psoriatic patients should be under a physician's care. The pharmacist's role in the management of psoriasis is that of a knowledgeable consultant. The pharmacist must consider the area to which the agent is to be applied, because response to topical medications shows striking anatomic regional variation.

Scalp. Previous guidelines for nonprescription therapy with a medicated shampoo for dandruff and seborrhea are applicable to the treatment of scalp psoriasis with regard to tar- as well as salicylic acid–based products. Sufficient contact time is essential. Although 1% hydrocortisone products for scalp itching and erythema may be used, significant lesions or widespread involvement dictates physician treatment.

Psoriasis of the Body, Arms, and Legs.   Emollients are widely used in mild as well as severe psoriasis.

Salicylic acid products may be more cosmetically acceptable than coal tar products and may encourage compliance. Such products are most useful if thick scales are present. Soaking the affected area in warm water for 10–20 minutes before applying a salicylic acid product enhances drug activity.

Coal tar products may be applied to the body, arms, and legs at bedtime. The patient should be advised to use appropriate bed linen and clothing during applications because coal tar stains most materials. The overnight application is followed by a bath in the morning.

Topical hydrocortisone ointment may be applied sparingly to lesions.

Intertriginous Psoriasis. Coal tar and salicylic acid should be used carefully, if at all, to treat psoriasis in areas such as the armpits and genitoanal region. Instead, hydrocortisone cream may be applied sparingly two or three times a day.

Skin Infections

Cutaneous infections may be caused by bacteria, fungi, viruses, or parasites. Many bacterial and fungal infections are amenable to topical therapy.

Bacterial Skin Infections

See Chapter 28, "First-Aid Products and Minor Wound Care."

Fungal Skin Infections

Fungal skin infections exhibit single or multiple lesions that may produce mild scaling or deep granulomas. Infections affect the hair, nails, and skin. They include:

- Tinea pedis, also known as athlete's foot or ringworm of the feet;
- Tinea capitis (ringworm of the scalp), which occurs primarily in children;
- Tinea cruris (jock itch) which occurs on the medial and upper parts of the thighs and the pubic area and is more common in males;
- Tinea corporis (ringworm of the skin), which is most common among persons living in humid climates and may be similar in appearance to noninfectious dermatitis.
- Moniliasis (candidiasis), which usually occurs in intertriginous areas such as the groin, axilla, interdigital spaces, under the breasts, and at the corners of the mouth; and
- Tinea versicolor, a fungal infection of the stratum corneum that is characterized by a change in pigmentation at the affected sites, ranging from white to medium brown.

Viral Skin Infections

Viral infections may occur in or on the skin and commonly present as warts, molluscum contagiosum, herpes simplex, or varicella-zoster infections (usually shingles [herpes zoster] in adults and varicella [chickenpox] in children).

Herpes Simplex

Herpes simplex virus (HSV) infection usually involves the skin and mucous membranes. Type 1 (HSV-1), causes fever blisters (cold sores) and is most commonly found in the perioral area, and type 2 (HSV-2) is most commonly seen as genital lesions. The virus is latent after the primary infection and may be reactivated by multiple factors. Lesions are characterized by grouped vesicles that are clear, may become pustular, and crust and heal within 7–10 days. There is often a painful, burning sensation associated with the lesions. Prior to the eruption, prodromal itching and tingling sensations at the site of the impending eruption is common.

Varicella-Zoster Infections

Herpes varicella (chickenpox) is acute, highly contagious, and generalized, and it develops in the nonimmune host; shingles (caused by the same virus) is localized and painful, and it develops in the partially immune host. The varicella-zoster virus is spread by respiratory droplets and direct contact with lesions. It is most common during winter and spring in children who are less than 10 years old.

Chickenpox erupts on the trunk and face as red macules and progresses to papules, vesicles, pustules, and crust formation. Severe pruritus may be present; fever and malaise are common.

Shingles probably results after reactivation of the latent virus. Patients usually have a past history of chickenpox. Neither shingles nor chickenpox is normally a recurrent disease. Lesions usually occur along a single dermatome; they appear as grouped vesicles on an erythematous base following the course of the nerve(s) involved. The involved area may coalesce to form larger plaquelike lesions that may be very painful. Appearance of lesions may be preceded by itching, tenderness, and pain in the involved region. Peripheral neuropathy (nerve pain), which may develop and persist for weeks or months, is treatable with the external analgesic agent capsaicin.

Molluscum Contagiosum

Molluscum contagiosum is a viral tumor caused by a poxvirus containing DNA. The disease is contracted by direct contact with an infected person, contact with a fomite, or autoinoculation.

The virus is manifested by one or more small, pink, slightly raised lesions that are usually found on the abdomen, inner thigh, or perianal area.

Assessment of Skin Infections

Before recommending a topical product for self-medication, the pharmacist should assess the nature of the patient's complaint. Noninfectious processes, including drug-induced eruptions, should be taken into account. In cases of infectious etiology or of a possible secondary infection, antimicrobial agents should be considered.

Referral to a physician should be considered if:

■ There is doubt as to the causative factor or organism.

■ Initial treatment has not been successful or the condition is worsening.

■ Applications of topical drug products have been used for prolonged periods over large areas, especially on denuded skin (creating a potential for systemic toxicity).

■ Exudate is excessive and continuous.

■ Infection is widespread.

■ There is a predisposing illness, such as diabetes, systemic infection, or an immune deficiency.

■ Fever, malaise, or both occur.

■ A primary dermatitis (allergic dermatitis, psoriasis, or seborrhea) exists and becomes secondarily infected.

■ Lesions are deep and extensive.

■ Lancing is needed to aid drainage of exudate or provide pain relief.

Treatment of Skin Infections

Viral Cutaneous Infections

There are no nonprescription products specifically used as antiviral agents for cutaneous viral infections. Most of the products used are antiseptic products for relieving symptoms and preventing secondary bacterial infection.

Topical preparations that enhance vesicular drying may reduce discomfort. For chickenpox, tepid oatmeal or starch baths, topical calamine lotion, and oral antihistamines may relieve pruritus. Oral acetaminophen may be given for fever.

For shingles, nonadherent dressings can be used to protect the lesional area from irritation. Soothing compresses may be used during the vesicular stages. Oral analgesics and occlusive dressings may help relieve pain; opioids may be necessary. Oral antihistamines may help relieve itching, and oral and topical antibiotics may be used for secondary infections. After resolution of the skin lesions, topical capsaicin may be used to relieve peripheral neuropathic pain. Topical antibacterial and antifungal products are often used to treat as well as to prevent secondary infection. Topical antiseptic drug products are used to help prevent cutaneous infections.

Cutaneous Antifungal Agents

Topical anti-infectives are used to treat and prevent fungal infection of various tissues (skin, hair, nails, and mucous membranes). Because this product classification is so broad, the present focus is on products for use in the prevention and self-treatment of fungal skin infections.

Clioquinol (3%), clotrimazole (1%), haloprogin (1%), miconazole nitrate (2%), povidone–iodine (10%), tolnaftate (1%), and various undecylenates (10%–25%) are the only topical antifungals considered safe and effective by the FDA for nonprescription use. These products are not recognized as safe and effective for diaper rash.

Creams or solutions are the most effective antifungal product forms for delivery of the active agent into the epidermis. Sprays and powders are useful as adjuncts to a cream or solution or as prophylactic agents.

The patient should clean the area first and then massage the product thoroughly into the entire affected area.

Haloprogin. Haloprogin is an effective alternative for the treatment of athlete's foot, jock itch, and ringworm. Side effects are relatively rare and include burning, itching, and scaling of the skin. Should they occur, use of the preparation should be discontinued.

Miconazole and Clotrimazole. Miconazole nitrate and clotrimazole are active against fungi and some gram-positive bacteria but not against gram-negative bacteria.

Treatment with miconazole and clotrimazole results in a low rate of recurrent infection when therapy is continued for 2 weeks or more. Allergic contact sensitization is rare, and other side effects are usually self-limiting on discontinuation of the preparation.

Selenium Sulfide. Selenium sulfide is usually effective in the treatment of tinea versicolor. Contact with the eyes and sensitive skin areas should be avoided. This treatment should be repeated daily for 2 weeks or until a response is noted; it should then be tapered to twice weekly and then once weekly according to response. Patients with recurrent tinea versicolor may use the product on a weekly basis indefinitely.

Tolnaftate. Tolnaftate is effective against most superficial dermatophytes but ineffective in the treatment of tinea versicolor and C albicans. Complete clearing of cutaneous lesions may take more than a month of therapy. Topically applied tolnaftate has a low incidence of toxicity.

Clioquinol. Clioquinol has antifungal and antibacterial properties. Its antifungal properties have been used to treat athlete's foot, jock itch, ringworm, and moniliasis. Clioquinol may cause transient stinging or pruritus as well as allergic contact dermatitis. If these symptoms persist, discontinuation of the product is recommended. Several prescription product forms (lotion, cream, and ointment) contain a combination of clioquinol and hydrocortisone. This product should not be used in children under 2 years of age or for diaper rash.

Patient Counseling

For viral and fungal infections, regular applications of medications throughout a complete course of therapy are important. Proper application technique should be described to the patient. If irritation occurs, the patient should be instructed to contact a physician. The pharmacist may also provide information that will help control or eradicate the infection and minimize the likelihood of recurrent infections. Such information should address proper care of the skin site, appropriate laundry techniques and products, minimal use of occlusive clothing, and avoidance of behavior that leads to recurring infections.

If there is not substantial improvement in 1 week, the patient should be referred to a physician. Recurring skin infections may be a sign of undiagnosed diabetes, immuno-deficiency, or other organic problems and should be referred to a physician.

Skin Hyperpigmentation

Although hyperpigmentation products serve a cosmetic function, they are drugs and have potential toxicity and side effects.

Assessment

Several types of hyperpigmentation, including freckles, melasma, and lentigines, are amenable to self-treatment. The pharmacist must inquire about concurrent drug therapy and systemic illnesses before recommending a nonprescription product. Diffuse pigmentation disorders and those caused by systemic factors should not be self-treated without prior evaluation by a physician. Similarly, patients with lesions that are changing in size, shape or color should be referred to a physician.

Treatment

Before selecting a nonprescription skin-bleaching product, the pharmacist should be sure that a physician has confirmed the patient's need for it. These products are intended to lighten only limited areas of hyperpigmented skin and should be used only in areas of brownish discoloration. Nevi (moles) and reddish or bluish areas, such as port wine discolorations, are not amenable to skin-bleaching treatment. These products should not be used on areas that are independently changing in size, shape, or color.

Freckles, melasma, and lentigines may be diminished by topical nonprescription skin-bleaching agents. Such products are directed at inhibiting melanin production. To avoid negating the effects of treatment, the pharmacist must emphasize the importance of avoiding even minimal exposure to sunlight and of using sunscreen agents as well as protective clothing on an indefinite basis, even after discontinuing the product. Systemic, physician-directed therapy is required for widespread pigmentation disorders.

Pharmacologic Agents for Hyperpigmentation

The FDA has recommended that only hydroquinone (*p*-dihydroxybenzene) in concen-trations of 1.5%–2.0% be available for nonprescription use.

The effectiveness of hydroquinone varies among patients, and treatment must usually be maintained faithfully on a prolonged basis to maintain the desired level of lightening. Results are best on lighter skin and lighter lesions.

Hydroquinone tends to overshoot the intended degree of hypopigmentation and may produce treated areas that are lighter than the surrounding normal skin color. Therefore, the patient must carefully observe the degree of lightening and decrease applications when sufficient lightening has occurred.

When treatment is begun, melanin production may increase briefly. A decrease in skin color usually becomes noticeable in about 4 weeks; however, the time of onset varies from 3 weeks to 3 months. Hypopigmentation lasts for 2–6 months but is reversible. Although sunscreens may help, even visible light may cause some darkening, and sun protection should preferably be opaque.

The appearance of mild inflammation need not be considered an indication to stop therapy except in the patient whose reaction increases in intensity. Topical hydrocortisone may be used to alleviate the inflammatory reaction.

Hydroquinone ingestion seldom produces serious systemic toxicity.

Reversible brown discoloration of nails has been reported following the application of 2% hydroquinone to the back of the hand. Discoloration of the cream is an indication of product deterioration.

Hydroquinone is dosed as a thin topical application of a 2% concentration rubbed gently but well into affected areas twice daily. Hydroquinone may be applied to a small area of unbroken skin and should be assessed at 24 hours to observe for irritation or allergic reactions. It should not be applied near the eyes or to damaged or sunburned skin. If no improvement is seen within 3 months, its use should be discontinued and the advice of a physician sought. Once the desired benefit is achieved, hydroquinone can be applied as often as needed in a once- or twice-daily regimen. Hydroquinone is not recommended for children under age 12 except under the supervision of a physician.

Hair Loss (Alopecia)

Hereditary hair loss (androgenetic alopecia) is the most common form of hair loss. In hereditary hair loss, the rate of progression and the pattern of hair loss appear to be genetically determined.

Nonhereditary hair loss can occur following a pregnancy or be induced by certain drugs or severe nutritional deficiencies. Iatrogenic causes of hair loss include chemotherapy and discontinuation of hormonal agents. Other pathophysiologic causes include autoimmune disorders, endocrine disorders such as hypothyroidism, and certain diseases that cause scarring of the scalp.

Treatment of Hair Loss

Topical minoxidil 2%, as a hydroalcoholic solution, is the only nonprescription agent currently approved by the FDA for use in regrowth of hair. Only hereditary hair loss in men and women is amenable to topical minoxidil treatment; this agent is not indicated for use in children.

In men, minoxidil is more likely to be effective when less than one fourth of the scalp surface has already experienced hair loss or thinning. Even with continued treatment, all of the hair usually does not grow back; however, progressive loss of hair is usually slowed.

Study data for males 18–49 years of age indicate that about one fourth of the patients experienced moderate or better hair regrowth after using topical minoxidil. One tenth of men receiving placebo experienced similar growth. In women, topical minoxidil is more effective if less than one third of the scalp is thinning. In studies, about one fifth of the women experienced moderate regrowth after using topical minoxidil. In the placebo group, 7% achieved a similar regrowth rate.

The most common side effect is local itching. Systemic side effects are rare. Scalp psoriasis, severe sunburn, or scalp abrasions may increase absorption of minoxidil. Additional precaution should be taken if corticosteroids or any agents known to increase cutaneous absorption of a drug are used concurrently with this product. Unstable cardiac patients should not use the product unless supervised by a physician.

Patient Counseling

Patients should be advised that most treatment regimens for hair loss do not alter its progression, especially if the hair loss has gone on for some time. With nonprescription minoxidil, beginning treatment early after the onset of thinning optimizes the therapeutic response and stops the progressing hair loss. The pharmacist should also emphasize that treatment must be continuous and indefinite to maintain regrowth.

Patients should be advised to apply 1 mL of the solution to the scalp twice daily, being careful not to allow the solution to come in contact with the eyes or mucous membranes. Such contact might result in burning or itching of these areas. After application of the solution, the scalp should be kept dry for 4 hours. Hair grooming and styling products (e.g., sprays, mousses, and gels) or permanents, coloring agents, or relaxing agents usually do not affect the efficacy of topical minoxidil and can be applied after the medication has dried.

The pharmacist should advise patients that it usually takes up to 12 months to assess whether an optimal response is being achieved. Patients should be cautioned that overuse will not achieve better regrowth or a more rapid response. They should also be cautioned to keep product containers out of the reach of children, because acute ingestion of minoxidil is hazardous.

CHAPTER 27

Acne Products

Questions to ask in patient assessment and counseling

- *How old are you?*
- *How long have you had acne?*
- *Is the acne a problem on areas other than your face (e.g., neck, shoulders, chest, back)?*
- *Have you consulted a physician about your acne? If so, what treatment was suggested? Are you following it?*
- *Are you using any prescription or nonprescription medications? If so, what are they?*
- *Have you already tried acne treatments? If so, which ones? How did you use them? How long did you use them? Were they effective?*
- *Do you prefer one type of acne treatment product (e.g., lotion, cream, gel, soap) over another?*
- *What type of cosmetics, including makeup, aftershave, or hair preparations, do you use? Do they seem to aggravate the acne?*
- *How often do you wash your face? How do you wash (e.g., with pads or washcloths)? What type of soap do you use?*
- *How often do you shampoo your hair? What type of shampoo do you use?*
- *Do you notice a seasonal change in the number or severity of acne lesions?*
- *Are you routinely exposed to environmental conditions such as heat or humidity or cooking oils in the air?*

Acne vulgaris, the most common adolescent skin disorder, is often linked to the onset of puberty. Approximately 85% of all people between the ages of 12 and 25 years will develop it to some degree. Although acne is not a physical threat, it may have a significant negative psychosocial impact on an adolescent.

Predisposing Factors

Many women with acne experience a premenstrual flare-up of symptoms. Hormonal changes associated with ovulation and pregnancy are also related to flare-ups. Oral contraceptives containing androgenic progestins with higher androgenic activity have been implicated, as have certain cyclic progestins used in menopausal hormone replacement therapy. Severe or prolonged stress or other emotional extremes may exacerbate the condition.

Hydration decreases the size of the pilosebaceous duct orifice, which explains why acne is exacerbated in conditions of high humidity or in situations that induce frequent and prolonged sweating. Local irritation may increase the incidence and severity of acne symptoms. Rough or occlusive clothing, headgear straps, athletic equipment, and other friction-producing devices can aggravate acne.

Editor's Note: This chapter is adapted from Joye Ann Billow, "Acne Products," in Covington, T.R., ed., *Handbook of Nonprescription Drugs*, 11th edition. For a more extensive discussion of the etiology, pathophysiology, and classification of acne, as well as information on treatment and patient counseling, readers are encouraged to consult Chapter 27 of the *Handbook*.

Acne cosmetica is a low-grade, mild form of acne on the face, cheek, and chin. It is more common in women than in men because women are more likely to use cosmetics. Oil-based cosmetics may be occlusive and plug the follicles, thus exacerbating or initiating acne. Pomade acne, most often seen in African Americans and manifested by comedones along the hairline on the forehead and temples, is reported to be caused by the long-term use of occlusive hair dressings.

Drugs can exacerbate acne. Corticosteroids may induce hypertrophic changes by sensitizing the follicle and producing "steroid acne." Other systemic drugs known to precipitate acne eruptions include androgens, iodides, bromides, ethionamide, azathioprine, dantrolene, haloperidol, halothane, isoniazid, lithium, phenytoin, thyroid preparations, and trimethadione.

Occupational exposure to dirt or certain industrial chemicals and vaporized oils may cause occupational acne.

There is little evidence to support a direct relationship between diet and acne. The practical approach is for patients to avoid any particular food that seems to exacerbate their acne.

Heredity may predispose a person to acne.

Treatment

Acne is rarely cured, but its symptoms can be controlled to varying degrees. The objectives of treatment should include the following:

- Ensuring patient compliance;
- Relieving physical and social discomfort;
- Removing excess sebum from the skin with proper cleansing;
- Preventing closure of the pilosebaceous orifice;
- Using irritants to unblock ducts;
- Reducing lipase activity;
- Minimizing conditions conducive to the development of acne (e.g., physical irritants, oil-based cleansers and cosmetics); and
- Educating the individual in the need for patience with the treatment regimen and how to follow it properly.

Self-Treatment versus Referral

Self-treatment should be limited to patients with noninflammatory acne of mild to moderate severity that is limited to observed whiteheads and blackheads. It is most appropriate if lesions are not extensive (i.e., fewer than 10 on one side of the face). Self-treatment is most effective in patients who are mature enough to understand that treatment will be long-term and that symptoms can be controlled but not cured.

Depending on the answers provided to the questions that introduce this chapter, the pharmacist may find the following pointers useful:

- If acne lesions are present where clothes, headbands, helmets, or other devices cause friction, preventing friction-induced irritation should be discussed.
- If oil-based cosmetic products are used, water-based products should be considered. If the hair is oily, frequent shampooing with a water-based shampoo is advisable.
- If face washing is frequent or a drying soap is used, gentle washing two to three times daily with a mild facial soap and soft washcloth is recommended. Medicated soaps are of equivocal value. Mild abrasive soaps help treat noninflammatory acne.

- If exposure to environmental factors (e.g., dirt, dust, oil, chemical irritants) seems to exacerbate the acne, the patient should be counseled on how to minimize or avoid these exposures.
- The patient should be advised never to squeeze, pinch, or pick at acne lesions.

Patients with inflammatory acne consisting of extensive papules, pustules, and nodules should be referred to a physician, preferably a dermatologist. If the acne is thought to be associated with the use of a drug with comedogenic (e.g., androgenic) activity, a physician should be contacted. If lesions persist beyond the mid-20s or develop in the mid-20s or later, they may signal rosacea rather than acne vulgaris.

Nondrug Measures

Appropriate nondrug measure include removal of excess sebum by washing the face at least twice daily with warm water and a medicated or unmedicated soap. No conclusive data support the use of antibacterial agents. Abrasives may be helpful for patients with inflammatory acne.

Pharmacologic Agents

The active topical antiacne ingredients recognized as safe and effective (Category I) by the Food and Drug Administration (FDA) include 0.5%–2% salicylic acid, 3%–8% sulfur, and a combination of 3%–8% sulfur with either 2% resorcinol or 3% resorcinol monoacetate. Benzoyl peroxide has been temporarily reclassified to Category III (current data are insufficient to classify it as safe as well as effective). The product remains on the market as an effective product, but a proposed FDA rule will require additional warning statements and directions on the label.

Salicylic Acid

Salicylic acid acts as a surface keratolytic. The use of salicylic acid in cleansing preparations is considered adjunctive acne treatment in reducing comedonal lesions and improving the overall condition. Its safety is questionable when used over large areas for prolonged periods.

Sulfur

Sulfur has met FDA criteria for nonprescription topical acne products, although the claim for its antibacterial effects was disallowed. In a precipitated or colloidal form, sulfur is included in acne products as a keratolytic in concentrations of 3%–10%. Sulfur is generally accepted as an effective agent for promoting the resolution of existing comedones, but continued use may have a comedogenic effect.

Sulfur-containing products are applied in a thin film to the affected area once or twice daily. They have a noticeable color and odor, characteristics that must be considered when they are being recommended. Compliance may be enhanced by recommending fleshtone products or suggesting use after school and at bedtime.

Sulfur Combined with Resorcinol or Resorcinol Monoacetate

The FDA includes the combination of 3%–8% sulfur with 2% resorcinol or 3% resorcinol monoacetate as safe and effective active ingredients for nonprescription acne products. The agents function primarily as keratolytics.

Sulfur–resorcinol products have the characteristic color and odor noted for the sulfur products. Resorcinol may produce a dark brown scale on some darker-skinned individuals, who should be forewarned and reassured that the reaction is reversible when the medication is discontinued.

Benzoyl Peroxide

Benzoyl peroxide is one of the most effective and widely used topical nonprescription medications available for treating acne.

At the instigation of the FDA, however, additional studies of the safety of benzoyl peroxide are under way. The reason for the reevaluation is the FDA's concern about the product's tumor-initiating and -promotion potential.

Benzoyl peroxide is available most commonly in concentrations of 2.5%, 5%, and 10% in such diverse dosage forms as lotions, gels, creams, cleansers, masks, and soaps. Clinical response to all concentrations is similar in terms of reducing the number of inflammatory lesions. However, the different formulations are not equivalent. The drying effect of the alcohol gel base enhances benzoyl peroxide's effectiveness; therefore, this form is superior to a lotion of the same concentration. Washes and cleansers containing benzoyl peroxide have been found to have little or no comedolytic effect.

Instructions for the proper use of topical nonprescription benzoyl peroxide products include the following:

- The affected area or area likely to be affected should be gently cleansed with a nonmedicated soap and patted dry, and a small quantity of the preparation should be smoothed over the area once or twice daily.

- Initial applications may be limited to one or two small areas at the 2.5% or 5% concentration.

- The initial application should be left on the skin for 15 minutes and washed off. The time benzoyl peroxide is left on the skin should then be increased in 15-minute increments as tolerance allows. Once it is tolerated for 2 hours, it can be left on the skin overnight. A morning dose may be applied if tolerated.

- Fair-skinned individuals should initiate therapy with the 2.5%, 4%, or 5% strength and apply it only once daily during the first few weeks of therapy.

- Benzoyl peroxide should be used with great care near the eyes, mouth, lips, and nose, as well as near cuts, scrapes, and other abrasions.

- The drug should not be used concurrently with other topical products unless recommended by a physician or pharmacist.

- The drug should be used externally only.

- Excessive dryness, marked peeling, some skin sloughing, erythema, or edema suggests that lower concentrations should be used for shorter periods of time. Cool compresses may relieve the discomfort of inflamed skin.

- The drug may bleach hair and clothing.

- The drug may cause transient stinging and burning. This is not a cause for alarm unless it persists or worsens.

- If excessive stinging and burning occur after application, the preparation should be removed with soap and water and not reapplied until the next day.

- Other sources of irritation, such as sunlamps and excessive exposure to the sun, should be avoided.

- The full therapeutic effect may not be experienced for 4–6 weeks.

Other Combination Products

Assorted nonprescription combinations of benzoyl peroxide, sulfur, salicylic acid, and resorcinol have been used to treat acne. The efficacy of these combination products over the single-ingredient products has not been demonstrated.

Other Treatments

Sunlight and artificial ultraviolet radiation are largely ineffective and not recommended. Sunlight can aggravate acne.

Formulation Considerations

The formulation that carries topical acne medication to the skin can influence the drug's effectiveness.

Cleansing bars, liquids, suspensions, lotions, creams, and gels are the vehicles generally used for antiacne preparations. Cleansing products alone are of little value since they leave little residue of active ingredient on the skin. Lotions and creams should have a low fat content so that they do not counteract drying and peeling. They are an acceptable alternative to the more effective gels, and are recommended for dry or sensitive skin and for use during dry winter weather. In general, gels are the most effective formulations because they are astringents and remain on the skin the longest. In general, cream formulations should be recommended for individuals with fair complexions and gels for those with dark complexions. The drying effect of volatile solvents such as ethyl and isopropyl alcohol may enhance the effectiveness of the various preparations, but the solvents' greater irritant effect may be unacceptable.

The solids in most preparations leave an invisible film that does not need coloring to blend in with the skin. However, some products are intended to hide blemishes by depositing an opaque film on the skin. These products rarely produce a satisfactory color match.

Patient Counseling

The patient's responses to the questions at the beginning of this chapter will provide essential information to aid the pharmacist in counseling. On the basis of these responses, the pharmacist should decide whether the condition merits self-treatment or physician referral.

Before recommending self-treatment, the pharmacist should evaluate the patient's attitude toward treatment and willingness to comply with a skin care program. The pharmacist should explain acne as a medical condition, describe the treatment, and correct any misconceptions the patient might have. The patient should be advised about scalp and hair care; use of cosmetics; and, above all, the need for long-term, conscientious care. The patient should also be advised of the following points when appropriate:

■ A proper diet is important in maintaining health, but many of the myths about diet and acne are unfounded.

■ Stressful situations may play a role in acne flare-ups but do not cause acne.

■ Sexual activity neither causes nor exacerbates acne.

Because acne cannot be cured but only controlled, reassurance and emotional support are often necessary.

CHAPTER 28

First-Aid Products and Minor Wound Care

Questions to ask in patient assessment and counseling

- *What type of wound is present? Is the wound acute (an abrasion, puncture, or laceration) or chronic (a pressure ulcer, arterial ulcer, or venous ulcer)?*
- *Where is the wound? How extensive is the area involved?*
- *Are foreign objects or dead tissue present at the wound site?*
- *What color is the wound bed? What is the condition of the wound margins and the surrounding skin?*
- *Is there redness, warmth, swelling, and/or pain in the affected area?*
- *Is pus present? If so, what color is it? Does it have an odor?*
- *Do you have a fever or any flulike symptoms?*
- *Do you have diabetes or any other medical conditions?*
- *Are you taking any medications?*
- *What measures or medications have you used to self-treat the wound? Were they effective?*
- *Do you have any allergies to topical medications? Do you have any other allergies?*

Factors Affecting Wound Healing

Several factors affect how efficiently and to what extent a wound will heal. They include tissue perfusion and oxygenation at the site of the wound; the patient's nutritional status, age, and weight; the presence or absence of local infection; coexisting diabetes mellitus; certain medications (topical and systemic corticosteroids, antineoplastic drugs and radiation therapy, and immunosuppressive agents and anticoagulants can interfere with healing); and wound characteristics.

Wound Classification and Type

Wounds can be classified according to their acuity and depth. Classification is essential in determining appropriate wound management.

Acute Wounds

Acute wounds include abrasions, punctures, lacerations, and burns. Burns are discussed in Chapter 31.

Editor's Note: This chapter is adapted from Edwina Chan and Raymond Benza, "First-Aid Products and Minor Wound Care," in Covington, T.R., ed., *Handbook of Nonprescription Drugs*, 11th edition, which is based, in part, on portions of two 10th edition chapters: "Topical Anti-Infective Products," written by Dennis P. West and Susan V. Maddux, and "Ostomy and Wound Care Products," written by Michael L. Kleinberg and Moya J. Vazquez. For a more extensive discussion of skin anatomy; wound healing, classification, and management; and superficial wound infections, readers are encouraged to consult Chapter 28 of the *Handbook*.

Abrasions

Abrasions usually result from a rubbing or friction injury to the epidermis and extend to the uppermost portion of the dermis. They should be cleansed with soap and water and covered with a sterile, semipermeable, nonadhering dressing.

Punctures

Punctures usually result from a sharp object that has pierced the epidermis and lodged in the dermis or deeper tissues. A physician should inspect these wounds to ensure that no foreign bodies are retained and to update tetanus prophylaxis, if necessary. The wounds should then be cleansed with water or sterile saline. They should be left open, elevated, and soaked daily with soapy water.

Lacerations

Lacerations result from sharp objects cutting through the skin. They should be inspected by a physician, debrided, and flushed. Tetanus prophylaxis is important. If these wounds are clean, they can be sutured. If they are grossly contaminated by foreign particles or inorganic matter or if they show evidence of early infection, they should be left open and covered with a sterile, nonadhering, semipermeable dressing.

Chronic Wounds

Pressure Ulcers

Pressure ulcers (decubitus ulcers) which are commonly encountered in bedbound or immobile patients, are initiated by pressure, shear, and friction. Common areas of involvement include the bony prominences, especially the sacrum, trochanters, heels, and elbows.

Pharmacists should counsel patients that decubiti should be closely supervised by individuals trained to treat these particular wounds.

Arterial and Venous Ulcers

Arterial ulcers are usually secondary to severe peripheral vascular occlusive disease. Venous ulcers are secondary to incompetent venous valves.

Wound Depth

Wound depth is classified into four stages on the basis of the extent or number of skin layers damaged. Stage I does not involve loss of any skin layers and consists primarily of reddened, unbroken skin. Stage II includes the development of a blister or partial-thickness skin loss involving all the epidermis and part of the dermis. Stage III, full-thickness skin loss, includes damage to the entire epidermis, dermis, and dermal appendages. Stage IV is an extension of stage III that involves the subcutaneous tissue and underlying muscle, tendon, and bone. Understanding these stages helps in the selection of appropriate dressings for wound closure (Figure 1).

Wound Management

Management depends on wound type, depth, location, and degree of contamination; the presence of comorbid conditions; and preexisting medical therapy. The goals of wound management include cleansing of the wound, selective use of antiseptics and antibiotics, and closure with an appropriate dressing.

Uncontaminated wounds require only basic supportive measures, including the use of mild soap and water for proper cleansing. To help prevent superficial skin infection in minor

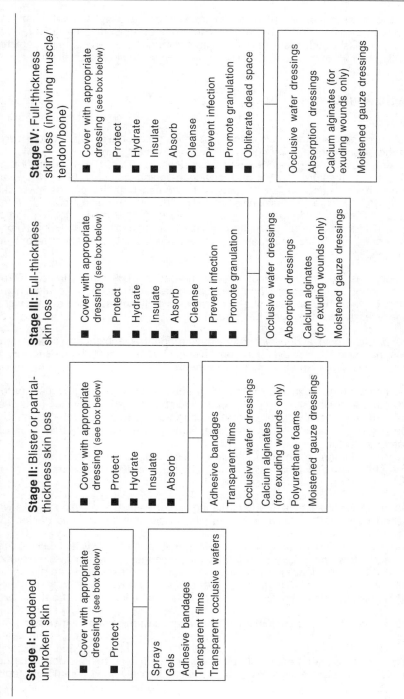

FIGURE 1 Guidelines for product selection based on wound severity. Adapted with permission from Jeter KF, Tintle TE. Wound dressings of the nineties: indications and contraindications. *Clin Podiatr Med Surg.* 1991; 8(4): 805.

cuts, scrapes, and burns, topical nonprescription antibiotic and antiseptic preparations can be useful; however, they should be viewed as extensions of supportive treatment. More serious or deeper tissue infection (e.g., puncture wounds, severe burns) requires consultation with a physician, who can assess the need for systemic or topical prescription antibiotics.

Pharmacologic Agents

First-Aid Antiseptics

The current recommendation is to avoid using antiseptics on open wounds and to reserve them for what they were originally intended: disinfection of intact skin.

Five ingredients—alcohol (60%–95%), isopropyl alcohol (50%–91.3%), iodine topical solution (USP), iodine tincture (USP), and povidone–iodine complex (5%–10%)—are recognized as safe and effective (i.e., Category I) for use both as preoperative skin preparations by health care professionals and as first-aid products. Two of these ingredients, alcohol and povidone–iodine, are considered safe and effective for all antiseptic uses. Other agents (e.g., hydrogen peroxide, phenolic compounds, hexyl-resorcinol, quaternary ammonium compounds) are considered safe and effective only for use as first-aid products.

Alcohol. Alcohol has good bactericidal activity in a 20%–70% concentration. Direct application of alcohol to the wound bed can cause tissue irritation. It is also highly flammable. Alcohol wash may be used one to three times daily and may be covered with a sterile bandage after the washed area has dried.

Isopropyl Alcohol. Isopropyl alcohol has somewhat stronger bactericidal activity and lower surface tension than alcohol. However, isopropyl alcohol has a greater potential for drying the skin (astringent action). Like alcohol, it is flammable.

Iodine. Iodine has a broad antimicrobial spectrum against bacteria, fungi, virus, spores, protozoa, and yeast. An iodine solution (USP) of 2% iodine and 2.5% sodium iodide is used as an antiseptic for superficial wounds. Iodine tincture (USP), which contains alcohol, is irritating to the tissue and therefore less desirable. Strong iodine solution (Lugol's) should not be used as an antiseptic.

To avoid tissue irritation, bandaging should be discouraged after iodine application. Iodine solutions stain skin, may irritate tissue, and may cause allergic sensitization in some people.

Povidone–Iodine. Povidone–iodine is a nonirritating, water-soluble complex of iodine with povidone. It contains 9%–12% available iodine, which accounts for its rapid bactericidal activity.

When used as a wound irrigant, povidone–iodine is absorbed systemically. When severe burns and large wounds are treated with povidone–iodine, iodine absorption through the skin and mucous membranes can result in excess systemic iodine concentrations. If renal function is normal, the absorbed iodine is rapidly excreted. Nonetheless, povidone–iodine should be used with discretion when treating large wounds.

Detergents formed by the combination of surfactants with povidone–iodine are not recommended.

Hydrogen Peroxide. Hydrogen peroxide (topical solution, USP), an antimicrobial oxidizing agent (along with sodium and zinc peroxides), is the most widely used first-aid antiseptic.

The duration of action is only as long as the period of active oxygen release. Using hydrogen peroxide on intact skin is of minimal value.

Hydrogen peroxide should be used where released gas can escape. For this reason, it should not be used in abscesses, and bandages should not be applied before the compound dries.

Phenolic Compounds. In very dilute solutions, phenol is an antiseptic and a disinfectant. It has local anesthetic activity and is claimed to be an antipruritic in concentrations of 1:100–1:200 (e.g., phenolated calamine lotion). In aqueous solutions of more than 1%, it is a primary irritant and should not be used on the skin except as a keratolytic agent.

Camphorated Phenol. Oily solutions of phenol and camphor contain relatively high concentrations of phenol (4%) and must be used with caution. To avoid damaging effects, these products should be applied only to dry skin.

Hexylresorcinol. As an antibacterial agent, hexylresorcinol (0.1%) is more effective and less toxic than phenol; however, it may be irritating.

Quaternary Ammonium Compounds. Quaternary ammonium compounds (benzalkonium chloride, benzethonium chloride, and methylbenzethonium chloride) are sometimes included in topical anti-infective products. In addition to their antiseptic properties, these agents are used for their cleansing properties.

These compounds are formulated as creams, dusting powders, and aqueous or alcoholic solutions. Used undiluted, these preparations may cause serious skin irritation. Quaternary compounds are irritating to the eyes, so caution must be used when applying them to skin near the eyes. For use on broken or diseased skin, concentrations of 1:5000–1:20,000 may be used. For use on intact skin and minor abrasions, a concentration of 1:750 is recommended.

First-Aid Antibiotics

When applied to dirty, contaminated wounds up to 4 hours after insult, topical antibiotic combinations have been demonstrated to reduce the likelihood of wound infection.

Topical antibiotic preparations should be applied to the infected wound bed after cleansing and before application of a sterile dressing. Caution should be taken when applying these preparations to large areas of denuded skin, because the potential for systemic toxicity can increase. Prolonged use may result in secondary fungal infection. If the wound does not heal within 5 days, the patient should consult a physician.

Six ingredients are considered to be generally safe and effective for use: bacitracin, neomycin, polymyxin B sulfate, tetracycline hydrochloride, chlortetracycline hydrochloride, and combination products containing oxytetracycline hydrochloride.

Bacitracin. Bacitracin inhibits cell wall synthesis in several gram-positive organisms. The development of resistance in previously sensitive organisms is rare. Minimal absorption occurs with topical administration. The frequency of allergic contact dermatitis is approximately 2%. Topical nonprescription preparations are applied one to three times a day.

Neomycin. Neomycin irreversibly binds to the 30S ribosomal subunit to inhibit protein synthesis in gram-negative organisms and some species of *Staphylococcus.* Applied topically, neomycin produces a relatively high rate of hypersensitivity (3.5%–6%). Resistant organisms may develop.

Because neomycin is a relatively common cause of allergic contact dermatitis and is not essential to topical antibacterial coverage of skin infections, it is rarely recommended. The combination of bacitracin and polymyxin B sulfate is more widely accepted than the combination of bacitracin, polymyxin B sulfate, and neomycin.

The concentration of neomycin commonly used in nonprescription products is 3.5 mg/g. Applications are made one to three times a day.

Polymyxin B Sulfate. Polymyxin B sulfate is effective against several gram-negative organisms. It is a rare sensitizer. Concentrations of 5000 U/g and 10,000 U/g are available in nonprescription combination preparations. Applications are usually made one to three times a day.

Tetracyclines. The tetracyclines have activity against gram-positive and most gram-negative bacteria, with the exception of *Proteus* and *Pseudomonas* species. Because of the high incidence of bacterial resistance, topical tetracycline and chlortetracycline are often ineffective for the treatment of primary bacterial infection. Toxicity is rare when applied topically; however, a hypersensitivity reaction may be triggered in allergic patients. If redness, irritation, swelling, or pain persists or increases in the applied area, tetracycline should be discontinued. Tetracycline products oxidize in the presence of light and may turn the skin a reversible yellow-brown color and may stain clothing.

Currently, 3% ointments of tetracycline and chlortetracycline are available as nonprescription agents, while oxytetracycline is available only in combination with polymyxin B. These products are usually applied one to three times daily and may be covered afterward with a sterile bandage.

Antimicrobial Selection Guidelines

Before recommending a topical product for self-medication of cutaneous infections, the pharmacist should assess the nature of the patient's complaint. Noninfectious processes, including drug-induced eruptions, should be considered. Antimicrobial agents should generally be recommended in cases of infectious etiology and where secondary infection may occur.

Referral to a physician should be considered if:

▪ There is doubt as to the causative factor or organism.

▪ Initial treatment has not been successful or the condition is worsening.

▪ Topical drug products have been applied for prolonged periods over large areas, especially on denuded skin (creating the potential for systemic toxicity).

▪ Exudate is excessive and continuous.

▪ Widespread infection has occurred.

▪ The patient has a predisposing illness, such as diabetes, systemic infection, or an immune deficiency.

▪ Fever, malaise, or both occur.

▪ A primary dermatitis (allergic dermatitis, psoriasis, or seborrhea) exists and becomes secondarily infected.

▪ Lesions are deep and extensive.

▪ Lancing is needed to aid drainage of exudate or relieve pain.

Wound Dressings

The goal of new wound treatment strategies is to create a moist environment that prevents eschar development, removes excess exudate without dehydration, and prevents bacterial invasion of the wound. This approach makes use of semipermeable dressings that promote optimal moisture, exudate removal, and gas exchange. This technique has been shown to accelerate healing and prevent scarring, reduce pain, and promote epithelialization and healing of chronic wounds.

Superficial abrasions and lacerations may simply require the application of adhesive bandages. Pharmacists should consider the various features of these bandages (e.g., contour, size, padding, allergenicity, impregnation with medication) in their recommendations for patients. More extensive wounds require referral to a physician or a wound care specialist.

Treatment of Acute Wounds

After performing an initial assessment of an acute wound (Figure 2), the pharmacist should counsel patients to:

- Position the wound above the level of the heart to slow bleeding and relieve throbbing pain.
- If it is dirty, clean the wound with mild soap and water or a mild wound cleanser.
- Cover the wound with a dressing that will keep the wound site moist and is an appropriate size and shape.
- Avoid disrupting the dressing unnecessarily; change it only if it is dirty or not intact.
- Use a mild analgesic to control pain.
- Observe the wound for signs of infection. (Redness, swelling, and exudate are a normal part of healing; foul odor is not.)
- Consult a physician if infection is suspected.
- Consult a physician if the wound occurred in dirty conditions and the patient's tetanus immunization status is uncertain.

Treatment of Chronic Wounds

Patients who have chronic wounds should be advised to seek medical advice. These patients should also:

- Consult a physician about any slow-healing wound;
- Prevent pressure ulcers by repositioning the body regularly and often and using pressure-relieving devices; and
- Watch for early signs of skin redness over bony prominences. Prompt intervention can prevent skin breakdown.

Superficial Skin Infections

Bacterial skin infection may occur secondary to a contaminated wound or as a primary infection. Pyoderma is a broad term that refers to cutaneous bacterial infection characterized by crusted, oozing lesions with variable amounts of purulence and tenderness. If the infection is deep or extensive, systemic toxicity may occur; manifestations include an elevation in temperature and leukocytosis. Pyodermic infection may be primary (no previous dermatoses) or secondary (a predisposing problem preceded the infection).

The risk of skin infection may be increased by a break in the intact skin surface, excessive scrubbing and irritation of the skin, excessive exposure to water, prolonged occlusion, excessively elevated skin temperature, or local injury.

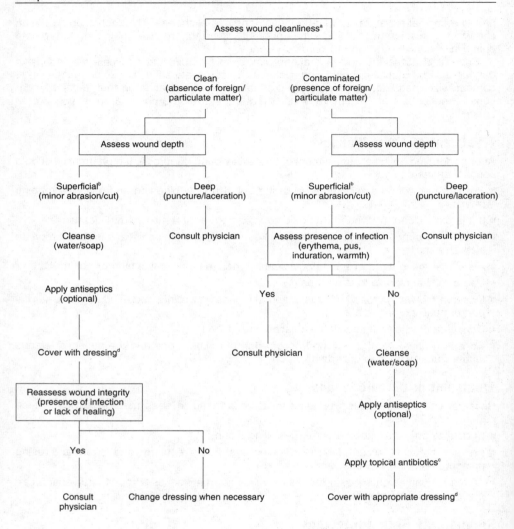

FIGURE 2 Initial assessment of acute wounds.

aEnsure that patient's tetanus immunization is up-to-date.

bConsider physician referral if affected area involves the face, mucous membrane, or genitalia or if patient has comorbid conditions.

cIf healing does not occur within 5 days, consult physician.

dRefer to Figure 1.

Types of Infection

The main pyodermic infections are impetigo, ecthyma, erysipeloid, folliculitis, furuncles and carbuncles, and erythrasma.

Impetigo (Primary)

Impetigo is a very superficial infection of the skin that is most common in preschool children and young adults. Direct contact with the infected exudate may result in transmission of the organisms. Lesions first appear as small red spots that may evolve into vesicles filled with amber fluid. Exudate accumulates and forms yellow or brown scabs that are often surrounded by erythematous skin. Lesions last for days, accompanied by variable pruritus. Satellite lesions occur by autoinoculation. The face, arms, legs, and buttocks are commonly affected.

Ecythma (Ulcerative Impetigo)

Ecythma is a lesion of neglect that develops in excoriations, insect bites, elderly patients who have sustained minor trauma, soldiers, sewage workers, alcoholics, and homeless people. The lesion usually begins as an erythematous pustule that rapidly erodes and becomes crusted. The lesions extend much deeper than those of impetigo. They commonly appear on the ankles, dorsa of feet, thighs, and buttocks. Lesions are pruritic and tender; they last for weeks and often heal with a scar.

Erysipeloid

Erysipeloid ("crab dermatitis") is an acute but slowly evolving cellulitis occurring at sites of inoculation, most commonly the hands. It is associated with handling fish, meat, poultry, hides, and bones. Infection follows an abrasion, scratch, or puncture wound while organic material containing *Erysipelothrix rhusiopathiae* is being handled. The incubation period is 1–4 days. The lesion is slightly tender and warm. Skin symptoms include itching, throbbing, and pain. Erysipeloid subsides in about 3 weeks. Should bacteremia develop, endocarditis or septic arthritis may be rare complications.

Folliculitis

Folliculitis is a superficial, often bacterial inflammation of hair follicles. Skin areas regularly exposed to tar, grease, mineral oil, adhesive plaster, and plastic occlusive dressings are most susceptible. The erythematous lesions, which appear dirty yellow or gray, last for days. Affected areas are nontender or slightly tender and pruritic.

Furuncles and Carbuncles

A furuncle is an acute, deep-seated, tender, erythematous, inflammatory nodule that evolves from a staphylococcal folliculitis. A carbuncle is a conglomerate of multiple coalescing furuncles. Children, adolescents, and young adults are frequently affected, and there is an increased incidence in boys. Chronic cases should be referred to a physician.

The fully established furuncle is bright red, indurated, and erythematous. These lesions commonly last for days, with associated skin symptoms of throbbing pain and exquisite tenderness. Constitutional symptoms include low-grade fever and malaise. Furunculosis may sometimes be complicated by bacteremia.

Erythrasma

Erythrasma is a chronic bacterial infection that affects the intertriginous areas of the toes, groin, and axillae. Adults are generally affected, with a higher incidence in obese, middle-aged blacks. Predisposing factors include diabetes and a warm, humid climate. The lesions are sharply marginated, brownish-red, and scaly. Eruptions may last for months to years. Irritation may be the only skin symptom.

Treatment of Skin Infections

For primary impetigo, a topical prescription antibiotic such as mupirocin is preferred. Topical nonprescription antibiotic preparations with neomycin, bacitracin, and polymyxin B sulfate seem to be most effective when lesions are superficial and are not extensive. Cleaning the area with mild soap and water and gently removing loose crusts should improve response to topical therapy. Because streptococcal infection can occur in other tissues (e.g., kidney, heart valve) concurrent with impetigo, most physicians treat impetigo infections with systemic as well as topical products.

For ecythma, folliculitis, and erysipeloid, a systemic antibiotic is usually indicated. The role of topical nonprescription antibiotics in these infections is limited, and their efficacy may be questionable. Furuncles and carbuncles may be resolved with incision, drainage, and systemic prescription antibiotics. Minor cases of erythrasma may respond to showers with povidone–iodine soap; however, systemic or topical prescription antibiotics are generally preferred.

CHAPTER 29

Diaper Rash, Prickly Heat, and Adult Incontinence Products

Questions to ask in patient assessment and counseling

Diaper Rash
- Do you use disposable diapers or a diaper service?
- Do you use cloth diapers? How do you launder them?
- Do you use double diapers or plastic pants?
- How often do you change the baby's diapers?
- How do you clean the baby's skin during a diaper change?
- What products have you tried for the rash?
- Does the baby have a fever?
- Has the baby had diarrhea recently?
- Has the baby ever had a yeast infection in the diaper area?
- Has any new type of food recently been added to the baby's diet?
- Is there a family history of allergic disorders?
- Is the baby being given any medication? If so, what product and by what route?

Prickly Heat
- Where is the rash? What does it look like?
- How long has the rash been present?
- Does the patient sleep in a warm, humid room?
- How much clothing does the patient wear during the day and night?
- What products have you tried for the rash?

Adult Urinary Incontinence
- Has the incontinence been evaluated by a physician?
- What type of urinary incontinence does the patient have?
- What time of the day is protection needed most? Least?
- Does the patient need assistance in changing or using absorbent materials?
- What products have been used to treat or prevent rash? Odor?

Editor's Note: This chapter is adapted from Gary H. Smith, Victor A. Elsberry, and Martin D. Higbee, "Diaper Rash, Prickly Heat, and Adult Incontinence Products," in Covington, T.R., ed., *Handbook of Nonprescription Drugs,* 11th edition, which is based, in part, on a chapter with a similar title that appeared in the 10th edition but was written by Gary H. Smith. For a more extensive discussion of these topics, readers are encouraged to consult Chapter 29 of the *Handbook.*

Diaper rash and prickly heat (miliaria rubra) are acute, transient, inflammatory skin conditions that occur in infants, children, and adults, especially those who are urine incontinent. Both conditions cause burning and itching that can result in restlessness, irritability, and sleep interruptions. Prevention is the best cure.

Although there are not many nonprescription products available for this medical problem, pharmacists nonetheless need to be familiar with this disease process to advise patients and caregivers appropriately.

Diaper Rash

The Food and Drug Administration (FDA) defines diaper rash as an inflammatory skin condition in the diaper area caused by moisture, occlusion, chafing, continued contact with urine or feces or both, or mechanical or chemical irritation.

Complications

Fungal and bacterial infections are the most common complications of diaper rash.

Fungal Infection

Fungal infections should be considered in all cases of severe diaper dermatitis. Candida albicans produces a bright red, sharply marginated rash with satellite pustules and erosions. The only precise method of diagnosis is culturing the organism.

In newborns younger than 2 weeks, candidal diaper dermatitis is usually accompanied by oral thrush. The lesions are usually erythematous and are surrounded by satellite pustules. They may become eroded and begin weeping. A physician should be consulted for appropriate treatment.

The systemic use of some broad-spectrum antibiotics may predispose the infant to diaper candidiases. Infants with severe diaper dermatitis who are concurrently receiving a broad-spectrum antibiotic should be evaluated for candidiasis by a physician.

Bacterial Infection

Bacterial infection of the diaper area is caused most commonly by *Staphylococcus aureus*. Lesions are follicular micropustules that coalesce with adjacent lesions to form lakes or pustules. An infant with a suspected bacterial infection in the diaper area should be referred to a physician.

Viral Infection

Herpetiform diaper dermatitis should be considered when a parent of an infant has an active herpes simplex infection. Jacquet's diaper dermatitis is characterized by well-demarcated ulcers or erosions with elevated borders. Its frequency has decreased with the increased use of disposable diapers. Cytomegalovirus diaper rash has been reported in infants born with human immunodeficiency virus (HIV).

Other Diaper Dermatitides

Other conditions that may present as diaper dermatitis include granuloma gluteale infantum, Kawasaki syndrome, atopic dermatitis, infantile seborrheic dermatitis, acute histiocytosis X, psoriasis vulgaris, congenital syphilis, acrodermatitis enteropathica, and biotin deficiency.

Ulceration of the penile meatus may be a painful complication of diaper rash in babies who are circumcised.

Assessment

The pharmacist may be able to determine the cause of many conditions by asking the parent questions such as those at the beginning of this chapter. In general, if diaper dermatitis is confined to the diaper area and does not present symptoms of fungal or bacterial infection, the pharmacist may recommend a nonprescription protectant product and also explain how to prevent recurrence. If diaper rash persists 1 week or more after the infant has been treated with protectants and diapers have been changed frequently, if the rash recurs often or is resistant to nonprescription treatment, if the rash occurs on areas outside the diaper area (e.g., groin, intergluteal fold, lower abdomen), or if the infant has had persistent diarrhea, appears irritable, or has a fever, a physician should be consulted.

Treatment

Primary Treatment

The area should be kept as dry and clean as possible; the diaper should be loose and well ventilated, and should be changed as quickly as possible after becoming soiled; and the diaper area should be dried completely before a new diaper is used. Plain water should be used to cleanse the diaper area. Cornstarch is a safe and effective dusting powder. Careful use of a hair blow-dryer on a low setting to dry the area is effective and safer than a heat lamp. The use of a protective agent, such as zinc oxide paste (Lassar's paste), Desitin, or white petrolatum, provides a barrier to protect the skin from moisture. Plastic pants should be avoided.

Pharmacologic Agents

External analgesics and antifungals. In 1992, the FDA declared that diaper rash claims should be removed from all nonprescription antifungals and external analgesics because of inadequate evidence of their safety and efficacy.

Antimicrobials. The FDA currently classifies no nonprescription antimicrobial ingredients in diaper rash products as Category I (safe and effective).

Protectants. Protectants help prevent or treat diaper rash by acting as a physical barrier to irritants and sealing out or absorbing moisture. Protectants classified as Category I include allantoin, calamine, and cod liver oil (in combination); dimethicone, kaolin, and lanolin (in combination); mineral oil; petrolatum; talc; topical cornstarch; white petrolatum; and zinc oxide.

Zinc oxide, an excellent protectant, is a mild astringent with weak antiseptic properties. Many preparations contain various concentrations of zinc oxide and petrolatum. Zinc oxide paste USP, the simplest of these formulations, contains 25% zinc oxide, 25% cornstarch, and 50% white petrolatum. Parents should be informed that this paste may easily be removed with mineral oil.

Petrolatum may trap moisture beneath it and keep the diaper area hydrated, a condition that is not desirable in cases of prickly heat. White petrolatum is also more irritating than zinc oxide paste. Of the two products, the one that will keep the diaper area driest and cause the least irritation is zinc oxide paste.

The powdered protectant agents that have been used most often in treating diaper rash and prickly heat are talc, magnesium stearate, calcium carbonate, cornstarch, kaolin, zinc stearate, and microporous cellulose. When applied after each diaper change, these products serve primarily to keep the diaper area dry. They should be applied with a cotton fluff to spread evenly. Powders should never be applied to an acute oozing dermatitis because they may promote secondary crusting and infection.

Inhalation of the dust by the infant may be harmful and could lead to chemical pneumonia. Parents should be instructed to use these agents cautiously and apply them carefully.

Hydrocortisone. Hydrocortisone is not recommended for use on children under 2 years of age except under supervision of a physician.

Treatment of Secondary Complications

The FDA believes that antimicrobial (antiseptic) drug products have significant limitations in treating the secondary infections that may accompany irritation caused by diaper rash. Such infections should not be treated with nonprescription drugs. Physician referral is advisable.

Product Selection Guidelines

Pharmacists should advise patients about the correct use of any product they recommend. Some general precautions should be mentioned, such as taking care in applying topical preparations that might sting already irritated skin. If powders are recommended, parents, caregivers, or patients should be instructed to apply them carefully to prevent accidental inhalation. When soaks and solutions are used, the unused portion should be discarded after each use.

Above all, pharmacists should caution parents about the general use of any medication for a baby's skin. The best therapy for diaper dermatitis (in adults as well as infants) is to keep the skin clean and dry. Parents should understand that using medications indiscriminately for diaper rash or prickly heat is ill-advised.

Prevention

Proper Hygiene

A diaper should be changed as soon as it is soiled. The apparently unsoiled part of the diaper should never be used to wipe the baby because this practice spreads microorganisms over the skin. Nondisposable cloth diapers should be made of soft material and fastened loosely. Plastic pants should be used as seldom as possible because they are occlusive. Changing the diaper within several hours after putting the child to bed is recommended because infants often urinate soon after they are put to sleep for the night.

The diaper area should be cleaned at each diaper change. Mild soap should be used for cleaning the diaper area and for bathing. Skin folds should be cleaned thoroughly and rinsed well with clean water. The various diaper wipe products should be used with care because irritants may be present and because a hypersensitivity reaction may occur. If such products must be used, unscented, hypoallergenic wipes are recommended.

Most babies who develop diaper rash respond to treatment and do not need prophylaxis. Babies who require continued prophylaxis should have it stopped periodically to determine whether it is still necessary.

Proper Washing of Cloth Diapers

Diapers should be washed with mild soap and rinsed thoroughly. If an automatic washing machine is used, repeating the rinse cycle is recommended. Air drying diapers in the sun helps kill bacteria. Ironing dry, washed diapers will reduce any surviving bacteria or fungi.

Adding laundry bleach during the washing cycle reduces the bacterial count. Acidification of diapers may also be helpful; this can be accomplished by rinsing the diapers a final time in a solution made by adding one cup of vinegar to a half-filled washing machine tub. The diapers are then added and soaked for 30 minutes.

Disposable versus Cloth Diapers

Several studies have compared the incidence of diaper rash in infants diapered with cloth versus disposable diapers. Cloth diapers cleaned by a diaper service were associated with the lowest incidence of diaper rash; disposable diapers showed a similar low incidence. Home-laundered diapers that were not rinsed with a bacteriostatic agent were associated with the highest incidence.

Infants who wear absorbent gelling material (AGM) diapers (Ultra Pampers) have been found to be substantially drier and to have significantly less diaper rash and less severe diaper rash than infants wearing either conventional disposable or home-laundered diapers.

Prickly Heat

The lesions associated with prickly heat result from obstruction of the sweat gland pores. Retained sweat causes the dilation and rupture of the epidermal sweat pores, producing swelling and inflammation of the dermis. The lesions usually produce some itching, but stinging is more common. Prickly heat occurs primarily during hot, humid weather or during a febrile illness with profuse sweating. It may also occur as a result of excessive clothing, polyester clothing, and overcovering, especially at night in warm, humid rooms.

In infants, the lesions most often appear in intertriginous areas and under plastic pants, diapers, and adhesive tape. In children and adults, the dermatitis is seen on areas of skin that have been heavily occluded with clothing. The lesions, which are erythematous papules, may become pustular and are usually localized to the sites of occlusion.

The primary treatment goal is to cool the patient to reduce sweating and, in patients with fever, to administer antipyretics. Light clothing and coverings are recommended to allow air to reach the skin. Air-conditioning the environment helps lower humidity and temperature. Maceration and irritants may be reduced with baths or sponge baths at least two times a day and the use of a bland talc dusting powder. Frequent diaper changes and the elimination of excessive soap or chemical irritants help reduce discomfort.

Adult Urinary Incontinence

Urinary incontinence is defined as the involuntary loss of urine sufficient in amount or frequency to be a social or health problem. The consequences of this problem, which primarily affects the elderly and is more common in women than in men, are considerable. The patient's social and psychologic well-being are compromised. Attempts to limit episodes of involuntary urine loss by restricting fluid intake cause dehydration and hypotension, while skin irritation and ulceration due to long exposure to urine result in "diaper rash" and even pressure ulcers. Often the loss of urine control leads to premature institutionalization or elder abuse. Urinary incontinence must always be medically evaluated, inasmuch as it can often be treated and resolved.

Types of Urinary Incontinence

The basic types of incontinence and their associated synonyms are as follows:

- *Detrusor instability:* detrusor hyperactivity, detrusor overactivity, detrusor hyperreflexia, unstable bladder, spastic bladder, uninhibited bladder, urge incontinence.

- *Stress incontinence:* sphincter insufficiency, outlet impotence.

- *Overflow incontinence:* detrusor areflexia, atonic bladder, impaired contractility, urge incontinence.

- *Functional incontinence:* reflex incontinence.

■ *Iatrogenic incontinence.*

■ *Mixed incontinence.*

Treatment of Incontinence

After medical evaluation has occurred and diagnosis has been established, treatment with appropriate agents and nonpharmacologic measures can be implemented. Most medications used to treat these disorders are prescription products. Most nonprescription items sold for urinary incontinence are medications to control or treat skin breakdown (diaper rash), agents to control odor, and absorbent products. Because some patients may attempt self-diagnosis, it is imperative that pharmacists inquire about a proper medical evaluation before recommending nonprescription products, including absorbent products.

Type-Specific Approaches

Detrusor Instability. Detrusor instability may be treated with anticholinergic medications (e.g., oxybutynin chloride, flavoxate hydrochloride, hyoscyamine), which facilitate urine storage by decreasing uninhibited detrusor contractions. Diphenhydramine is occasionally used as initial drug therapy. Pharmacists should counsel patients about potential side effects, which include sedation, dry mouth (a problem in patients who wear dentures), constipation, and confusion. These side effects occur more often with diphenhydramine than with the other three products. The patient should be instructed to do pelvic floor muscle exercises and to adhere to a "timed voiding" schedule to increase the efficacy of treatment. Contraindications to the use of diphenhydramine and other anticholinergic medications include many conditions that occur more often in elderly individuals (e.g., narrow-angle glaucoma, peptic ulcer, urinary tract obstruction, hyperthyroidism) than in other patients.

Stress Incontinence. Stress incontinence is often treated with nonprescription agents such as ephedrine, pseudoephedrine, phenylephrine, and phenylpropanolamine, which increase outflow resistance. Caution should be used when initiating such therapy in patients with hypertension and/or cardiac arrhythmias, and the patient should be advised to monitor blood pressure and pulse, and to report any new occurrences of heart palpitations or fainting. The use of pelvic floor muscle exercises and a timed voiding schedule will assist in controlling this type of incontinence.

In women, estrogen therapy may also be used; benefits are seen in 4–6 weeks. Pharmacists should counsel about the common side effects of estrogen therapy, such as weight gain, fluid retention, increased blood pressure, and vaginal spotting. Should medical treatment fail, surgical correction may be possible.

Overflow Incontinence. The treatment of overflow incontinence is directed by the cause. Surgery is often necessary. Bethanechol chloride, with or without metoclopramide, may be initiated where the bladder has insufficient contractile strength. Catheterization is a last resort.

Functional and Iatrogenic Incontinence. Functional and iatrogenic incontinence require evaluation of the patient's entire medical status and medication history to determine the underlying cause.

Absorbent Products

The use of protective undergarments and pads is aimed at protecting clothing, bedding, and furniture while allowing independence and mobility. They should be used only after a thorough and complete examination. If patients or caregivers prematurely initiate the use of absorbent protective products, they treat the symptom and obscure the cause.

Selection Factors. The type of absorbent product used depends on several factors, including type and severity of incontinence, functional status, sex, availability of caregivers, patient preference, and convenience. Pharmacists should discuss such factors with patients and their caregivers when helping select absorbent products.

The capacity of each disposable product corresponds to the needs of the patient:

- *Guards/shields:* 2–12 oz (60–360 mL), light to heavy capacity;
- *Briefs:* 28–36 oz (840–1100 mL), moderate to heavy capacity;
- *Undergarments:* 12–18 oz (360–540 mL), moderate to heavy capacity.

Another important issue is the functional capacity of the patient. Does the patient use the toilet and change undergarments independently? Is the patient limited in mobility so that the heaviest protection is needed during the night? Will the patient need assistance in changing the products? If so, briefs or diapers with roll-on bed application and adhesive closures may be useful for a caregiver.

Securing the product may be an important issue. Some garments or shields have adhesive strips or belts to hold them in place. Belts may require assistance from a caregiver. Comfort and security from leakage are important. The anatomic differences between men and women are another consideration; products designed with these differences in mind should be considered when large-capacity products are used.

Protective underpads are often used in conjunction with briefs and undergarments for extended duration activities, such as sleeping and sitting. Both bed and chair pads are available, and the pharmacist should inquire about the need for additional protection. The underpad should have a known capacity, a waterproof duration of several hours, and the ability to remain intact when wet.

Complications from Absorbent Products. Because the use of absorbent products increases the risk of skin irritation and maceration, such products should be checked every 2 hours. With continual urine loss, it is recommended that the absorbent material be changed every 2–4 hours. The use of skin protectants (barrier creams and ointments) as in diaper rash is appropriate. Should a rash occur, the same treatment is indicated as was described for infants.

Pressure ulcers may occur if the patient is immobile. Any skin breakdown with development of a lesion should be reported to the primary care provider.

Since most pharmacies do not carry a full line of products for the urine incontinent patient, the pharmacist can direct patients to Help for Incontinent People (HIP) Inc., PO Box 544, Union, SC 29379; 803–579–7900, 800–BLADDER, or fax 803–579–7902.

CHAPTER 30

Sunscreen and Suntan Products

Questions to ask in patient assessment and counseling

- *Do you sunburn easily?*
- *How long can you stay in full sun before your skin turns red?*
- *How well do you tan?*
- *Do you spend much time outdoors because of your job, sports, or other activities?*
- *Are you using a sun protection product?*
- *What products have you used in the past?*
- *Has your physician or other health professional ever told you that a growth on your skin or lip was caused by the sun?*
- *Have you ever had a reaction to a prescription or nonprescription drug?*
- *Have you ever had a reaction to any sunscreen product?*
- *Are you taking a tetracycline, diuretic, or sulfa drug?*
- *Will you be using the product while swimming, skiing, participating in strenuous activities, or working?*

Within the last 20 years, research has proved that ultraviolet (UV) radiation is harmful. It is clear that avoiding excessive exposure to UV radiation will reduce the incidence of premature aging of the skin, skin cancer, and other long-term dermatologic effects.

Ultraviolet Radiation

The UV spectrum is divided into three major bands: UVC, UVB, and UVA. Although UVC does not stimulate tanning, it can cause some erythema (redness) of the skin. Cutaneous UVB exposure is responsible for vitamin D_3 synthesis in the skin. Its therapeutic benefit notwithstanding, however, UVB is considered to be primarily responsible for inducing skin cancer, and its carcinogenic effects are believed to be augmented by UVA. In addition, UVB is primarily responsible for wrinkling of the skin, epidermal hyperplasia, elastosis (loss of skin elasticity), and collagen damage.

UVA radiation penetrates deeper into the skin than UVB. This can cause both histologic and vascular damage. Based on current research into the effects of UVA on the skin and underlying structures, the UVA band has been divided into two subsets: UVA I and UVA II. UVA II is more damaging to the skin than UVA I. This has significant implications for sunscreen products and the type of protection they offer.

Editor's Note: This chapter is adapted from Edward M. DeSimone II, "Sunscreen and Suntan Products," in Covington, T.R., ed., *Handbook of Nonprescription Drugs,* 11th edition. For a more extensive discussion of burning and tanning, skin disorders induced by exposure to ultraviolet radiation, and sunscreen products, readers are encouraged to consult Chapter 30 of the *Handbook.*

Burning and Tanning

A sunburn is the result of an inflammatory reaction involving a number of mediators. It is, in fact, a burn. It is most often seen as a first-degree (superficial) burn, with a reaction ranging from mild erythema to tenderness, pain, and edema. The intensity of the UVB-induced erythema peaks at 12–24 hours after exposure. Severe reactions to excessive UV exposure can sometimes produce a second-degree burn, with the development of vesicles (blisters) or bullae (large blisters) as well as the constitutional symptoms of fever, chills, weakness, and shock.

A tan is produced when UV radiation stimulates the melanocytes in the germinating skin layer to generate more melanin and oxidizes the melanin already in the epidermis. Both processes serve as protective mechanisms by diffusing and absorbing additional UV radiation.

UV-Induced Skin Disorders

Consumers use sunscreens primarily to prevent sunburn and to aid in the development of a tan. Sunscreens are also effective in protecting against drug-related UV-induced photosensitivity and other types of photodermatoses. They can also be used to protect exposed areas of the body from premature photoaging and the long-term hazards of skin cancer.

Drug Photosensitivity

Photosensitivity encompasses two types of conditions: photoallergy and phototoxicity. Drug photoallergy, a relatively uncommon immunologic response, involves an increased, chemically induced reactivity of the skin to UV radiation and/or visible light. UV radiation (primarily UVA) triggers an antigenic reaction in the skin, which is characterized by urticaria, bullae, and/or sunburn. This reaction, which is not dose related, is usually seen after at least one prior exposure to the involved chemical agent or drug.

Phototoxicity is also an increased, chemically induced reactivity of the skin to UV radiation and/or visible light. However, this reaction is not immunologic. It is often seen on first exposure to a chemical agent or drug. It is dose related and usually exhibits no drug cross-sensitivity. It is most likely to appear as an exaggerated sunburn. Drugs associated with phototoxicity are listed in Table 2 of Chapter 31. This type of reaction is not limited to drugs but is also associated with plants, cosmetics, and soaps.

It seems reasonable to assume that, because UVA radiation is primarily responsible for triggering a photosensitivity reaction, a sunscreen effective throughout the entire UVA range, especially above 360 nm, would help prevent a large number of cases of photosensitivity. Since UVB can also produce photosensitivity, it would be best to use a broad-spectrum sunscreen that also protects throughout the entire UVB range.

Photodermatoses

Photodermatoses are skin eruptions that are idiopathic (self-originated) or exacerbated (photoaggravated) by radiation of varying wavelengths. UVB is most often responsible for the reactions. More than 20 known disorders are classified as photodermatoses (Table 1).

Avoidance of UV radiation is the best way to prevent the occurrence or exacerbation of photodermatoses. Sunscreens with the widest range of UV absorbance may afford the next best protection.

TABLE 1 Most common photodermatoses	
Idiopathic disorders Actinic prurigo Chronic actinic dermatitis Polymorphic light eruption Solar urticaria **Photoaggravated disorders** Acne vulgaris Atopic dermatitis Atopic eczema Bullous pemphigoid	Chloasma Dermatomyositis Drug photosensitivity Erythema multiforme Herpes simplex labialis Lichen planus Psoriasis Rosacea Seborrheic dermatitis Systemic lupus erythematosus

Source:

Pathak MA, Fitzpatrick TB, Parrish JA. In: Fitzpatrick TB et al, eds. *Dermatology in General Medicine*. 3rd ed. New York: McGraw-Hill; 1987: 254–62.

Guercio-Hauer C, Macfarlane DF, Deleo VA. Photodamage, photoaging and photoprotection of the skin. *Am Fam Phys*. 1994 Aug; 50: 327–32.

Kligman LH, Kligman AM. In: Fitzpatrick TB et al, eds. *Dermatology in General Medicine*. 3rd ed. New York: McGraw-Hill; 1987: 1470–5.

Premature Aging

One of the long-term hazards of radiation is premature photoaging of the skin. This type of aging is genetically determined; for example, Caucasians are more susceptible than African Americans. The condition is most easily characterized by wrinkling and yellowing of the skin. Prolonged exposure to UV radiation in susceptible individuals results in elastosis (degeneration of the skin due to breakdown of the skin's elastic fibers). Pronounced drying, thickening, and wrinkling of the skin may also result. Other physical changes include cracking, telangiectasia (spider vessels), solar keratoses (growths), and ecchymoses (subcutaneous hemorrhagic lesions).

There is some evidence that, in certain cases, sun protection allows for repair of existing damage. Sunscreens appear to help by keeping additional UV radiation from reaching the skin structures. This not only helps prevent a worsening of the condition but also appears to aid in the reversal of some of the skin damage. Patients should be counseled to use a sunscreen product of no less than sun protection factor (SPF) 15 during treatment.

Skin Cancer

The two most common types of nonmelanoma skin cancer are basal cell carcinoma and squamous cell carcinoma. Other UV-induced disorders include premalignant actinic keratosis (which usually develops into squamous cell carcinoma if left untreated), keratoacanthoma, and malignant melanoma.

During the 1980s, a large number of studies linking skin cancer with UV exposure were reported. It has been shown that the incidence of skin cancer increases steadily in populations closer to the equator. Skin cancer occurs more often in Caucasians than in other ethnic groups. Another risk factor is a history of severe sunburn. Avoidance of the sun as an adult may not alter the chances of developing basal cell carcinoma later in life.

Until all the other major factors affecting skin cancer are conclusively identified, it is recommended that avoidance of UV radiation exposure, the use of hats and other coverings, and the use of sunscreens be the norm.

Sunscreen Products

FDA Review of Sunscreen Agents

The Food and Drug Administration (FDA) has not issued its final monograph on sunscreen agents. Confusion may arise concerning the best product to use, given that product formulation and labeling may now follow FDA's advance notice of proposed rulemaking or tentative final monograph (TFM). The TFM allows for the following labeling claims on sunscreen product packaging:

- Helps prevent sunburn;
- Helps prevent lip damage;
- Helps prevent skin damage;
- Helps prevent freckling;
- Helps prevent uneven coloration; and
- Permits tanning.

Each claim and the specific language used depend on the SPF of the product.

Classification as Drug Products

Prior to FDA review, sunscreens were considered to be cosmetics. The TFM stipulates that sunscreen products will be classified as drugs rather than cosmetics because they are intended to be used therapeutically. However, cosmetics that contain sunscreen agents will be classified as cosmetics so long as the terms *sunscreen* or *SPF* or an SPF value do not appear on the label and no therapeutic claims are made.

Official Names of Sunscreen Agents

The FDA's policy is that drug names "will ordinarily be either the compendial name of the active ingredient or, if there is no compendial name, the common and usual name of the active ingredient." If no official name exists, the name published in the *USP Dictionary of USAN and International Drug Names* will be considered the established name.

Sunscreen Efficacy

Minimal Erythema Dose

It is difficult to ascertain the efficacy of sunscreens on humans because individual responsiveness to UV radiation varies greatly. The standardized measure that is used is the minimal erythema dose (MED), defined as the "minimum UV radiation dose that produces clearly marginated erythema in the irradiated site, given as a single exposure." The MED is indicative not only of the amount of energy reaching the skin but also of the responsiveness of the skin to the radiation. There may be different MEDs on different parts of the body. In addition, the MED for African Americans with heavy pigmentation has been estimated to be up to 33 times higher than that for Caucasians with light pigmentation.

Sun Protection Factor

The SPF is derived by dividing the MED of protected skin by the MED of unprotected skin. The higher the SPF, the more effective the agent in preventing sunburn. If it normally takes

60 minutes for someone to experience 2 MEDs (a bright erythematous sunburn), a sunscreen with an SPF of 6 will allow that individual to stay in the sun six times longer (or 6 hours) before receiving this same sunburn (assuming the sunscreen is reapplied at the recommended intervals).

Table 2 presents the revised skin type classifications and relationships of sunburn and tanning history to SPF and product category designations, as set forth in the TFM.

Substantivity

The efficacy of a sunscreen is related to its ability to remain effective during prolonged exercise, sweating, and swimming. This property can be a function of the active sunscreen, the vehicle, or both. Products with cream-based (water in oil) vehicles appear more resistant to removal by water than those with alcohol bases. Oil-based products have traditionally been the most popular and are the easiest to apply. However, they tend to have lower SPF values.

The TFM guidelines for sunscreen product substantivity are *water resistant* (i.e., retains its sun protection for at least 40 minutes in water) and *very water resistant* (retains its sun protection for at least 80 minutes in water). The latter category is intended to replace *waterproof,* which is currently in use.

Types of Sunscreen Agents

Two definitions for therapeutic sunscreen types have been proposed: *sunscreen active ingredient* and *sunscreen opaque sunblock.* Based on these definitions, topical sunscreens can be divided into two major subgroups: chemical and physical. Chemical sunscreens work by absorbing and thus blocking the transmission of UV radiation to the epidermis. Physical sunscreens are generally opaque and act by reflecting and scattering UV radiation. Many sunscreen products contain a combination of sunscreen agents.

TABLE 2 Sunburn and tanning history

Skin type[a]	Sunburn/tanning history	Recommended SPF	Recommended PCD[a,b]
I	Always burns easily; never tans	20–30	Ultra high
II	Always burns easily; tans minimally	12–<20	Very high
III	Burns moderately; tans gradually	8–<12	High
IV	Burns minimally; always tans well	4–<8	Moderate
V	Rarely burns; tans profusely	2–<4	Minimal
VI[c]	Never burns; deeply pigmented (insensitive)	—	—

[a]Optional labeling information according to the TFM.

[b]Product category designation (PCD).

[c]Skin type VI, which is not part of the proposed *Recommended Sunscreen Product Guide,* is included in this table because the TFM addresses it with the other skin types; however, this skin type is used only under the general testing procedures for the selection of test subjects.

Adapted from *Federal Register.* 1993 May; 58: 28194–302.

Chemical Sunscreens

Aminobenzoic Acid (ABA) and Derivatives. ABA is an effective UVB sunscreen, especially when formulated in a hydroalcoholic base (maximum of 50%–60% alcohol). The SPF of such formulations increases proportionally as the concentration of ABA increases from 2% to 5%. There is evidence that some UVA is also blocked at the 5% or higher level.

One advantage of ABA is its ability to penetrate into the horny layer of the skin and provide lasting protection. It has significant substantivity on sweating skin. The primary advantage of ABA derivatives over ABA is that they do not stain clothing.

The disadvantages of alcoholic solutions of ABA include contact dermatitis, photosensitivity, stinging and drying of the skin, and yellow staining of clothes upon exposure to the sun. Drugs that may induce cross-sensitivity to ABA and its derivatives include thiazide diuretics, sulfonamides, and "caine" anesthetics such as lidocaine and benzocaine. Patients who have experienced a photosensitivity reaction to any of these drugs should not use a sunscreen containing ABA or any of its derivatives.

Anthranilates. Menthyl anthranilate is a weak UV sunscreen with maximal absorbance in the UVA range. It is usually found in combination with other sunscreen agents.

Benzophenones. There are three agents in the benzophenone group: dioxybenzone, oxybenzone (benzophenone-3), and sulisobenzone (benzophenone-4). These agents are primarily UVB absorbers; however, their absorbance extends well into the UVA range. Benzophenones are often found in combination with other sunscreens.

Cinnamates. There are four sunscreens in this group. Three of the four agents—cinoxate, diethanolamine methoxycinnamate, and octyl methoxycinnamate—have similar absorbance ranges as well as maximum absorbances. The exception is octocrylene, which has an absorbance range well into the UVA range. Octocrylene is currently found in many more commercial sunscreen preparations than it was in the past, possibly reflecting its broader spectrum of absorbance. Unfortunately, cinnamates do not adhere well to the skin and must rely on the vehicle in a given formulation for their substantivity.

Salicylates. Salicylic acid derivatives are weak sunscreens. They do not adhere well to the skin and are easily removed by perspiration or swimming.

Physical Sunscreens

Physical sunscreens scatter rather than absorb UV and visible radiation. They are most often used on small and prominently exposed areas by people who cannot limit or control their exposure to the sun (e.g., lifeguards). The nose and tops of the ears are often coated with a white or colored substance containing zinc oxide or titanium dioxide. The effectiveness of physical sunscreens is related to the thickness with which they are applied. Their disadvantages are that they can discolor clothing and may occlude the skin. Because titanium dioxide increases the effective SPF of a product and extends the spectrum of protection well into the UVA range, the number of commercial products containing this agent has increased.

UVA Sunscreens

Dibenzoylmethane derivatives are the first of a new class of sunscreen agents effective throughout the entire UVA range. The first of these new agents is avobenzone. Although avobenzone absorbs UV radiation through all of the UVA spectrum, its absorbance falls off sharply at 370 nm.

Combination Products

The FDA has not recommended any limits on the number of sunscreen agents that may be used together in a nonprescription product. Since the SPF is product specific and not dependent on the sunscreen active agent alone, the TFM has eliminated a required minimum strength for single active ingredient sunscreen products.

Suntan Products and Devices

Two types of products fall under the heading of suntan products: those that contain a sunscreen and those that do not. Products without a sunscreen are easily identified by the absence of an SPF value on the label. These products are considered cosmetics and are used for coloring the skin rather than for any therapeutic indications. They provide no protection against the short- and long-term hazards of UV radiation exposure. However, all suntan products that contain sunscreen active ingredients can be considered suntan products. Thus, the TFM allows the claim of "permits tanning" on products with an SPF of 2 to <12, while a product with an SPF of 12 to <20 "limits tanning."

Pigmenting Agents

Oral Agents

A number of products claim to be effective oral tanning compounds. Their active ingredients are the dyes canthaxanthin and beta-carotene. The dyes alter skin tone by coloring the fat cells under the epidermal layer.

The FDA has not approved either beta-carotene or canthaxanthin for artificial tanning. One major concern is the discoloration of the feces to brick red, which could mask gastrointestinal bleeding. A second concern is the long-term adverse effects that may be associated with the large doses recommended.

Topical Dyes

For years, dihydroxyacetone (DHA) has been the major ingredient in products that claim to tan without sun. The intensity of the tan is related to the thickness of the skin. The color fades after 5–7 days with desquamation of the stratum corneum.

The FDA has determined that DHA alone is ineffective as a sunscreen and that it should be classified as a cosmetic. However, in combination with lawsone, a major dye component of henna, the combination is classified as a weak sunscreen. Several sunless tanning products combine DHA with various sunscreen agents, which at least helps prevent photodamage for persons who intend to spend some time in the sun.

Tan Accelerators

Tan accelerators are cosmetic products that claim to stimulate a faster, deeper tan. Their major ingredient is tyrosine, an amino acid necessary for the production of melanin. The TFM states that "any product containing tyrosine or its derivatives and claiming to accelerate the tanning process is an unapproved new drug."

Melanotropins

A hormone known as alpha-melanotropin or alpha-melanocyte-stimulating hormone (ALPHA-MSH) has been shown to affect skin color through its action on melanocytes. Alpha-melanotropin is currently under investigation to determine whether it can affect skin tanning.

Tanning Booths and Sunbeds

The newer types of tanning devices use UV radiation sources composed of more than 96% UVA and less than 4% UVB, a considerably different mix of UV radiation than that obtained from natural sunlight. It would appear that UVA, used properly, could generate a tan without producing an erythematous sunburn. However, it is believed that even 1% UVB emission can cause a significant increase in the incidence of skin cancer. There is a small but growing body of evidence that the use of sunlamps and sunbeds is related to the rising incidence of malignant melanoma worldwide.

UVA radiation may trigger the eruption of cold sores. In addition, it can produce a photosensitivity reaction in patients who have ingested or applied photosensitizing agents. Moreover, because UVA is less likely to produce the overt burning (erythema) of UVB, patients may become complacent and forgo the use of eye goggles; this practice will produce eye burns and may increase the risk of subsequently developing cataracts.

Patients should be advised that the possibility of long-term hazards related to UVA has not yet been fully assessed and that there are currently no accepted health benefits from tanning devices.

Sunglasses

Many patients erroneously believe that all sunglasses screen out UV radiation. In response, the Sunglass Association of America, working with the FDA, has developed a voluntary labeling program. Based on its UV radiation filtration properties, each pair of sunglasses is placed in one of three categories:

- *Cosmetic* sunglasses block at least 70% of UVB, 20% of UVA, and less than 60% of visible light. They are recommended for activities in nonharsh sunlight.

- *General-purpose* sunglasses block at least 95% of UVB, at least 60% of UVA, and 60%–92% of visible light. With shades that range from medium to dark, they are recommended for most activities in sunny environments, such as boating, driving, flying, or hiking.

- *Special-purpose* sunglasses block at least 99% of UVB, 60% of UVA, and 20%–97% of visible light. They are recommended for activities in very bright environments, such as ski slopes and tropical beaches.

Product Selection Guidelines

The most important thing a pharmacist needs to know before recommending a sunscreen product is the patient's natural skin type and tanning history. The pharmacist should also find out how much time is normally spent out of doors. Other questions the pharmacist might ask are presented at the beginning of this chapter. Using this information, as well as knowing both the active and inactive ingredients in the various products and the products' SPFs, the pharmacist can recommend a sunscreen product.

Efficacy Considerations

Sun Protection Factor

Patients with less natural skin protection should use products with higher SPFs. A product with an SPF-15 will prevent sunburn while also allowing for a gradually developing tan. A product of SPF-30 should be recommended for patients who burn easily, cannot tan, or cannot afford any degree of sunburn or overexposure to UV radiation of any type. Patients who have a personal or family history of certain dermatologic problems, such as atopic dermatitis or sunburn with short exposure, or who have any type of skin cancer or precancerous dermatologic lesion should use a total blocking agent or a sunscreen with an SPF of 30 or higher when prolonged exposure to sunlight is expected.

In the vast majority of cases, an SPF of 30 is the best choice. However, for patients with UV-induced disorders or taking photosensitizing drugs, a sunscreen that absorbs throughout the UVA range is probably a better choice than the highest SPF product. A broad-spectrum sunscreen, while effective throughout the UVB range, is required to have absorption activity only through 360 nm and not through 400 nm. Therefore, it may not provide complete protection, especially against photosensitivity.

Broad-Spectrum Sunscreens

A number of commercial products claim to be broad spectrum; the TFM allows such claims if the product contains ingredients that absorb or reflect UVB (290–320 nm) *and* absorb up to 360 nm. Products with equal SPFs may still differ significantly in total UV protection, depending on the absorbances of the various sunscreens they contain. Most broad-spectrum products have a minimum of two sunscreen ingredients.

There is no one generally accepted measure to evaluate the efficacy of a product that claims to provide UVA protection. The best recommendation would be to select a product that contains a combination of sunscreen agents that protect throughout the entire UVB range and across the widest possible UVA range. A product that contains avobenzone, claims to be broad spectrum, and has an SPF of at least 15 is an excellent choice for patients with UV-induced disorders or taking photosensitizing drugs. Currently, Shade UVAGuard is the only such product on the market. A very broad spectrum of coverage can also be obtained by using an ABA derivative combined with one of the benzophenones, octocrylene, or menthyl anthranilate.

Substantivity

Given three products of equal SPF, the best and most cost-effective selection is the product that is most substantive. The less substantive a product, the more likely it is to be rubbed off by any type of contact.

Lip Protection

One of the most common locations for oral cancer is the lips. More than a dozen sunscreen products are on the market to prevent burning of the lips (or nose). Although they differ in ingredients and UVA and UVB spectrum, these products carry virtually the same labeling, including the SPF, as do the sunscreen lotions (with the exception that they do not require "for external use only"). Lip protection not only helps prevent drying and burning of the lips but also helps prevent the development of cold sores (fever blisters) triggered by the herpes simplex virus in patients who are susceptible to recurrent cold sores.

Sunscreens for Children

Special consideration is needed when recommending a sunscreen product for young children. Absorptive characteristics of human skin in children under 6 months of age are different from those of adult skin. Moreover, the metabolic and excretory systems of children under 6 months of age are not fully developed to handle any sunscreen agent absorbed through the skin. Guidelines for use of sunscreens in children are as follows:

■ Unless otherwise instructed by a physician, sunscreens should not be used in children under 6 months of age.

■ Children under 2 years of age should use sunscreen products with a minimum SPF of 4.

Caregivers should be extremely wary regarding sun exposure in children, especially those under 6 months old. Regular use of an SPF-15 product starting after 6 months of age and continuing through age 18 can reduce the incidence of skin cancer over a lifetime by up to 78%.

Precautions

Staining

Sunscreen products containing ABA should be allowed to dry before the skin comes into contact with clothing, vinyl, or fiberglass. This is probably a good rule to follow regardless of the sunscreen used. The only other sunscreen ingredient that has potential for staining is DHA.

Contact Dermatitis and Other Skin Considerations

Photosensitivity and contact dermatitis are more likely to occur with ABA and its esters. Other sunscreens, including the benzophenones, the cinnamates, homosalate, avobenzone, and menthyl anthranilate, have been reported to produce both conditions, although to a lesser degree. In addition, patients who are allergy-prone and have allergies to various drugs, such as benzocaine, thiazides, or sulfonamides, may develop an allergic reaction to ABA or its esters.

Many products are labeled noncomedogenic, fragrance-free, and hypoallergenic. Products that are noncomedogenic are those that do not plug the pores and therefore do not exacerbate acne. Many individuals are sensitive to various ingredients, including fragrances, emulsifiers, and preservatives. Ethyl and isopropyl alcohols, which are included in a number of sunscreen products, should be avoided by patients with dry skin.

Patient Counseling

Pharmacists can provide a great service by counseling consumers about the suntanning process and the proper selection and use of sunscreens.

The rays of the sun are the most direct and damaging between 10 AM and 3 PM. It is best to avoid sunning during this period. Very little UV radiation is filtered by clouds; thus, an overcast day gives a false sense of security against sunburn. In addition, the intensity of exposure increases as one moves closer to the equator.

Another potential problem is that UV radiation reflects off of various surfaces. Fresh snow reflects 85%–100% of the light and radiation that strikes it, creating the need for sunglasses when one is skiing on a sunny day. Similarly, sand, white-painted surfaces, and water reflect a significant amount of the radiation striking them. A person sitting in the shade of a beach umbrella may still be bombarded by UV radiation reflecting off the sand.

If properly applied, products with an SPF of 15–30 allow an individual to stay out in the sun for long periods and slowly develop a tan over several days to weeks. It is important to remember, however, that as an individual tans, a natural protection against burning also develops. Therefore, an individual who insists on tanning should begin the summer using a product with an SPF of at least 15 and switch to products with lower SPFs as the natural tan progresses.

The two major causes of poor sun protection with sunscreen use are application of inadequate amounts and infrequent reapplication. Sunscreens must be liberally applied to all exposed areas of the body and reapplied as often as the label recommends for maximum effectiveness.

Reapplying a sunscreen does not extend the amount of time a person can spend in the sun. Outdoor exposure to UV radiation should be within the limits of the SPF value of the sunscreen. Moreover, although some sunscreen products now have an SPF of 50, the use of an SPF-30 offers adequate protection to the average person. The best all-purpose, general recommendation for providing optimal protection from immediate as well as long-term injury from sun exposure is a product with an SPF of 30. Children should use SPF-30 sunscreens whenever they play outdoors, not just when swimming.

Under hot, humid conditions, there is increased sweating but poor evaporation. When the humidity is low, overheating during exercise may occur in persons who have applied sun screens, possibly because the oily vehicle of the sunscreen may block the pores. Sunbathers should be cautious when exercising in hot weather after applying a sunscreen product.

Oral ingestion of ABA has been associated with a lowered white blood cell count, drug fever, and organ damage, and thus should be vigorously discouraged.

The TFM also proposed that labeling of all sunscreens contain the following warnings:

- For external use only, not to be swallowed.

- Avoid contact with eyes. If contact occurs, rinse eyes thoroughly with water.

- Discontinue use if signs of irritation or rash appear. If irritation or rash persists, consult a doctor.

Consumers should be advised that if itching, redness, or a rash develops while using a particular product, they should discontinue using the product and contact a pharmacist.

CHAPTER 31

Burn and Sunburn Products

Questions to ask in patient assessment and counseling

- What caused the burn—chemicals, sun exposure, electricity, or heat?
- How severe is the burn? Is the skin broken or blistered?
- When did the burn occur?
- Where is the burn? How large is the burned area?
- Is the burn oozing?
- Is the burn painful?
- What treatment have you used on the burn?
- How long have you been using this treatment?
- What effect has this treatment had?
- Do you have any other injuries or symptoms?
- Do you have any other medical problems?
- Are you taking any oral prescription or nonprescription medication?
- Are you now, or have you recently been, using any topical medication for a condition other than the burn?

Classification of Burns

The depth of a burn has traditionally been described as first, second, or third degree. A classification of fourth degree is used to describe burns affecting all layers of the skin as well as underlying muscle. Today, the terms *superficial, partial thickness,* and *full thickness* are used with greater frequency. The inflammatory response to a burn injury evolves over the first 24–48 hours, so the initial appearance of the injury can lead to an underestimation of its actual severity. Table 1 presents a classification of burns by depth and lists the corresponding characteristics.

Complications of Burn Injuries

The two major complications of burn injuries are infection and scar contracture. A burn wound infection may increase the depth of the original injury, delay healing, and invade the host, thereby causing systemic infection. Prophylaxis with topical antimicrobial therapy has been universally adopted by burn treatment facilities for patients with moderate to severe burns. Systemic antibiotics are not used unless symptoms warrant.

Editor's Note: This chapter is adapted from Robert H. Moore III and John D. Bowman, "Burn and Sunburn Products," in Covington, T.R., ed., *Handbook of Nonprescription Drugs,* 11th edition. For a more extensive discussion of burn etiology and categorization, complications of burn injuries, sunburn, and self-treatment of minor burns, readers are encouraged to consult Chapter 31 of the *Handbook.*

TABLE 1 Classification of burn by depth

Type	Tissue affected	Characteristics
First degree	Epidermis	Superficial, erythematous, local pain, no blistering, no scarring, little epidermal alteration. Heals within 3–10 days.
Second degree	Epidermis and the most superficial portion of dermis	Erythematous, local pain, elevated vesicle (blister) formation, little or no irreversible damage to dermis, depigmentation in some cases. Usually heals fully in 3–4 weeks with no scarring. Considered a partial-thickness burn.
Third degree	Entire depth of dermis and epidermis; may penetrate into subcutaneous tissue	Extensive and partially irreversible damage to entire depth of dermis and epidermis (and possibly subcutaneous tissue), leathery/white mottled appearance, too severe to blister. Less painful than some first- or second-degree burns because of destruction of nerve endings. Infection a significant risk. Heals over several months. Scarring probable; skin grafting may be necessary to minimize scarring. Considered a full-thickness burn.
Fourth degree	All layers of skin (full thickness) and underlying tissue, including muscle	Charred, dry. Great risk of severe gram-positive or gram-negative infection. Takes months to heal. Skin grafting necessary.

Scar contracture can be minimized by prolonged splinting, range-of-motion exercises, application of pressure such as the wearing of pressure garments, skin grafting of wounds with full-thickness skin, proper surgical incision across joints, and surgical release of formed contractures.

Sunburn

Signs and symptoms of sunburn are seen in 1–24 hours following exposure. With mild exposure, erythema with subsequent scaling and exfoliation of the skin occurs. Pain and low-grade fever may accompany the erythema. More prolonged exposure causes pain, edema, skin tenderness, and possibly blistering. Systemic symptoms similar to those of thermal burn, such as fever, chills, weakness, and shock, may be seen in persons in whom a large portion of the body surface area (BSA) has been affected.

Photosensitization

Some drugs can produce photosensitivity reactions. The drugs alone pose no hazard, but when the patient comes into contact with ultraviolet (UV) radiation, photosensitivity reactions may occur. These can be manifested as photoallergy or phototoxicity. Table 2 lists medications associated with photosensitivity reactions.

TABLE 2 Selected groups of medications associated with photosensitivity reactions

Antidepressants
Amitriptyline
Amoxapine
Clomipramine
Desipramine
Doxepin
Imipramine
Isocarboxazid
Maprotiline
Nortriptyline
Phenelzine
Protriptyline
Trazodone
Trimipramine

Antihistamines
Astemizole
Azatadine
Brompheniramine
Buclizine
Carbinoxamine
Chlorpheniramine
Clemastine
Cyclizine
Cyproheptadine
Dexchlorpheniramine
Dimenhydrinate
Diphenhydramine
Doxylamine
Hydroxyzine
Meclizine
Methapyrilene
Methdilazine
Pheniramine
Promethazine
Pyrilamine
Terfenadine
Trimeprazine
Tripelennamine
Triprolidine

Antihypertensives
Captopril
Diltiazem
Enalapril
Labetalol
Lisinopril
Methyldopa
Minoxidil
Nifedipine

Antipsychotics
Acetophenazine
Chlorpromazine
Fluphenazine
Haloperidol
Mesoridazine
Perphenazine
Prochlorperazine
Promazine
Thioridazine
Thiothixene
Trifluoperazine
Triflupromazine

Coal tar and derivatives (selected brand name products)
Denorex Medicated
　Shampoo
DHS Tar Gel Shampoo
Doak Tar Shampoo
Estar Gel
Ionil T Plus Shampoo
Neutrogena T/Derm
　Body Oil
Neutrogena T/Gel Extra
　Strength Therapeutic
　Shampoo
Tegrin Shampoo
Zetar Shampoo

Diuretics (thiazides)
Bendroflumethiazide
Benzthiazide
Chlorothiazide
Chlorthalidone
Cyclothiazide
Hydrochlorothiazide
Hydroflumethiazide
Methyclothiazide
Polythiazide
Trichlormethiazide

Estrogens/progestins (includes ingredients in oral contraceptives)

Estrogens
Chlorotrianisene
Diethylstilbestrol
Estradiol
Estrogens, conjugated
Estrogens, esterified
Estropipate
Ethinyl estradiol
Megestrol

Progestins
Medroxyprogesterone
Norethindrone
Norgestrel

Hypoglycemics
Acetohexamide
Chlorpropamide
Glipizide
Glyburide
Tolazamide
Tolbutamide

Continued on next page

TABLE 2 *continued*

Nonsteroidal anti-inflammatory drugs

Diclofenac
Diflunisal
Fenoprofen
Flurbiprofen
Ibuprofen
Indomethacin
Ketoprofen
Meclofenamate
Nabumetone
Naproxen
Piroxicam
Sulindac
Tolmetin

Psoralens

Methoxsalen
Trioxsalen

Sulfonamides

Sulfadiazine
Sulfamethizole
Sulfamethoxazole
Sulfapyridine
Sulfasalazine
Sulfinpyrazone
Sulfisoxazole

Tetracyclines

Chlortetracycline
Demeclocycline
Doxycycline
Methacycline
Minocycline
Oxytetracycline
Tetracycline

Other agents

Anticancer drugs

Dacarbazine
Fluorouracil
Flutamide
Methotrexate
Procarbazine
Vinblastine

Anti-infectives (other)

Ciprofloxacin
Dapsone
Enoxacin
Ethionamide
Flucytosine
Gentamicin
Griseofulvin
Lomefloxacin
Nalidixic acid
Norfloxacin
Ofloxacin
Pyrazinamide
Sulfonamides
Trimethoprim

Antiparasitic drugs

Bithionol
Chloroquine
Quinine
Thiabendazole

Diuretics (other)

Acetazolamide
Amiloride
Furosemide
Metolazone
Triamterene

Sunscreens

Benzophenones
Cinnamates
Homosalate
Menthyl anthranilate
Oxybenzone
PABA esters
Para-aminobenzoic acid

Miscellaneous

Amiodarone
  (antiarrhythmic)
Benzocaine (local
  anesthetic)
Benzyl peroxide
Carbamazepine
  (anticonvulsant)
Disopyramide
  (antiarrhythmic)
Etretinate (antipsoriatic)
Gold salts (antiarthritic)
Isotretinoin (antiacne)
Lamotrigine
  (anticonvulsant)
Lovastatin
  (antihyperlipidemic)
Nabilone (antiemetic)
Phenytoin (anticonvulsant)
Quinidine sulfate
  (antiarrhythmic)
Selegiline
  (antiparkinsonism)
Tretinoin (antiacne)

Sources: *Med Lett.* 1993; 37: 946.

Medications That Increase Sensitivity to Light: A 1990 Listing. FDA Pub No 91-8280. Washington, DC: US Department of Health and Human Services, Public Health Service; 1995.

Drug Facts and Comparisons. St. Louis: JB Lippincott Co; 1993.

Photoallergy

Photoallergic reactions, which are immunologic, are most commonly caused by exposure to UV radiation. A drug or other chemical absorbs UV radiation. This combination is then acted upon by the immune system as an antigen, eliciting antibody formation. With future use of the drug and exposure to UV radiation, a hypersensitive immunologic response can occur. Usual reactions include erythema, edema, and warmth. Eczema may occur. Topical preparations cause more photoallergic responses than do systemic agents.

Phototoxicity

Phototoxicity is more common than photoallergy. Phototoxicity does not produce an immune response, so it may occur the first time an offending or precipitating drug is used. Such a reaction occurs within minutes to hours following exposure to UV radiation. An exaggerated erythema is seen. The effects are maximal within a few hours to a few days.

Patient Assessment

The cause, depth, and location of the burn; the BSA involved; and when the burn occurred should be taken into consideration. The degree of pain, as well as the presence of elevated body temperature and dehydration, should be assessed. If the cause of the burn is unclear, a careful drug history is important because drug photosensitivity or contact dermatitis may be implicated.

It is important to assess the depth of the burn correctly and to reassess it at 24–48 hours, when the true depth may become apparent.

Age should also be taken into account. Newborns, young children, and elderly people do not tolerate the effects of burns as well as young adults. Individuals with chronic illnesses, such as diabetes, cardiovascular disease, alcoholism, renal disease, or immunosuppression are more likely to develop complications than normal persons.

The pharmacist should feel confident in recommending treatment for minor first-degree burns that do not cover an extensive area and do not involve the eyes, ears, face, feet, or perineum, as well as for minor second-degree burns that cover less than 1% of the BSA. All burns greater than first degree should be evaluated by a physician to prevent complications, particularly infections. All second-degree burns covering a more extensive area should be referred to a physician. Extreme care should be taken when the burn is electrical, occurs by inhalation, or occurs in a high-risk patient. If the degree or severity of the burn is difficult to determine, the patient should be referred to a physician immediately.

Patients who have received burns to the genitalia, the perineum, and the eye are prone to more serious symptoms and complications. Facial burns may be associated with respiratory injuries due to inhalation. Burns of the hands and feet deserve special attention, not only because they are often quite painful but also because healing may be delayed in these areas, particularly in patients with a circulatory disorder. All such patients should be referred to a physician.

Self-Treatment of Minor Burns

The goals in treating first- and second-degree burns are to relieve pain associated with the burn, avoid tissue maceration, prevent dryness, and provide a favorable environment for healing.

Thermal Burns

Thermal burns include flame, heat, sun, and scald burns. The initial treatment of minor thermal burns is to cool the affected area in cool tap water for 10–30 minutes. This treatment may help prevent blister formation. If blisters form, medical referral should be made. Aspirin, ibuprofen, naproxen, or acetaminophen may be given to reduce pain.

Electrical Burns

The only visible signs of electrical burns may be the points of entrance and exit. The superficial extent of these points may mask extensive underlying tissue damage. Only when an electrical burn is very minor should self-medication be attempted.

Chemical Burns

In the case of chemical burns, any clothing on or near the affected area should be immediately removed. The affected area should be washed with tap water for 15 minutes to 2 hours until the offending agent has been removed. If the eye is involved, the eyelid should be pulled back and the eye irrigated with tap water for at least 15–30 minutes. The irrigation fluid should flow from the nasal side of the eye to the outside corner to prevent washing the contaminant into the other eye. The area poison information center should be contacted immediately for treatment guidelines. In most cases of chemical burns and chemical contact with the eye, medical attention should be sought as soon as possible.

Sunburn

Minor sunburn can be relieved with cool compresses or a cool bath. Nonprescription analgesics (e.g., aspirin, ibuprofen, naproxen, acetaminophen) are recommended for treatment of pain.

Heat stroke may occur with excessive exposure to sunlight in a hot or humid environment. Patients exhibiting hyperpyrexia, confusion, weakness, or convulsions should be referred to a physician immediately.

Cleansing of Burns

After cool moisture is applied to the burned area to help stop the progression of the burn injury, reduce local edema, and relieve pain, the area should be gently cleansed with water and a bland soap, such as a baby wash or a surfactant (e.g., Shur-Clens). Alcohol-containing preparations should not be used. A nonadherent, hypoallergenic dressing may be applied if the area is small; a skin protectant/lubricant may be applied if the burn is extensive. If the burn is weeping, soaking it in warm tap water three to six times a day for 15–30 minutes will provide a soothing effect and diminish the weeping.

Minor burns usually heal without additional treatment. For second-degree burns, once- or twice-daily cleansing to remove dead skin is recommended. Patients should be advised to avoid pulling at loose skin or peeling off the burned skin since viable skin may be removed in the process and healing delayed.

Dressings for Burns

The following is the recommended sequence for dressing a small burn (normally necessary only with second-degree burns):

■ A nonadherent primary layer of sterile, fine-mesh gauze lightly impregnated with sterile petrolatum should be applied over the burn.

- An absorbent intermediate layer of piled-up gauze should be applied over the petrolatum gauze. This layer should be applied loosely.

- A supportive layer of rolled gauze bandage should be applied over the primary and intermediate gauze layers to hold these layers in place and mildly restrict movement.

The dressing should be changed every 24–48 hours. If the dressing sticks to the wound, soaking in warm water will loosen it. The wound should be examined for signs of infection at each dressing change. The earliest signs of infection may be inflamed wound edges, new blistering, or intensified pain. If the affected skin begins to become macerated (i.e., if it feels or looks wet, wrinkled, or fissured), dressing the wound should be temporarily discontinued, and the wound should be exposed to air. Once the pain subsides and healing begins (usually in 4–10 days), wound dressings may be discontinued.

Pharmacologic Agents

Most first- and minor second-degree burns heal without complications. The purposes of pharmacotherapy are to make the patient more comfortable and to allow the skin to heal normally. The pharmacist should not recommend a product for extensive or deep second-, third-, or fourth-degree burns because this may cause the patient to delay seeking medical evaluation and treatment.

Protectants

Based on recommendations of its advisory panel, the Food and Drug Administration (FDA) has recognized the agents in Table 3 as safe and effective for the temporary protection of minor burns and sunburn. Skin protectants protect the burn from mechanical irritation and prevent drying.

Liver oils have been used for many years as folk remedies for wound healing. Shark liver oil contains a high concentration of vitamin A. Vitamin A and D ointment has been used to treat minor skin burns and abrasions. The FDA recommends that the restriction preventing the use of these products on children under 2 years of age be waived except for those products containing live yeast-cell derivatives, shark liver oil, and zinc acetate. The patient with minor burns may apply a skin protectant as often as needed. If the burn has not improved in 7 days or if it worsens, the patient should consult a physician immediately.

TABLE 3 Topical protectant agents used in the treatment of minor burns

Ingredient	Approved concentrations (%)
Allantoin	0.5–2
Cocoa butter	50–100
Petrolatum	30–100
Shark liver oil	3
White petrolatum	30–100

Adapted from *Federal Register.* 1983; 48: 6832.

Analgesics

Aspirin, naproxen, and ibuprofen may be used to alleviate the pain associated with minor burns. These drugs may decrease the erythema and edema in the burned area. For patients who cannot tolerate aspirin, naproxen, or ibuprofen, acetaminophen can provide pain relief.

The use of various systemic nonsteroidal anti-inflammatory drugs (NSAIDs) has been shown to decrease inflammation caused by exposure to UV radiation; however, this effect lasts only about 24 hours. The combined use of a topical corticosteroid and oral ibuprofen or another NSAID may produce more relief than either agent used alone.

Local Anesthetics

The pain of minor burns and sunburn can be attenuated by the judicious use of local anesthetics. The agents that the FDA has approved as safe and effective for the temporary relief of pain associated with minor burns are found in Table 4.

The higher concentrations of the local anesthetics are appropriate for burns in which the skin is intact; the lower concentrations are better for skin that has been broken.

Benzocaine produces a hypersensitivity reaction in about 1% of patients. This is a higher incidence than that seen with lidocaine. Benzocaine is essentially devoid of systemic toxicity. Systemic toxicities due to lidocaine are rare if the product is used on intact skin, on localized areas, and for short periods.

Local anesthetics should be applied no more than three or four times daily. Since their duration of action is short (15 to 45 minutes), continuous pain relief cannot be obtained with these agents. Local anesthetics should not be used to treat serious burns.

Topical Hydrocortisone

Although not FDA-approved for use in treating minor burns, 1% topical hydrocortisone is often used in the first-aid treatment of minor burns covering a small area. It should be used with caution if the skin is broken.

Antimicrobials

Antimicrobial therapy is crucial in major burns; however, nonprescription first-aid antibiotic or antiseptic drugs are of limited value, especially when the skin is intact. These drugs may be used on minor burns in which the skin has been broken. Preparations that may be used to help prevent infection in minor burns or sunburn are presented in Chapter 28.

Any patient in whom infection is evident or whose burn is so severe that a bacterial infection is likely should be referred to a physician immediately. Prophylactic application of a double or triple antibiotic ointment to minor burns should be done with caution; such use can aggravate burns should the patient develop a topical fungal infection or allergic contact dermatitis to one of the antibiotics.

Counterirritants

Although counterirritants such as camphor, menthol, and ichthammol are approved for use in minor burn treatment, they should not generally be used for such purposes because they may further irritate the already sensitized or damaged skin. The FDA is still evaluating these agents.

TABLE 4 Topical ingredients approved by the FDA in the treatment of minor burns

Types	Approved concentrations (%)
Amine and "caine"-type local anesthetics	
Benzocaine	5–20
Butamben picrate	1
Dibucaine	0.25–1
Dibucaine hydrochloride	0.25–1
Dimethisoquin hydrochloride	0.3–0.5
Dyclonine hydrochloride	0.5–1
Lidocaine	0.5–4
Lidocaine hydrochloride	0.5–4
Pramoxine hydrochloride	0.5–1
Tetracaine	1–2
Tetracaine hydrochloride	1–2
Alcohol and ketone counterirritants	
Benzyl alcohol	10–33
Camphor	0.1–3
Camphor	3–10.8[a]
Camphorated metacresol	
Camphor	3–10.8
Metacresol	1–5
Juniper tar	1–5
Menthol	0.1–1
Phenol	4.7[a]
Phenolate sodium	0.5–1.5
Resorcinol	0.5–3
Antihistamines	
Diphenhydramine hydrochloride	1–2
Tripelennamine hydrochloride	0.5–2

[a]When combined in a light mineral oil, USP vehicle. Adapted from *Federal Register*. 1983; 48: 5867–8.

Miscellaneous Agents

The ability of topical agents such as aloe vera, vitamin E, and shark liver oil to aid in the healing of minor burns and sunburn has not been substantiated. Neosporin Ointment, Silvadene Cream, and benzoyl peroxide lotion 10% and 20% have increased the rate of healing.

Product Selection Guidelines

An initial step in treating the patient with a minor burn is to recommend the short-term administration of an oral analgesic, preferably one with anti-inflammatory activity, such as aspirin, naproxen, or ibuprofen. If the patient cannot tolerate these agents, acetaminophen would be a short-term alternative. Aspirin, naproxen, or ibuprofen may be especially beneficial in the patient with mild sunburn.

If a local anesthetic or topical hydrocortisone is appropriate therapy, the pharmacist should recommend the most appropriate products.

Ointments provide a protective film that impedes the evaporation of water from the wound area. If the skin is broken, an ointment may not be appropriate. Creams allow some fluid to pass through the film, so they provide less of a medium for bacterial growth and are best applied to broken skin. Creams are also less messy and easier to apply than ointments. To prevent contamination of the preparation, ointments and creams should not be applied directly onto the burns from the container.

Lotions can be easily spread and may be more easily applied when the area of the burn is large. Lotions that produce a powdery cover should not be used on a burn. They tend to dry the area, are difficult to remove, and provide a medium for bacterial growth under the caked particles.

Aerosol and pump sprays are more costly than other topical dosage forms. Sprays offer the advantage of precluding the need to touch the injured area, so there is less pain associated with applying the medication. Sprays are not usually protective in that the aerosol is typically water- or alcohol-based and will evaporate.

CHAPTER 32

Poison Ivy, Oak, and Sumac Products

Questions to ask in patient assessment and counseling

- How long have you had the rash?
- Where is the rash? How extensive is it?
- Would you describe the rash or affected skin?
- Do the skin lesions contain fluid? Are they oozing?
- Have you recently been camping, walking in the woods, or working in the garden?
- Have you ever had a rash from poison ivy, poison oak, or poison sumac?
- What treatments have you tried? Were they effective?
- Are you allergic to any medication or product ingredient?

Rhus dermatitis (a topical reaction caused by exposure to poison ivy, poison oak, or poison sumac) is often treated with nonprescription drugs. The condition may be acute or chronic, depending on the extent of the patient's exposure and the degree of the patient's sensitivity to the allergens.

Etiology

Causative Plants

Poison ivy (Figure 1), which grows as a shrub or trailing vine, is identified by its clusters of three lobe-shaped leaflets, each 3–15 cm long, and its white, ball-shaped berries that appear in the fall. It grows everywhere in the United States except at altitudes above 4000 feet and in Alaska, Hawaii, and the desert areas of California and Nevada. Poison oak (Figure 2) commonly appears as a bush or vine. The center leaf of the cluster resembles an oak leaf. Western poison oak grows along the Pacific Coast. Eastern poison oak is indigenous to regions from New Jersey to Florida and from central Texas to Kansas, growing primarily in sandy soil. Poison sumac (Figure 3), also known as poison dogwood or poison elder, has pointed, pale-green leaves that are about 10 cm long. A woody shrub or small tree, poison sumac is found in swamps and along ponds and streams of the southern and eastern United States.

The following discussions pertain to all three plants.

Allergenic Constituents

Toxicodendrol, a phenolic oily resin, is present in all the poisonous species and contains a complex active principle, urushiol. Urushiol is distributed in the roots, stems, leaves, and fruit of the plant, but not in the flowers, pollen, or epidermis. Contact with the intact epidermis of the plant is harmless; dermatitis occurs only after contact with a damaged plant or its sap.

Editor's Note: This chapter is adapted from Henry Wormser, "Poison Ivy, Oak, and Sumac Products," in Covington, T.R., ed., *Handbook of Nonprescription Drugs,* 11th edition. For a more extensive discussion of this topic, readers are encouraged to consult Chapter 32 of the *Handbook.*

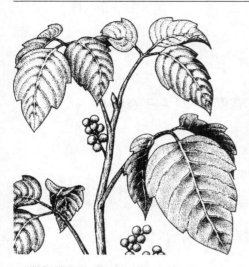

FIGURE 1 Poison ivy.

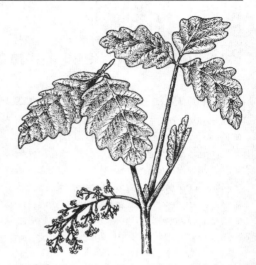

FIGURE 2 Poison oak.

Direct contact with the plant is not necessary; contact may be made with the allergens via an article that injured the plant or via soot particles that contain allergenic material from the plant. The highest incidence of dermatitis occurs in spring and summer. The urushiol may remain active for months on tools, sports equipment, shoes, and clothing, especially in a dry atmosphere. Stroking a pet whose fur is contaminated is a common cause of allergic reaction.

The dermatitis cannot be contracted through the air unless the plants are burned. Smoke from burning plants carries a substantial amount of the oleoresin and may cause serious external and systemic reactions. Inhalation may produce severe trauma to the oral and nasal mucosa and lung tissue.

Mechanism of Contact Dermatitis

Contact dermatitis has two phases: a *sensitization* phase, during which a specific hypersensitivity to the allergen is acquired, and an *elicitation* phase, during which subsequent contact with the allergen elicits a visible dermatologic response.

The degree of hypersensitivity to the toxic agent varies. Dark-skinned people seem less susceptible than light-skinned individuals. Young people are more susceptible than the elderly, and newborns are readily sensitized. The interval between contact with the allergen and appearance of symptoms varies. Reaction time is usually 2–3 days but not less than 12 hours.

Dermatologic lesions vary from simple maculae to vesicles and bullae. Fluid in the vesicles and bullae is not antigenic. Premature bursting of the vesicles may lead to secondary bacterial infection.

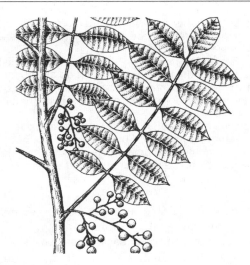

FIGURE 3 Poison sumac.

Patient Assessment

Signs and Symptoms

All skin areas that come in contact with the allergen may be affected. Distribution of lesions may be erratic. The dermatitis may appear early in one area of the body and later in another. Linear streaking is common.

The initial reaction after exposure to the antigen is erythema or rash. The development of raised lesions follows, and finally, fluid accumulates in the raised lesions of the epidermis, forming vesicles and bullae. The initial lesions are usually marked by mild to intensive itching and burning. The affected area, often hot and swollen, oozes, dries, and crusts. Secondary bacterial infections may occur. The rash is not photoactivated. Most cases disappear in 14–20 days.

Treatment

Preventive Measures

People should learn to recognize and avoid poison ivy and related plants. They should observe the terrain carefully when hiking and choosing a picnic area or campsite. Susceptible individuals should wear protective clothing when exposure to the offending agents is probable. After an outing, they should launder their clothing with a detergent and hot water. They should also wash with alcohol or another suitable organic solvent any object that may have come in contact with the plants.

When a poisonous plant is in a garden or yard, it should be destroyed chemically or removed physically. Herbicide sprays may be used any time the plant is in full leaf. Spraying should begin no later than mid-August because the plants begin to go dormant then and the herbicides are ineffective. At least three to four sprayings at intervals of 2–8 weeks are necessary.

Pulling up the plants by the roots may sometimes be the only satisfactory method of removal. Regardless of the removal method chosen, individuals should wear protective gear. Roots, stems, and leaves should be buried.

Once contact with poison ivy is made, the antigen enters the skin rapidly. Thorough washing with an alkaline soap or organic solvents such as alcohol or acetone within 5–10 minutes of exposure is necessary to prevent absorption of the antigen. Another topical preventive measure is the application of barrier creams prior to contact; however, many clinicians question their effectiveness.

Although anecdotal claims have been made for zirconium oxide, tests have found it to be ineffective for preventing the dermatitis. Some success has been obtained with some formulations of organoclay (a quaternary ammonium salt of bentonite), polyamine salts of linoleic acid dimer (Stokoguard), and a product marketed under the name Ivy Shield.

Topical Treatment

Simplicity and safety are key elements of treatment. In most cases, the contact dermatitis is self-resolving. Objectives of therapy are to:

■ Protect the damaged tissue until the acute reaction has subsided;

■ Prevent excessive accumulation of debris and complications resulting from oozing, scaling, and crusting, without disturbing normal tissue; and

■ Relieve itching and thus prevent scratching, excoriation, and secondary bacterial infection.

Mild Dermatitis

Linear streaks of papules and vesicles characterize mild rhus dermatitis. They can be treated by an antipruritic lotion such as calamine or zinc oxide. A combination of 1% menthol and equal parts of calamine, zinc oxide, and rubbing alcohol can be soothing.

Soaks, baths, or wet dressings can also be effective in soothing pain and itching. A diluted (1:40) aluminum acetate solution (Burow's solution), saline solution, or sodium bicarbonate solution can be used for 30 minutes, three or four times a day. The application of warm or very cold water may provide relief. Parents of children with rhus dermatitis should clip their child's fingernails. Good hygiene will help prevent secondary infections.

Use of topical preparations containing local anesthetics or antihistamines is controversial because of their sensitizing capabilities. Nonprescription topical steroids such as hydrocortisone have proven safe and effective for mild dermatitis. Greasy ointments should not be used when vesicles are oozing.

Moderately Severe Dermatitis

Moderately severe rhus dermatitis is characterized by bullae and edematous swelling in addition to the papules and vesicles present in milder cases. Large bullae may be drained by a trained medical professional. Application of cool compresses of Burow's solution (1:10) to edematous areas may be helpful.

Facial lesions can be treated by wet dressings. If the eyelids are affected, cold compresses of a dilute boric acid solution can be used. Lotions should be avoided because they tend to cake. Shaving, although uncomfortable, prevents accumulation of crust and debris in the beard.

During the healing phase, application of a soothing cream helps prevent crusting, scaling, and thickening of the lesions. Any cream that is recommended should be of neutral pH.

Tepid tub baths using oatmeal or a commercially available colloidal preparation may be soothing. Because these preparations make the bathtub slick, patients who use them should be warned to place a nonskid mat in the tub. They also should be reminded to follow the package instructions carefully.

Severe Dermatitis

A patient experiencing a widespread reaction over the body that is associated with major swelling or eye involvement should be referred to a physician. Topical treatment of severe rhus dermatitis is similar to that recommended for moderately severe dermatitis. Systemic treatment usually involves prescription drugs such as anti-inflammatory steroids. Corticosteroids are administered orally over 7 days to 3 weeks in a gradually descending dosage schedule. Pharmacists must counsel patients to adhere to the directions and complete the entire course of therapy.

Oral antihistamines may be useful for their systemic antipruritic effects. However, their anticholinergic side effects could exacerbate preexisting conditions of patients who have prostatic hypertrophy, narrow-angle glaucoma, stenosing peptic ulcer, bladder neck obstruction, and a tendency toward constipation. Histamine plays only a minor role in contact dermatitis allergic reactions, so the benefits of these agents may be less than the risks.

Pharmacologic Agents

Four types of agents—local anesthetics, antipruritics, antiseptics, and astringents—are used as topical nonprescription products for rhus dermatitis.

Local Anesthetics

Benzocaine and pramoxine hydrochloride are the most common local anesthetics found in nonprescription products for rhus dermatitis. Poorly soluble local anesthetics (e.g., benzocaine) are less likely to be absorbed and to produce systemic toxicity than are more soluble local anesthetics (e.g., tetracaine hydrochloride). Regardless of the agent selected, the high serum concentrations necessary to produce systemic toxicity are difficult to achieve with nonprescription topical anesthetics. If a contact dermatitis worsens after the topical application of a local anesthetic, the affected area should be washed thoroughly, and use of the anesthetic should be discontinued.

Antipruritics

Antihistamines

Antihistamines such as diphenhydramine (Benadryl) relieve itching and produce a mild local anesthetic effect. The topical use of antihistamines does not produce anticholinergic adverse effects or systemic toxicity. Antihistamines may act as sensitizers and aggravate a contact dermatitis.

Antihistamines are more effective as antipruritics when taken orally, particularly when itching is generalized. An individual who is sensitized to a topical agent should not take it orally.

Counterirritants

Low concentrations of these drugs (i.e., 0.1%), particularly menthol, relieve irritation by the depression of cutaneous receptors. Other counterirritants include phenol and camphor.

Hydrocortisone

The effectiveness of topical corticosteroids on rhus dermatitis is acknowledged by the FDA. Short-term use of 0.5%–1% hydrocortisone is unlikely to exacerbate cutaneous bacterial, fungal, or viral infections, and allergic reactions to hydrocortisone at these concentrations are rare. Prolonged administration does not appear to cause toxic effects by systemic absorption, even when applied to large areas of damaged or abraded skin.

Recommended dosage for adults and children 2 years of age and above is 1% hydrocortisone applied to the affected area three or four times a day. Children under 2 years of age should be treated only under supervision of a physician.

Antiseptics

Antiseptics in products for rhus dermatitis are intended for prophylaxis against secondary bacterial infections. Their effectiveness is questionable. Of the available antiseptics (e.g., phenols, alcohols, oxidizing agents) and quaternary ammonium compounds (e.g., benzalkonium chloride), the latter seem to be more effective.

Astringents

Astringents (e.g., witch hazel, aluminum acetate, tannic acid, zinc and iron oxides) are used to stop oozing, reduce inflammation, and promote healing.

Burow's solution is diluted with water to produce a 1:10 or 1:40 solution and used as a wet dressing three or four times a day. Therapy may be continued for 5–7 days. Continuous or prolonged use may be inflammatory. The pharmacist should make sure that the patient understands how to dilute Burow's solution.

Zinc oxide lotion (15%–25%) has mild astringent, protective, and antiseptic actions. Because of its color, calamine plus zinc oxide is often preferred over zinc oxide alone.

Product Selection Guidelines

Although patients with severe rhus dermatitis should be referred to a physician, mild to moderately severe cases can usually be self-treated. Systemic use of antihistamines may be combined with application of topical agents to relieve itching. Preparations that contain benzocaine or other local anesthetics should be used with caution.

Lotions, which may contain phenol or menthol, provide prompt relief from itching. The pharmacist should caution against their frequent or excessive use. They pile layers of material on the skin, which may produce discomfort and can be difficult to remove.

The pharmacist should inform individuals who are sensitive to toxicodendron plants that certain cosmetics, hair dyes, bleaches, and other topical commercial products contain compounds related to 3-PDC and could cause cross-sensitivity. Such patients should reduce their use of these products.

CHAPTER 33

Insect Sting and Bite Products

Questions to ask in patient assessment and counseling

- How extensive are the bites or stings?
- Is the reaction limited to the site of the bite or sting?
- Have you developed hives, excessive swelling, dizziness, vomiting, or difficulty in breathing since being bitten or stung?
- Have you ever been previously stung by a honeybee, wasp, or hornet?
- Have you previously had severe reactions to insect bites or stings?
- Have you ever consulted a physician because of a bite or sting?
- What, if anything, have you tried so far to treat the reaction?
- Have you ever had adverse reactions to topically applied products?
- Do you have a personal or family history of allergic reactions such as hay fever?
- If a child, what is the patient's age and approximate weight?

For about 90% of Americans, reactions to insect stings or bites are mild and local in nature. About 1% of the population is allergic to the insect venom. For them, the reaction can be severe and possibly life-threatening.

Biting Insects and Arachnids

Insects such as mosquitoes, fleas, bedbugs, lice, and arachnids such as ticks and chiggers (red bugs) insert their biting organs into the skin to feed by sucking blood from their hosts. In sensitive individuals, the salivary secretions, which contain antigenic substances, produce local erythematous, itching papules with central puncta.

Mosquitoes

Mosquitoes are found worldwide, particularly in humid, warm climates. Although they usually attack exposed parts of the body, they can bite through thin clothing.

Fleas

Fleas are tiny (1.5–4 mm long), bloodsucking, wingless, parasites with strongly developed posterior legs used for leaping. Fleas parasitize various avian and mammalian hosts. Most people are bitten about the legs and ankles; bites usually are multiple and grouped. Each lesion is characterized by an erythematous region around the puncture and causes intense itching.

Editor's Note: This chapter is adapted from Farid Sadik, "Insect Sting and Bite Products," in Covington, T.R., ed., *Handbook of Nonprescription Drugs,* 11th edition. For a more extensive discussion of insect stings and bites and the products used to treat them, readers are encouraged to consult Chapter 33 of the *Handbook.*

Bedbugs

Bedbugs have a short head and a broad, flat body (4–5 mm long and 3 mm wide). The reaction to a bedbug bite may range from irritation at the site of the bite to a small dermal hemorrhage.

Bedbugs deposit their eggs in crevices of walls, floors, bedding, and furniture. They normally hide during the day and become active at night. Persons may be bitten in subdued light while sitting in theaters or other public places.

Lice

Lice are wingless parasites with well-developed legs. They do not jump or fly. Each leg has a claw that helps the louse cling firmly to hair or clothing fibers while sucking blood. The host may receive hundreds of bites each day. The bites produce papular dermatitis and cause the host to scratch constantly.

Lice infestations (pediculosis) in the United States are common. Three types of lice infest humans: head lice, body lice, and pubic lice.

Head Lice

Head lice is the most common lice infestation. The majority of cases involve children. Outbreaks are common in crowded places such as schools, day care centers, and nursing homes.

Transmission of head lice occurs directly through physical contact with an infested individual or indirectly through the sharing of articles such as combs, towels, and hats. Awareness and action by health officials, school authorities, and parents are essential in stopping the spread of lice. Pharmacists can obtain information on safe treatments and preventive measures for head lice from the National Pediculosis Association, PO Box 610189, Newton, MA 02161; 617-449-NITS.

Assessment of Head Lice. Head lice may be assessed by examining the hair for nits, nymphs, or crawling adults. Examination is best done under strong light; a magnifying glass may be used. Parting the hair with a comb or with fingers protected by gloves may reveal the nits.

Scratching the irritation may result in excoriation of the scalp tissue and, possibly, a secondary bacterial or fungal infection.

Treatment of Head Lice. A 1% permethrin cream rinse is the drug of choice for treating head lice in adults and in children 2 years of age and older. Before permethrin cream rinse is applied, the hair should be shampooed with regular shampoo, rinsed, and dried. Approximately 25–30 mL of the undiluted liquid is then applied to saturate the hair and scalp and allowed to remain for 10 minutes. Next, the medication is rinsed out with water, and the hair is towel dried. A special comb, included in the package, may be used to remove the nits and nits' shells. The main adverse reaction to permethrin is transient pruritus, burning, stinging, and irritation to the scalp. Permethrin should not be used on infants under 2 years of age or on individuals who are sensitive to pyrethroid, pyrethrin, or chrysanthemums.

Pyrethrins are insecticides. A combination of pyrethrins (0.17%–0.33%) with piperonyl butoxide (2%–4%) in a nonaerosol product formulation has been generally recognized as safe and effective by the Food and Drug Administration (FDA) in its tentative final monograph. The medication is applied to the infested area and allowed to remain in place for 10 minutes; it is then thoroughly washed out with warm water. Pyrethrins rarely produce adverse reactions; however, contact with eyes and mucous membranes should be avoided.

Prescription products used for head lice include gamma benzene hexachloride and malathion.

Body Lice

Body lice live and lay their eggs in clothing, particularly in the seams and folds of underclothing. Infestations occur in individuals who do not change clothing frequently. These insects are larger than head lice. Diagnosis can be made by identifying the adult lice and nits in the seams of clothing. Intense body itching and scratching should also provide a clue to the presence of an infestation.

Treatment of body lice is similar to that of head lice. However, body lice may be eradicated by measures other than medications. Washing clothing with hot water (125°F [52°C]) or disinfecting them with dry cleaning is effective. Changing clothing and underclothing daily, as well as bathing daily, should then rid the body of the lice. To relieve itching, an antipruritic lotion may be applied.

Pubic Lice

Pubic lice, commonly called crab lice because of their crablike appearance, may be encountered in all persons, including those with high standards of hygiene. An infestation is identified by the presence of the parasite and its nits. Pubic lice may also infest armpits and occasionally eyelashes, mustaches, beards, and eyebrows. They may be transmitted through sexual contact, toilet seats, or shared undergarments and sheets. Treatment is similar to that of head lice.

Sarcoptes scabiei

Scabies, commonly called "the itch," is a contagious parasitic skin infestation caused by Sarcoptes scabiei, a very small and rarely seen arachnid mite. It burrows beneath the stratum corneum but neither bites nor stings. Characterized by secondary inflammation and intense itching, this infestation is associated with poor hygiene, crowded conditions, and venereal disease. Scabies is transmitted through bodily contact with an infested host, clothing, or bed linen. It is possible to acquire scabies from a toilet seat. The most common infestation sites are the interdigital spaces of the fingers, the flexor surface of the wrists, the male genitalia, the buttocks, and the anterior axillary folds. The head and neck are not affected, except in infants. When the mite first burrows in the skin, there is no local reaction; within a month, however, sensitization begins. Intense itching occurs, especially at night, at the infestation site. Unrestrained scratching may cause secondary bacterial infections. Diagnosis may be made by identifying the mite under a microscope and the burrow in the skin. The burrow is visible to the naked eye and appears as a narrow, dark line on a raised bump or blister.

Scabies may be controlled by using 25% benzyl benzoate lotion, 1% gamma benzene hexachloride cream or lotion, or 10% crotamiton lotion or cream. Nonprescription 5% permethrin cream is also effective. Before applying the medication, the patient should bathe and vigorously scrub the infested area. The preparation should then be applied to the entire body except the face and should remain in place for a specified period of time, after which the patient should bathe again. A second application is usually unnecessary. Clothing and bedding of infested individuals should be washed in hot water. Since the incubation period of scabies is delayed, it is recommended that other members of the household undergo treatment.

Ticks and Lyme Disease

Ticks are parasites that feed on the blood of humans and of wild and domesticated animals. The local reaction to tick bites consists of itching papules, which disappear within 1 week.

Ticks should be removed from the skin intact by using fine tweezers. If fingers are used, they should be protected by gloves and washed afterwards. Fingernail polish or mineral oil may be applied on the tick to facilitate its removal.

The deer tick, which is responsible for Lyme disease, lives in wooded areas and parasitizes white-tailed deer (the primary carrier), mice, dogs, squirrels, and other mammals. It is one eighth of an inch in diameter.

Most acute stages of the infection are heralded by a skin rash and flulike symptoms. The rash appears as a papule at the bite site and may become an enlarged circle with a clear center, referred to as a "bull's eye." The infection then gradually spreads. The lesions are usually urticarial and tender. They appear 3–30 days after the bite and disappear spontaneously within 3–4 weeks. The flulike symptoms include fever, headache, fatigue, muscle and joint pain, and, in severe cases, conjunctivitis.

Lyme disease can be diagnosed by studying the medical history of the patient and by laboratory examinations. Prompt treatment of Lyme disease can prevent neurologic, cardiac, and rheumatologic manifestations. It is treated with antibiotics (e.g., tetracyclines, amoxicillin, cephalosporins).

Lyme disease can be prevented by avoiding areas that may be infested with deer ticks; applying insect repellent containing *N,N*-diethyl-*m*-toluamide (DEET) on the skin as well as on shoe tops and socks; applying the pesticide permethrin on clothes; and treating pets regularly with insecticides.

Chiggers

Chiggers, or red bugs, cause cellular disintegration of the affected area, a red papule, and intense itching. Chiggers are prevalent in the southern United States mainly during summer and fall. Chigger infestation may be prevented by using insect repellent and wearing protective clothing. Bathing immediately after exposure is helpful. Removing brush, mowing grass, and spraying the area with lawn pest insecticide are also useful. Treatment consists of antipruritic topical medications.

Stinging Insects

Stinging insects belonging to the order Hymenoptera are most often responsible for insect sting hypersensitivity. They include honeybees, bumblebees, paper wasps, yellow jackets, hornets, fire ants, and harvester ants. Death from an insect sting is usually due to allergic hypersensitivity, which can lead to an anaphylactic reaction within 5–30 minutes after the sting.

Some ants only bite; others bite and sting simultaneously. Fire ants are now found in the southern and western United States. They live in underground colonies, forming large raised mounds. Fire ants are considered a health hazard. Their sting causes intense itching, burning (hence the name), vesiculation, necrosis, and anaphylactic reaction in hypersensitive persons.

It appears that there is very limited or no cross-sensitivity between the venom of fire ants and that of bees, wasps, hornets, and yellow jackets.

Reactions to Insect Bites and Stings

An insect bite or sting is an injury to the skin caused by penetration of the biting or stinging organ of an insect. The reactions are produced mainly by substances contained in the saliva of biting insects or in the venom of stinging insects. The aftereffects vary according to the degree of exposure and hypersensitivity.

Insect Bites

Reactions to biting insects are usually local and vary in intensity. Wheal formation, erythema, papular reaction, and itching are characteristic reactions to mosquito bites. The lesions may have a rapid or slow onset and may persist for weeks. Hypersensitivity to mosquito bites aggravated by scratching causes papule and nodule formations that may persist and lead to secondary infections such as impetigo, furunculosis, or infectious eczematoid dermatitis. Systemic reactions such as fever and malaise may occur.

Insect Stings

Reactions may be divided into three categories: local, unusual, and anaphylactic.

Local Reactions

Most allergic reactions to insect stings are cutaneous and local. They include erythema, pruritus, urticaria (hives), or angioedema. Symptoms last from several hours to several days. Swelling may cover an extensive area.

Unusual Reactions

Neurologic reactions, renal involvement, serum sickness reactions, encephalopathy, and delayed hypersensitivity skin reactions have been reported. The mechanisms for these reactions have not been elucidated.

Anaphylactic Reactions

The most serious sequelae from stings are systemic anaphylactic reactions. These reactions are immunologically mediated and usually occur within 15 minutes after the sting. In severe cases, hypotension, laryngeal edema, bronchospasm, and respiratory distress may occur, leading to a shocklike state. If these reactions are not treated promptly, death may ensue. Less common anaphylactic reactions may produce nausea, vomiting, or diarrhea.

Treatment of Systemic Reactions

For local reactions, a nonprescription product that minimizes scratching by relieving discomfort, itching, and pain may be recommended. Nonprescription drugs are of no value in systemic reactions; such cases are considered medical emergencies.

The pharmacist should advise hypersensitive individuals of the following:

- If symptomatic, the victim must seek medical attention immediately after an insect sting or bite.
- Basic first aid, such as applying ice to the sting and removing the stinger, is helpful.
- Emergency kits for insect stings are available by prescription. Kits containing epinephrine are preferable to those containing antihistamines for treating allergic reactions.
- Receiving injections of venom extract for protection against systemic reactions (desensitization) is useful.
- Insect repellents are not effective against stinging insects.

First Aid

Prompt application of ice packs to the sting site helps slow absorption and reduce itching, swelling, and pain. The benefits of prompt removal of the honeybee's stinger and venom sac, which usually are left in the skin, should be explained, particularly to allergic individuals. The sac should not be squeezed; rubbing, scratching, or grasping it releases more venom. Scraping the stinger with tweezers or a fingernail minimizes the venom flow. After the stinger is removed, an antiseptic should be applied.

Emergency Kits

Emergency kits for individuals hypersensitive to insect stings are available by prescription. In addition to tweezers for removing the honeybee stinger, the typical kit includes epinephrine hydrochloride and antihistamines. Kits containing autoinjectable epinephrine syringes are also available. Kits must be stored in the dark at room temperature. A kit should not be left in the glove compartment of a car, where heat may become excessive.

Epinephrine Hydrochloride

Epinephrine hydrochloride (1:1000) injection is used to counteract the bronchoconstriction associated with anaphylaxis. It should be administered subcutaneously immediately after stinging. Some insect sting emergency kits have a preloaded (0.3-mL) sterile syringe. Generally, a 0.25-mL dose is injected subcutaneously. After 15 minutes, another dose is injected if necessary. For individuals with cardiovascular disease, diabetes, hypertension, or hyperthyroidism, the injection should be administered with caution.

Antihistamines

Although they are slow in onset of action and may be ineffective in severe reactions, antihistamines often are used in conjunction with epinephrine hydrochloride. They are administered orally or parenterally.

Preventive Measures

Avoidance of Exposure

Individuals who are hypersensitive to insect stings should take precautions to avoid exposure to these insects. Foods and odors attract insects; therefore, outdoor activities such as picnicking should be engaged in cautiously. Keeping food covered will help keep insects away. Shoes should always be worn outdoors. Perfumes and brightly colored clothes attract stinging insects and should not be worn outdoors. Destroying hives of stinging insects located in the vicinity of homes is recommended.

Venom Immunotherapy (Desensitization)

Hymenoptera venom, administered by subcutaneous injection, is used prophylactically to treat patients who have had reactions to stings. Patients should be advised that if they stop the immunotherapy, they may again be at high risk for anaphylaxis following a sting.

Nonprescription Pharmacologic Agents

External Analgesics/Antipruritics

This category includes agents with analgesic activity derived from the stimulation of cutaneous sensory receptors (counterirritants), the depression of cutaneous sensory receptors (anesthetics and antihistamines), and the reduction of inflammation (hydrocortisone). These agents are considered safe and effective when used as recommended for adults and children over 2 years of age. They are not recommended for children under 2 years of age except under the advice or supervision of a physician.

Counterirritants

Counterirritants reduce pain and itching by stimulating cutaneous sensory receptors to provide a feeling of warmth, coolness, or milder pain, which obscures the more severe pain of the injury. The activity of these agents depends on the concentration.

Camphor. At concentrations of 3%–11%, camphor stimulates cutaneous receptors and therefore acts as a counterirritant. Camphor is safe and effective for use as an external analgesic at these concentrations when applied to the affected area no more than three or four times a day. Camphor-containing products can be very dangerous if ingested. Patients should be warned to keep them out of the reach of children and to contact a physician or poison control center immediately if ingestion is suspected.

Cresol. Camphor complex (camphorated metacresol) is not classified by the FDA as effective in treating insect bites and stings.

Ichthammol. The effectiveness of ichthammol for insect stings is difficult to assess in concentrations used in nonprescription products.

Menthol. Menthol is considered a safe and effective antipruritic when applied to the affected area in concentrations of 0.1%–1%.

Methyl Salicylate. Methyl salicylate stimulates cutaneous receptors when used in concentrations of 10%–60%.

Peppermint and Clove Oils. Applied externally, peppermint and clove oils act as mild counterirritants.

Local Anesthetics

Benzocaine and dibucaine are safe and effective when used according to label directions in persons 2 years of age and older. Any dermatitis that may occur is caused by frequent contact, and patients should be warned against continued applications for prolonged periods.

Benzocaine. The concentrations of benzocaine available in nonprescription products range from 5% to 20%. It is applied to the affected area no more than three or four times a day.

Cyclomethycaine Sulfate. The FDA concluded that cyclomethycaine sulfate is safe but that available data are insufficient to permit final classification of its effectiveness for use as a nonprescription external analgesic.

Dibucaine. Although in the same class as benzocaine, dibucaine products carry additional labeling warning patients not to use them in large quantities, particularly over raw surfaces or blistered areas. This is because convulsions, myocardial depression, and death have been reported from systemic absorption. The recommended dosage is a 0.25%–1% solution applied to the affected area no more than three or four times a day.

Phenol. Phenol is considered safe and effective when applied to the affected area no more than three or four times a day in concentrations of 0.5%–1.5% for adults and children 2 years of age and older. Higher concentrations are irritating and may cause skin sloughing. The product should not be applied to extensive areas of the body or under compresses or bandages.

Ammonium Hydroxide and Trimethanolamine. These agents have been claimed to have a neutralizing effect on insect bites and stings. The FDA regards ammonium hydroxide as Category I.

Antihistamines

Topical antihistamines relieve pain and itching by depressing cutaneous sensory receptors. They are not absorbed in sufficient quantities to cause systemic side effects, even when applied to damaged skin. However, antihistamines are capable of producing hypersensitivity reactions.

Use of any of these agents over 3–4 weeks increases the possibility of allergic contact dermatitis. Their antipruritic action over a period of time is questionable. The FDA recommends that these agents be used for no longer than 7 days except under the advice of a physician. They are not recommended for children under 2 years of age.

Diphenhydramine. Products containing diphenhydramine are Category I in concentrations of 1%–2% and may be applied three or four times a day.

Tripelennamine. Tripelennamine in concentrations of 0.55%–2% may be applied three or four times a day.

Hydrocortisone

Hydrocortisone relieves pain and itching by reducing inflammation. Preparations containing hydrocortisone in concentrations of up to 1% are considered safe and effective for nonprescription use. They should be applied three or four times a day for adults and children 2 years of age and older. Patients should be warned against using topically applied hydrocortisone if they have scabies, tinea, bacterial infections, and moniliasis.

Aspirin

The FDA concluded that aspirin is safe, but available data are insufficient to permit final classification of its effectiveness for use as a nonprescription external analgesic. Aspirin possesses no direct topical anesthetic activity.

Skin Protectants

Agents in this category include aluminum acetate (2.5%–5%), glycerin, hamamelis water (witch hazel), zinc oxide, and calamine.

Antibacterials

The most commonly used antibacterial agents in nonprescription products for insect stings and bites are benzalkonium chloride, benzethonium chloride, and methylbenzethonium chloride. These compounds, which are included to prevent and treat secondary infection that may result from scratching, are classified as safe and effective.

Insect Repellents

The vapor of insect repellents discourages the approach of insects and prevent them from alighting.

The best all-purpose repellent is *N,N*-diethyl-*m*-toluamide, commonly called DEET. Use of products containing DEET is discouraged in children under 2 years of age because of possible toxicity to the central nervous system. Ethohexadiol dimethyl phthalate, dimethyl ethyl hexanediol carbate, and butopyronoxyl are effective repellents. A mixture of two or more of these repellents is more effective against a greater variety of insects than is a single repellent. Local reactions to the application of insect repellents have been reported.

Repellents may be toxic if taken internally. People who are sensitive to these chemicals may develop skin reactions. Repellents cause smarting when they are applied to broken skin or mucous membranes. They should be applied carefully around the eyes. Permethrin may be used as a clothing spray for protection against mosquitoes and ticks.

The FDA's final rule on insect repellents for nonprescription oral use in humans indicates that these products are not recognized as safe and effective and are misbranded.

Product Selection Guidelines

It is important to determine what symptoms appeared following the sting or bite, how soon the symptoms appeared, how severe the symptoms are, and what other drugs are being used.

Nonprescription products are of minimal value to hypersensitive individuals. The pharmacist should record all information on such individuals and recommend that the person wear a tag or carry a card showing the nature of their allergy. If the symptoms are minor, an appropriate nonprescription product may be recommended. Topical lotions, creams, ointments, and sprays are the main nonprescription product forms used for symptomatic relief of local reactions to insect stings and bites. The main considerations in product selection are reducing the possibility of additional stings or bites, protecting the affected skin, preventing secondary infection, and relieving itching and irritation. The pharmacist may also advise patients of several nonpharmacologic measures to relieve itching and irritation:

■ Avoid wearing rough and irritating clothing, especially wool, over the affected area;

■ Avoid using strong or highly perfumed and harsh detergents;

■ Apply an occlusive skin protectant to the affected area after bathing;

■ Bathe in cool (never warm) water for 10–20 minutes; and

■ Avoid scratching the affected area and keep fingernails trimmed short and filed smooth.

Although they are capable of producing topical or systemic adverse reactions, external analgesics and antipruritics are relatively safe and effective for adults and children 2 years of age and older. They should be applied no more than three or four times a day. Children under 2 years of age should use these products only under supervision of a physician. Patients should be instructed that if the condition worsens or symptoms persist for more than 7 days, they should discontinue use of these products and consult a physician.

CHAPTER 34

Foot Care Products

Questions to ask in patient assessment and counseling

General Foot Conditions

- *Where is the sore located (on or between the toes or on the sole of the foot)? Is the toenail involved?*
- *Is there any redness, itching, blistering, oozing, scaling, or bleeding from the lesion?*
- *Is the condition painful? Is it too uncomfortable to walk? Do your feet hurt or ache at the end of the day?*
- *During which activities do you notice the pain?*
- *How long have you had the problem? Did it develop gradually?*
- *Did the problem begin with the use of new shoes, socks, or soap?*
- *Do your shoes seem tighter than they have been in the past? Do they feel particularly tight at the end of the day?*
- *Can you associate the symptom with a particular type/pair of shoe(s)?*
- *Have you tried to treat this problem yourself? If so, how?*
- *Did you see your physician about this problem? If so, what did he or she tell you to do? What have you done? Did it help?*
- *Do your feet sweat a lot? Do you notice an odor when you take off your shoes? Do your feet sweat more when you wear socks or hosiery made of nylon or other synthetic material?*
- *Do you have allergies, asthma, or skin problems?*
- *What is your occupation?*
- *Have you recently increased repetitive weight-bearing activity? Do you plan to continue this activity?*
- *Do you have a history of a fracture, dislocation, or surgery in the legs or feet?*
- *Did you wear corrective shoes or braces on your legs or feet as a child?*
- *Did you ever injure your foot? If so, do the current symptoms seem to be related to the prior injury?*
- *How often and in what manner do you trim your toenails?*
- *Is a physician treating you for any medical condition, such as diabetes, heart trouble, or circulatory problems?*
- *Do you take insulin? What prescription or nonprescription medications, if any, do you take on a routine basis?*
- *Have you ever had vascular surgery or been treated for circulatory problems?*

Editor's Note: This chapter is adapted from Nicholas G. Popovich and Gail D. Newton, "Foot Care Products," in Covington, T.R., ed., *Handbook of Nonprescription Drugs,* 11th edition, which is based, in part, on the chapter with the same title that appeared in the 10th edition but was written by Nicholas G. Popovich. For a more extensive discussion of specific foot conditions and their treatment, readers are encouraged to consult Chapter 34 of the *Handbook.*

- *Can a family member or other caregiver assist you with the recommended treatment?*
- *Do you participate in a regular exercise program such as jogging or aerobics?*

Foot Conditions Related to Running/Jogging

- *Is the discomfort worsening?*
- *Has the discomfort reached a constant level that continues to affect your running?*
- *Is the discomfort more frequent and severe while running? Is it present while not running?*
- *Is the discomfort causing you to compensate and develop additional injuries?*
- *Have attempts at self-treatment (e.g., new shoes, a change of running surface, a change in training intensity) failed to relieve the symptoms?*

Corns, Calluses, and Warts

Corns and Calluses

A corn (clavus) is a small, raised, sharply demarcated, hyperkeratotic lesion with a central core. It is yellowish-gray and ranges from a few millimeters to 1 cm or more in diameter. The base of the corn is on the skin surface; the apex points inward and presses on the nerve endings in the dermis, causing pain. Corns may be hard or soft. Hard corns occur on the surface of the toes and appear shiny. Soft corns are whitish thickenings of the skin that are usually found on the webs between the fourth and fifth toes. Hard corns (usually) and soft corns (less frequently) are caused by underlying bony prominences.

Pressure from tight-fitting shoes is the most frequent cause of pain from corns. The fifth toe is the usual site of a hard corn. Pain may be severe and sharp.

A callus may be broad based or have a central core with sharply circumscribed margins and diffuse thickening of the skin. It has indefinite borders and ranges from a few millimeters to several centimeters in diameter. It is usually raised and yellow, and it has a normal pattern of skin ridges on its surface. Calluses form on joints and weight-bearing areas, such as sides and soles of the feet.

Friction (caused by loose-fitting shoes or tight-fitting hosiery), walking barefoot, and structural biomechanical problems contribute to the development of calluses. Calluses are usually asymptomatic, causing pain only when pressure is applied.

Warts

Warts (verrucae) are common viral infections of the skin and mucous membranes. They are caused by human papillomaviruses (HPVs). The pharmacist should be aware that warts may be confused with more serious conditions, such as squamous cell carcinoma and deep fungal infections.

Warts have a rough, cauliflower-like appearance. They are slightly scaly, rough papules or nodules that appear alone or grouped. Various types of warts may appear at different sites on the body. Plantar warts (verrucae plantaris) are common on the soles of the feet. They may be confined to the weight-bearing areas of the foot (the sole of the heel, the great toe, the areas below the heads of the metatarsal bones, and the ball) or may occur in non–weight-bearing areas of the sole of the foot.

Plantar warts, if located on weight-bearing portions of the foot, are under constant pressure and are usually not raised above the skin surface. The wart itself is in the center of the lesion and is roughly circular, with a diameter of 0.5–3.0 cm. The surface is grayish and friable, and the surrounding skin is thick and heaped. Several warts may coalesce, giving the appearance of one large wart (mosaic wart).

Because of their smooth keratotic surfaces, calluses may resemble isolated plantar warts. However, unlike a callus, a plantar wart is tender with pressure and interrupts the footprint pattern. Optimally, a podiatrist or dermatologist will have the opportunity to assess the condition and make a differential diagnosis.

Susceptibility

Three criteria must be met for an individual to develop a wart:

■ The papillomavirus must be present.

■ There must be an open avenue such as an abrasion through which the virus can enter the skin.

■ The individual's immune system must be susceptible to the virus.

Immunodeficient patients (e.g., those maintained on systemic or topical glucocorticoids), once infected, develop widespread and highly resistant warts.

Warts are most common in children and young adults. Warts may spread by direct person-to-person contact, by autoinoculation to another body area, or indirectly through public shower floors or swimming pools. The incubation period is 1–20 months, with an average of 3–4 months.

Mechanism

Warts begin as minute, smooth-surfaced, skin-colored lesions that enlarge over time. Repeated irritation causes them to continue enlarging. Plantar warts are usually asymptomatic when small. However, if they are large or occur on the heel or ball of the foot, they may cause severe discomfort and limitation of function.

Warts are not usually permanent; approximately 30% clear spontaneously in 6 months, 65% clear in 2 years, and most warts clear in 5 years.

Evaluation

The pharmacist should ask questions such as those at the beginning of this chapter. In general, medical referral is indicated if:

■ Diabetes mellitus, a peripheral circulatory disease, or another medical condition for which the patient is already under a physician's care exists;

■ Hemorrhaging or oozing of purulent material occurs;

■ Corns and calluses indicate an anatomical defect or fault in body weight distribution;

■ Corns and calluses are extensive, painful, and debilitating;

■ Extensive warts exist at one site;

■ Proper self-medication for warts has been tried for an adequate period without success; or

■ The patient has a history of rheumatoid arthritis and complains of painful metatarsal heads or deviation of the great toe.

Self-treatment is appropriate if:

■ Chronic, debilitating diseases do not contraindicate the use of foot care products;

■ The patient is not diabetic;

■ The patient can follow directions for use of the products with no difficulty;

■ No concurrent medication (e.g., immunosuppressives) is being taken that contraindicates the use of these products;

- Corns and calluses are minor;
- Predisposing factors (e.g., ill-fitting footwear or hosiery) of corns and calluses are removed;
- Neither an anatomical defect nor faulty weight distribution is indicated by corns or calluses; and
- Plantar warts have not spread extensively.

Treatment

Pharmacologic Approaches

Corns and Calluses. Successful treatment of corns and calluses with nonprescription products depends on eliminating the causes: pressure and friction. This entails wearing well-fitting, nonbinding footwear that evenly distributes body weight. For anatomical foot deformities, orthopedic corrections must be made. Before beginning self-treatment, a patient should consult a doctor or a pharmacist.

In the final monograph for over-the-counter (OTC) drug products that remove corns and calluses, the Food and Drug Administration (FDA) recommends that only salicylic acid be categorized as safe and effective for this purpose. The monograph dictates that products containing salicylic acid in a plaster, pad, disk, or collodion vehicle must be classified as Category I.

Warts. Many practitioners recommend early and vigorous treatment of warts. Choice of treatment type depends on the location, size, and type of wart, and on the extent and number of lesions. It should also take into account the patient's age, immunologic status, and expected compliance with treatment. Other pretreatment considerations are the degree of pain, the inconvenience of treatment, and the risk of scarring.

No effective medication for curing warts is available, although topical agents and procedures can help in their removal and relieve the pain. Topical salicylic acid is the only drug that is safe and effective for self-treatment of common or plantar warts. However, the FDA recommended that the drug be labeled for treating *only* common and plantar warts. Painful plantar warts, as well as multiple flat warts, facial warts, periungual warts, and venereal warts, should be treated by a physician. Warts may reappear several months after they have been "cured."

Pharmacologic Agents

Salicylic Acid. Salicylic acid, the only nonprescription drug found by the FDA to be both safe and effective as a keratolytic agent for the treatment of corns, calluses, and plantar warts, is formulated in many strengths (Table 1).

Significant percutaneous absorption may occur when salicylic acid is applied over large body areas. Although occlusive vehicles can enhance such absorption, it is highly unlikely that salicylism will result during therapy with recommended dosages.

The patient should thoroughly wash and dry the affected area before applying the product. Soaking prior to using the product is no longer felt to be helpful. For corns and calluses, the solution is applied once or twice daily as needed for up to 14 days or until the corn or callus is removed. For warts, it is applied once or twice daily as needed for up to 12 weeks or until the wart is removed. For all three conditions, the product is applied one drop at a time until the affected area is well covered. It is suggested that the patient keep the adjacent healthy skin dry and clean, and that the collodion film be peeled away every 2 or 3 days to remove keratotic debris.

Salicylic acid may also be delivered to the skin through a plaster disc or pad. This system provides direct and prolonged contact of the drug with the affected area. The patient selects

---

> **TABLE 1 FDA final monographs on foot care products for corns, calluses, and warts**
>
> ### Corn and callus remover drug products[a]
> Salicylic acid, 12–40% in a plaster vehicle
> Salicylic acid, 12–17.6% in a collodion-like vehicle
>
> ### Wart remover drug products[b]
> Salicylic acid, 12–40% in a plaster vehicle
> Salicylic acid, 5–17% in a collodion-like vehicle
> Salicylic acid, 15% in a karaya gum, glycol plaster vehicle
>
> [a]*Federal Register*. 1990 Aug 14; 55 (157): 33258–62.
> [b]*Federal Register*. 1990 Aug 14; 55 (157): 33246–56.

---

the appropriately sized disk, places it on the affected area, and covers it with the pad.

For corns and calluses, salicylic acid plasters or discs are generally applied and removed within 48 hours, with a maximum of five treatments over a 2-week period. For warts, these products are applied and removed every 48 hours for a maximum of 12 weeks. The karaya gum, glycol plaster with 15% salicylic acid for wart removal is designed to be applied at bedtime and left on for at least 8 hours; in the morning, it is removed and discarded. This procedure is repeated every 24 hours as needed for up to 12 weeks. If the wart remains, a physician should be consulted.

Collodion Vehicles. Topical keratolytics used in treating corns, calluses, and warts are generally formulated in flexible, collodionlike delivery systems containing pyroxylin; various combinations of volatile solvents such as ether, acetone, or alcohol; or a plasticizer, usually castor oil. Collodions help the active ingredient penetrate the affected tissue and result in sustained local action of the drug. They may be mechanically irritating. The collodion's occlusive nature allows systemic absorption of some drugs.

Adjunctive Therapy

In addition to nonprescription drugs, self-therapy measures include daily soaking of the affected area throughout treatment for at least 5 minutes in warm water. Dead tissue should be removed gently with a rough towel, callus file, or pumice stone. Knives or razor blades should not be used because they may cause bacterial contamination and infection.

To relieve painful pressure emanating from inflamed tissue and irritated or hypertrophied bones underneath a corn or callus, patients may use a pad with an aperture for the corn or callus. They may be used for 1 week or longer. To prevent the pads from adhering to hosiery, patients may wax them with paraffin or a candle, and then powder them daily with a hygienic foot powder or cover them with an adhesive bandage. If, despite these measures, friction causes the pads to peel at the edge and stick to hosiery, patients may cover their toes with the forefoot of an old stocking or pantyhose before putting on hosiery. Many of the disadvantages associated with pads have been overcome by a new cushioning material, Cushlin.

If the pad begins to cause itching, burning, or pain, it should be removed and a physician or podiatrist be consulted. These pads will provide only temporary relief and will rarely cure a corn or callus.

To avoid the spread of warts, patients should wash their hands before and after treating or touching wart tissue. A specific towel should be used only for drying the affected area after cleaning. Patients should not probe, poke, or cut the wart tissue. If warts are present on the sole of the foot, patients should not walk in bare feet unless the wart is securely covered.

Patient Education and Consultation

The containers of liquid products should be kept tightly capped. The volatile delivery systems are flammable and should be stored in amber or light-resistant containers away from direct sunlight or heat.

All foot-care products should be stored out of children's reach. Collodion-containing products are volatile, have an odor similar to that of airplane glue, and may be subject to abuse by inhalation.

Nonprescription corn, callus, and wart removal products are not recommended for patients with diabetes or circulatory problems. Pharmacists should reinforce contraindications, warnings, and precautions with all patients to avoid the inadvertent use of these products by individuals who have such conditions.

Bunions

Bunions are swellings of the bursae, exostoses, or both. They can be caused by various conditions, including friction on the toes from bone malformations and a hereditary predisposition. Pressure may result from the manner in which a person sits, walks, or stands. Pressure from a tight-fitting shoe over a period of time generally aggravates the condition. Bunions are usually asymptomatic but may become quite painful, swollen, and tender. The patient should correct the etiologic condition by wearing properly fitting shoes or should seek the advice of a podiatrist or orthopedist.

Topical nonprescription padding (e.g., moleskin) may be all that is necessary to decrease the irritation of footwear. Padding can help decrease inflammation around the bunion area.

Larger footwear may be necessary to compensate for the space taken up by the pad; not increasing shoe size appropriately may cause pressure in other areas. Protective pads should not be used on bunions when the skin is broken or blistered. Abraded skin should receive palliative treatment before pads are applied. If symptoms persist, particularly in diabetic patients, the pharmacist should recommend consultation with a podiatrist or an orthopedist.

Athlete's Foot

The clinical spectrum of athlete's foot (tinea pedis) ranges from mild itching and scaling to a severe, exudative inflammatory process characterized by fissuring and denudation. The prevalent type of athlete's foot, midway between these two extremes, is characterized by maceration, hyperkeratosis, pruritus, malodor, itching, and a stinging sensation of the feet.

Etiology

In addition to specific microorganisms, environmental factors contribute to the disease. Footwear is a key variable, as illustrated by the incidence of the disease in individuals who wear occlusive footwear, especially in hot, humid weather.

The infection is acquired most often by walking barefoot on infected floors (e.g., hotel bathrooms, swimming pools, locker rooms) and may be spread within families by exposure to bathroom floors, mats, or rugs.

Types

There are four variants of tinea pedis; two or more of these types may overlap. The most common is the chronic, intertriginous type, characterized by fissuring, scaling, or maceration in the interdigital spaces. Typically, the infection involves the lateral toe webs. From these sites, the infection spreads to the sole or instep of the foot but rarely to the dorsum. Warmth and humidity aggravate this condition.

The second variant, the chronic, papulosquamous pattern, is usually found on both feet and is characterized by mild inflammation and diffuse scaling on the soles of the feet. Ringworm of one or more toenails may also be present. The toenails must first be cured with oral drug therapy, such as griseofulvin, itraconazole, or ketoconazole, or removed surgically to rid the area of the offending fungus.

The third variant is the vesicular type. Small vesicles or vesicopustules are observed near the instep and on the midanterior plantar surface.

The acute ulcerative type is the fourth variant of tinea pedis. It is often associated with macerated, denuded, weeping ulcerations of the sole of the foot. It may produce an extremely painful, erosive, purulent interspace that can be disabling.

Susceptibility

Trauma to the skin, especially that which produces blisters (from wearing ill-fitting footwear), may be significantly more important to the occurrence of human fungal infections than is simple exposure to the offending pathogens. Although tinea pedis may occur at all ages, it is more common in adults. Individual susceptibility is affected by concomitant disease processes.

Evaluation

The most common complaint is pruritus. Painful burning and stinging may also occur. There may be weeping or oozing. Some patients may merely note bothersome scaling of dry skin. Small vesicular lesions may combine to form a larger bullous eruption marked by pain and irritation. The only symptoms may be brittleness and discoloration of a hypertrophied toenail. The true determinant of a fungal foot infection is the clinical laboratory evaluation of tissue scrapings from the foot.

The pharmacist should question the patient regarding the condition to determine symptoms, the extent of disease, previous compliance with medications, and any mitigating circumstances such as diabetes or obesity. It is appropriate to inspect the foot if privacy and sanitary conditions allow, and it is especially appropriate with diabetes patients.

The pharmacist should seek to distinguish tinea pedis from diseases with similar symptoms, such as dermatitis, allergic contact dermatitis, and atopic dermatitis. In children, peridigital dermatitis or atopic dermatitis is more common than tinea pedis. Shoe dermatitis is perhaps the most common form of allergic contact dermatitis from clothing.

Hyperhidrosis of interdigital spaces and the sole of the foot is common, as is infection of the toe webs by gram-negative bacteria. In hyperhidrosis, vesicles cover the sole of the foot and toes and may be quite painful. The skin generally turns white, erodes, and becomes macerated. This condition is accompanied by a foul odor.

Severe tinea pedis may progress to disintegration and denudation of the affected skin and to profuse, serous, purulent discharge. When the disease is out of control, its progression is observed on the dorsum of the foot and the calf in the form of tiny red follicular crusts.

If the patient has used a nonprescription antifungal product appropriately for 4 weeks without satisfactory results, a disease other than tinea pedis may be involved. Persons suffering from such an infection or from hyperhidrosis, allergic contact dermatitis, or atopic dermatitis need referral.

The pharmacist should be aware of the implications of the following conditions and be able to recommend to the patient the appropriate course of action:

- If the toenail is involved, topical treatment will not allay the condition until the disease's primary focus is treated with oral griseofulvin, itraconazole, or ketoconazole or until other preventive measures are instituted (e.g., surgical avulsion of the nail).
- If vesicular eruptions are oozing purulent material that could indicate a secondary bacterial infection, topical astringent therapy and/or antibiotic therapy may be appropriate.
- If the interspace between the toes is foul-smelling, whitish, painful, soggy, or characterized by erosions, oozing, or serious inflammation, and especially if the condition is disabling, the patient should be referred to a physician.
- If the foot is seriously inflamed or swollen and a major portion of it is involved, supportive therapy must be instituted before an antifungal agent may be applied.
- If the patient is a child who presents with an eczematous eruption of the feet, including that complicated by blisters and/or pyoderma, self-treatment should not be recommended.
- If the patient is under a physician's supervision for a disease such as diabetes or asthma, in which normal host defense mechanisms may be deficient, nonprescription products should not be recommended before medical consultation.

Pharmacologic Treatment

Hydrocortisone, in conjunction with clioquinol (formerly iodochlorhydroxyquin), has demonstrated favorable results toward resolving uncomplicated cutaneous fungal infections, including tinea pedis. However, their indiscriminate use could complicate and delay appropriate medical care. Topical hydrocortisone by itself is contraindicated in the presence of fungal infections because it may complicate and delay healing.

Self-treatment is effective only if the patient understands the importance of compliance with the entire treatment plan. Specific antifungal products must be used appropriately in conjunction with other treatment measures, including hygienic measures and local drying.

The FDA has stated that a nonprescription product must provide more than temporary symptomatic relief of athlete's foot and related infections. Such products must contain a Category I antifungal ingredient capable of killing the fungus (Table 2).

TABLE 2 FDA-approved topical antifungal drugs for over-the-counter use[a]

Drug	Concentration (%)
Haloprogin	1
Clioquinol	3
Miconazole nitrate	2
Tolnaftate	1
Undecylenic acid and its salts	10–25
Povidone–Iodine	10

[a]*Federal Register.* 1993 Sep 23; 58 (183): 49890–9.

Clioquinol

Clioquinol has a low incidence of side effects; however, it may cause itching, redness, and irritation. It may interfere with thyroid function tests. Patients undergoing these tests must be questioned carefully to assess their prior use of iodine-containing clioquinol.

Clotrimazole and Miconazole Nitrate

Both of these drugs are suggested for application twice daily. They are indicated when tolnaftate fails to cure tinea pedis and when patient factors have been ruled out as a cause. Rare cases of mild skin irritation, burning, and stinging have occurred with their use.

Tolnaftate

Tolnaftate is the only nonprescription drug approved for both the prevention and treatment of athlete's foot. It does not have antibacterial properties. It is valuable primarily in the dry, scaly type of athlete's foot. For treatment of tinea pedis, concomitant administration of oral griseofulvin, itraconazole, or ketoconazole is often necessary.

Tolnaftate is well tolerated when applied to intact or broken skin, although it usually stings slightly when applied. Delayed hypersensitivity reactions are unlikely. Discontinuation is warranted if irritation, sensitization, or worsening of the skin condition occurs.

Tolnaftate (1% solution, cream, gel, powder, spray powder, or spray liquid) is applied sparingly twice daily after the affected area is cleaned thoroughly. Effective therapy takes at least 2–4 weeks. When medication is applied to pressure areas of the foot, where the horny skin layer is thicker than normal, concomitant use of a keratolytic agent (e.g., Whitfield's ointment) may be advisable. If weeping lesions are present, the inflammation should be treated before tolnaftate is applied.

The 1% solution may be more effective than the cream. The topical powder formulation uses cornstarch-talc as the vehicle. This vehicle not only is an effective drug delivery system but also offers a therapeutic advantage, because the two agents retain water.

Undecylenic Acid–Zinc Undecylenate

This combination may be effective for mild superficial fungal infections, excluding those involving nails or hairy parts of the body.

Applied as an ointment, diluted solution, or dusting powder, undecylenic acid–zinc undecylenate is relatively nonirritating, and hypersensitivity reactions are rare. The undiluted solution may cause transient stinging when applied to broken skin. Caution must be exercised to ensure that these ingredients do not come into contact with the eye and that the powder is not inhaled.

The product is applied twice daily after the affected area is cleansed. When the solution is sprayed or applied to the affected area, the area should be allowed to air dry. The odor of undecylenic acid may be objectionable to some patients, possibly promoting noncompliance. If improvement does not occur in 2–4 weeks, the condition should be reevaluated and an alternative medication used.

Salts of Aluminum

Aluminum salts do not have any direct antifungal activity; however, their possible use in athlete's foot merits their inclusion in this chapter. These compounds act as astringents; in concentrations greater than 20%, they possess antibacterial activity.

Aluminum acetate for use in tinea pedis is generally diluted with 10–40 parts of water. The patient may immerse the foot in the solution for 20 minutes up to three times a day (every 6–8 hours) or apply the solution to the affected area in the form of a wet dressing.

For patient convenience, aluminum acetate solution (Burow's solution) or modified Burow's solution is available for immediate use in solution. It is also available in forms that may be diluted in water (powder packets, powder, and effervescent tablets). In the acute inflammatory state of tinea pedis, this solution should be used for less than 1 week. The patient should discontinue use if inflammatory lesions appear or worsen.

Concentrations of 20%–30% aluminum chloride have been the most beneficial for the wet, soggy type of athlete's foot. Twice-daily applications are used until the signs and symptoms abate; after that, once-daily applications control the symptoms. The use of concentrated aluminum salt solutions is contraindicated on severely eroded or deeply fissured skin.

Aluminum salts do not cure athlete's foot but are useful when combined with other topical antifungal drugs. In hot, humid weather, the condition may return within 7–10 days after the application is stopped.

Product Ingredients and Formulations

The primary drug delivery systems used in treating tinea pedis are creams, solutions, and powders. Powders, including those in aerosol forms, are generally indicated for adjunctive use with solutions and creams. In very mild conditions, powders alone may suffice.

Solution and cream forms should be formulated in a vehicle that is nonocclusive, anhydrous, spreadable, water miscible, nonsensitizing, nontoxic, and capable of efficient drug delivery. Criteria for the powder form (shaker or aerosol) are basically the same as those for solutions and creams.

Product Selection Guidelines

Elderly patients may require a preparation that is easy to use; obese patients, in whom excessive sweating may contribute to the disease, should use topical talcum powders as adjunctive therapy.

Before recommending a nonprescription product, the pharmacist should review the patient's medical history. Persons with diabetes should have their blood glucose levels moderately controlled because increased glucose in perspiration may promote fungal growth. Patients with allergic dermatitides usually have a history of asthma, hay fever, or atopic dermatitis and thus are extremely sensitive to most oral and topical agents. By acquiring a good history, the pharmacist may be able to distinguish a tinea infection from atopic dermatitis and avoid recommending a product that may cause skin irritation.

Prescription drugs may sometimes be more beneficial than nonprescription products. In the soggy, macerated athlete's foot complicated by bacterial infection, the broad-spectrum antifungal agents (e.g., econazole nitrate) are the agents of choice.

Product line extensions that have the same brand name do not necessarily have the same active ingredient(s). For example, the cream and solution formulations of Lotrimin AF contain clotrimazole, 1%, whereas the topical spray and powder formulations contain miconazole nitrate, 2%. Similarly, Desenex Maximum Strength Antifungal cream contains miconazole nitrate, 2%, whereas the traditional Desenex Cream contains undecylenic acid and zinc undecylenate in a 25% concentration.

Patient Education and Counseling

Pharmacists should advise patients not to expect dramatic remission of the condition. Medication should be used for a minimum of 2–4 weeks. If there is no improvement, the patient should consult a physician. Patients should also be told of the necessity to adhere strictly to the dosage regimen or the directions for use. Pharmacists may advise patients or caregivers to continue the medication for a few days beyond the recommended time to decrease the risk of relapse.

Patients should be advised to discontinue the product if itching, swelling, or exacerbation of the disease occurs. In addition, patients should avoid contact of the product with the eyes. After applying the product, patients should thoroughly wash their hands with soap and water.

Pharmacists should inform patients of the need for proper hygiene before effective drug therapy can begin. The feet should be cleansed with soap and water and thoroughly patted dry each day. Patients should be cautioned against overzealous cleansing and drying between the toes so as not to further irritate the area. Patients should have their own washcloths and towels. After bathing, the feet should be dried last so the towel does not spread the infection to other sites.

General measures should be taken to eliminate the predisposing factors of heat and perspiration. Shoes and light cotton socks that allow ventilation should be worn; wool and some synthetic fabrics interfere with foot moisture dissipation. Occlusive footwear, including canvas, leather, or rubber-soled athletic shoes, should not be worn for prolonged periods. Shoes should be alternated as often as possible so that the inside can dry, and they should be dusted with foot powders. Socks should be changed daily and washed thoroughly after use.

Contaminated clothing and towels should be laundered in hot water. The feet, particularly the area between the toes, should be dusted with a medicated or unmedicated drying powder at every change of socks. Whenever possible, the feet should be aired. Cotton balls may be placed between the tips of the toes to keep the web spaces open. Nonocclusive protective footwear (e.g., rubber or wooden sandals) may be worn in areas of family or public use.

Individuals whose feet perspire excessively may find odor-controlling insoles useful. Patients must be advised to change insoles every 3–4 months or more often.

Nail Fungus

Nail fungus (tinea unguium) causes nails to become discolored, rough, and thick. There is no approved nonprescription treatment. Patients can use Fungal Nail Revitalizer, which is intended to reduce nail discoloration and smooth out the thick, rough nail. The patient applies the cream over the entire surface of the infected nail, scrubs it for at least 1 minute with the provided nailbrush, and then washes and dries the nail completely. This procedure should be done daily for 3 weeks.

Tired, Aching Feet

The first way to avoid tired, aching feet is to use well-fitted footwear that has sufficient padding and cushioning. Second, full shoe inserts, which can provide cushioning and absorb shock, are available in a variety of sizes and thicknesses. The patient must realize that the insert should conform to the type of shoe worn. Partial insoles are preferred when cushioning or support is desired in a certain portion of the shoe. If the patient has heel pain, a heel cup or heel cushion may be indicated.

Potentially Serious Conditions

Selected chronic diseases predispose certain patients to foot problems. Most noteworthy is the diabetic patient with poor circulation and diminished limb sensitivity (Chapter 18). These factors make this patient vulnerable to infectious foot problems. Other vulnerable patients include those with peripheral circulatory disease or arthritis. The pharmacist can identify these patients by asking questions about daily medication use or reviewing the patient's drug profile.

Pharmacists are also in a position to advise patients on self-treatment and prevention of the following conditions.

Poor Circulation

Patients with poor circulation of the feet and legs may complain of feelings of cold, numbness, tingling, burning, or fatigue. Other symptoms include discolored skin, dry skin, absence of hair on the feet or legs, or a cramping or tightness in the leg muscles. The most discriminating questions a pharmacist can ask are "Do you experience aching in your calves when you walk?" and "Do you have to hang your feet over the edge of the bed during sleep to relieve the soreness in your calves?" A positive response to either question warrants referral to a physician or podiatrist.

If a patient complains of coldness in only one foot, there may be a blockage (clot) of circulation to the foot. Sometimes the involved foot or lower leg will appear larger than the other, be red or waxy, have no hair growth on the toes, and exhibit thickened nails. If a review of the patient's medication history does not indicate the use of medications intended to relieve these symptoms, the patient should be advised to consult a physician or podiatrist.

A daily footbath is a simple measure that will assist these patients. After the foot is patted dry, an emollient foot cream can be applied. The feet should be kept warm and moderately exercised every day.

Arthritis

Proper foot care is especially important for arthritic patients. These patients should wear properly fitted shoes, pad their shoes with insoles to protect their feet from the shock of hard surfaces, and undergo regular podiatric or medical examinations.

Ingrown Toenails

An ingrown toenail occurs when a section of nail presses into the soft tissue of the nail groove. The nail curves into the flesh of the toe corners and becomes embedded in the surrounding soft tissue of the toe, causing pain. Swelling, inflammation, and ulceration are secondary complications.

The most frequent cause of ingrown toenails is incorrect trimming of the nails. The correct method is to cut the nail straight across without tapering the corners. Wearing pointed-toe or tight shoes, as well as hosiery that is too tight, has also been implicated.

In the early stages, therapy is directed at providing room for the nail to resume its normal position. This is accomplished by relieving the external source of pressure and applying medications that will harden the nail groove or help shrink the soft tissue. The patient should be referred to a podiatrist or physician if the condition is recurrent or gives rise to an oozing discharge, pain, or severe inflammation.

In its final rule for ingrown toenail relief products, the FDA did not propose any OTC active ingredient for ingrown toenail relief as safe and effective. Previously approved drugs, tannic acid and sodium sulfide, were withdrawn from the market. The pharmacist must be aware of product reformulations to accommodate this rule. For example, Outgro Pain-Relieving Formula, which formerly contained tannic acid for the treatment of ingrown toenails, now contains benzocaine, 20%, for the relief of pain associated with ingrown toenails.

Patients with ingrown toenails often fail to realize that they may also be helped by oral medication intended to allay pain and inflammation. The pharmacist may recommend aspirin, ibuprofen, ketoprofen, or naproxen, provided there are no contraindications to their use for a particular patient.

Frostbite

Frostbite is defined as the freezing of tissues by excessive exposure to low temperatures. Minor frostbite may cause only blanching of the skin; severe frostbite may result in the loss of fingers and toes. Predisposing factors to the development of frostbite include low temperatures (especially with high winds), long periods of exposure to cold, lack of proper clothing, wet clothing, poor nutrition, exhaustion, dehydration, smoking, circulatory disease, immobility, direct contact with metal or petroleum products at low temperatures, and individual susceptibility to cold.

Frostbite is not amenable to therapy with nonprescription drug products. The frostbitten part should be promptly and thoroughly rewarmed in water heated to 104°–108°F (45.6°– 47.8°C). The container of water should be large enough for the frozen part to move freely without bumping against the sides. Rewarming should be continued until a flush returns to the most distal tip of the thawed part. This usually takes about 20–30 minutes. Dry heat (e.g., a heating pad) should be avoided. Once the injured part has been warmed, it should be soaked for about 20 minutes in a whirlpool bath once or twice daily until healing is complete.

The best treatment for frostbite is prevention. Pharmacists should provide a few simple rules:

- Dress to maintain body warmth, taking into account the face, neck, and head as well as the extremities.
- Avoid exposure to cold during times of sickness or exhaustion.
- Do not exceed the body's tolerance to cold exposure.
- Avoid tight-fitting garments; wear layered clothing.
- Wear clothing that allows ventilation and prevents perspiration buildup.
- Wear insulated boots or shoes and socks (preferably wool) that fit snugly but are not tight.
- Wear mittens instead of gloves in severe cold.
- Never touch objects (especially cold metal or petroleum products) that facilitate heat loss.

When given the opportunity, the pharmacist should seek to correct a few misconceptions. It is dangerous to rub the affected area with ice or snow; this can result in prolonged contact with the cold, and the ice crystals may lacerate cells. Persons should refrain from drinking alcohol. Alcohol can induce a loss of body heat even though it may give the person a feeling of warmth when ingested. Finally, frostbite victims should avoid smoking because nicotine can induce peripheral vasoconstriction and further reduce the blood supply to the frostbitten extremity.

Exercise-Induced Foot Problems

The pharmacist should be aware of the problem of exercise-induced foot injuries, particularly those caused by running, jogging, or other high-impact physical activities. A misconception among runners is that they can "work out" the problem by continuing to jog. Individuals must be instructed that pain is the body's communication mechanism to indicate that something is abnormal.

Specific Injuries

Shin Splints

The term *shin splint* describes pain emanating from below the knee and above the ankle. Shin splint is an overuse phenomenon that occurs in runners or walkers who use hard surfaces. The typical complaint is pain in the medial lower third of the shin that increases gradually with exercise. If the discomfort is located on the anterior lateral aspect of the skin; is described as a cramping, burning tightness; and repeatedly occurs at the same distance or time during a run, self-treatment may be ill-advised. The runner should be referred to a physician, podiatrist, or physical therapist.

Rest and application of ice (e.g., an ice bag, a cold compression wrap) to the painful area are good initial treatments. It is best to alternate compresses (10 minutes applied, 10 minutes off). To ensure greater contact with the injured part, the patient should use crushed or shaved ice. Aspirin or ibuprofen can be used to relieve pain and reduce tissue inflammation. Using analgesics to suppress pain or increase endurance during a workout is not recommended.

Stress Fracture

Stress fracture (also known as march, army, or fatigue fracture) may be encountered in runners, especially those who run repetitively on hard surfaces. This injury usually involves the long bones of the foot or leg. It is not an overt break but an alteration in the architecture of the normal bone.

The onset of pain is associated with runners who drastically change aspects of their training routine (e.g., running surface, speed, distance). The person will often complain of deep pain in the lower leg with an area of extreme tenderness.

Treatment is complete rest from running, sometimes for 4–6 weeks or longer.

Achilles Tendinitis

Running on hills or the beach, wearing improper footwear, and moving with excessive pronation (rolling in of the feet) are common causes of Achilles tendinitis. Typical symptoms are posterior heel pain that is worse in the morning when getting out of bed, at the beginning of an exercise session, and when walking after prolonged sitting. This condition may also be an early sign of arthritis or rupture of a tendon. Achilles tendinitis should be referred to a physician, podiatrist, or physical therapist.

The best treatment is prevention, which entails careful progression of training and replacement of worn footwear. Bony malalignments leading to excessive pronation should be accounted for with orthotic therapy. Shoe inserts can be custom-made or purchased off the shelf.

Symptomatic self-treatment may consist of rest, new shoes, ice applications, appropriate use of nonsteroidal anti-inflammatory agents, physician-prescribed temporary heel lifts, and careful calf-stretching exercises.

Blisters

Ill-fitting footwear and inappropriate hosiery can cause or contribute to the development of blisters.

Prevention is the key to treating blisters. Cotton or woolen socks are preferred for running. The runner can wear two pairs of socks with talcum powder sprinkled between them. Some individuals with soft skin continue to suffer from blisters until their skin toughens enough to withstand friction during running. Application of compound tincture of benzoin or of a flexible collodion product will help toughen the skin.

Ankle Sprains

The typical mechanism of lateral ligament injury to the ankle is through rotation of the body over the fixed foot. The incidence of ankle sprains during jogging and running is low, because runners usually do not take sharp diagonal cuts. However, stepping on an unnoticed stone or curb edge may result in an ankle sprain.

The differential diagnosis of an ankle fracture from a sprained ankle requires an x-ray.

Ice, compression, elevation (ICE) therapy is well accepted as the most appropriate immediate treatment for an ankle sprain. It remains controversial whether cold application without elevation is helpful or harmful. If possible, the ankle should be bound with a wet elastic wrap while the cold is being applied; the wet wrap facilitates temperature transfer so that the ankle benefits most from the cold application. The use of alternating cold applications should continue for 24–72 hours, depending on injury severity. Treatment should be initiated as soon as possible.

Intermetatarsal Neuritis

Intermetatarsal neuritis is characterized by pain and numbness between the toes, most often within the third interspace. The cause is linked to the foot jamming forward into the shoe without enough space to accommodate the foot. The solution is correct-fitting shoes with a metatarsal pad or orthotic device. Lacing of the shoe can be modified by skipping the bottom two eyelets.

Toenail Loss

Blisters under the toenail occur as a result of not keeping the toenails trimmed and of running in poorly fitted shoes. This condition is very painful and can result in the temporary loss of the toenail.

Runner's Bunion

In runners, a bunion can gradually enlarge and cause increasing discomfort. See the discussion of Bunions earlier in this chapter.

Heel Pain

The common diagnosis of heel pain in runners is plantar fasciitis (heel spur). The cause is excessive running or rapid gain in body weight. The pain is worse when getting out of bed or when standing up after sitting. Self-treatment includes replacing worn shoes or heel pads, using a night splint, strapping or taping the arch, decreasing the amount of weight-bearing activity, and, if necessary, entering a weight-reduction program. Anti-inflammatory treatment, including ice applications, is appropriate. If self-treatment fails, referral is indicated.

Treatment

Responses to the questions listed at the beginning of this chapter may indicate that the person has had a number of continuous days of high-intensity workouts. The pharmacist should emphasize that a good training program entails "hard-easy" days, with extended mileage on 3 or 4 days per week and light, easy workouts on the remaining days.

If the runner or jogger has an injured leg or foot, that activity must be interrupted to allow the injured leg or foot to rest. Relative rest (i.e., avoiding activities that produce the symptoms) is often indicated. The pharmacist should encourage alternative exercise modes, such as swimming or bicycling (stationary or outdoor).

Preventive Measures

Proper Footwear

Injuries and problems often develop when sport-specific shoes are used for the inappropriate activity; for example, the heel on tennis shoes is too low for jogging. Pharmacists should advise individuals to use proper equipment.

Shoes are designed to provide stability and cushioning. As soon as a shoe becomes worn, it should be replaced. Individuals with a history of stress fractures, osteoarthritis, or rigid high arches should not wait until the outer sole wears through before replacing shoes. It is wise to replace shoes early and often.

The Running Surface

The ideal running or walking surface is relatively smooth, level, and resilient. A walker who wants to increase energy expenditure may try walking on dirt or sand; these surfaces can boost energy expenditure by as much as one third. Similarly, walking on a mild, 14-degree slope requires more muscle power than walking on a straight, flat surface. Walkers who become overzealous on these surfaces can encounter the same problems as runners do.

Patient Education and Consultation

When self-treatment is appropriate, the pharmacist can assist the patient in selecting nonprescription drugs (e.g., aspirin, ibuprofen, topical antibiotic ointments) and make recommendations for their administration. The pharmacist can also assist in selecting prescription accessories (e.g., a compression ice wrap, ice bags, Ace bandages, arch supports, heel cushions).

If an ice bag is used, the English type, which is identified by its commercial cloth material, is preferred because the patient does not have to wrap a towel around it to protect the skin. The ice should be broken into walnut-sized pieces with no jagged edges and should fill the bag to one-half to two-thirds capacity. Once the bag has been filled, trapped air should be squeezed out, the outside dried, and the bag checked for leaks. The bag should then be applied to the specific body area. Ice should be replaced every 2–4 hours. Alternate applications (10 minutes applied, 10 minutes off) up to three to four times per day are suggested to avoid tissue damage. Because maximal swelling from an ankle sprain occurs within 48 hours of the injury, patients should continue applying ice for 2–3 days. After the ice bag is used, the patient should drain it and allow it to air dry. The bag should be turned inside out for more efficient drying. After this, the cap should be placed on the bag and the whole accessory stored in a cool, dry place.

Cold wraps are also useful. These can be one-use or multiple-use products. The patient activates the one-use product by squeezing the middle of the pack to burst the bubble, which initiates an endothermic reaction of ammonium nitrate, water, and additives. Reusable products consist of a cold pack or gel pack that is stored in the freezer and a cloth cover that is kept at room temperature. Once placed in the freezer, the cold pack reaches optimal temperature within 2 hours. The patient removes the cold pack from the freezer, inserts it in the cloth cover, and applies it to the specific body area. The patient should be instructed that the cold pack should not be uncomfortable; if it is, it should be removed for a minute or two and then reapplied. After use, the cold pack is stored again in the freezer. All cold packs should be kept out of the reach of children.

An Ace bandage is typically used for an ankle or knee sprain. The pharmacist must consider whether the patient will understand how to use the bandage in conjunction with an ice application so that additional damage is not incurred. If there is reason to believe the patient may cause further injury with a compression bandage through inappropriate use, the pharmacist should recommend simply elevating the body part and applying an ice pack or, if warranted by the severity of the injury, consulting a physician.

If an Ace bandage is to be used, its width depends on the injury site. A foot or an ankle requires a 2.5- to 3-in. bandage. The pharmacist should review with the patient the correct procedure for wrapping. The patient should be advised to unwind about 12–18 in. of bandage at a time and to allow the bandage to relax. After the bandage is unwound, it can be soaked in water: when applied with ice, a wet elastic bandage facilitates the transfer of cold. The injured area should be wrapped by overlapping the previous layer of bandage by about one third to one half its width. The point just above the toes should be tightly wrapped, with decreasing tightness as the bandage is wrapped upward. Foot circulation should not be impaired (i.e., no cold toes). The patient should assess the degree of discomfort after wrapping the injury. If the bandage feels tight, it should be removed and rewrapped. After use, it should be washed in lukewarm, soapy water, thoroughly rinsed, allowed to air dry on a flat surface, and rolled. It should not be ironed.

CHAPTER 35

Herbs and Phytomedicinal Products

Questions to ask in patient assessment and counseling

- *Have you used this product before?*
- *Are you allergic to any plant materials? If so, which specific materials or products?*
- *Is this product for personal use or for someone else (e.g., a child)?*
- *Are you pregnant or breast-feeding?*
- *Are you aware of the importance of closely following label instructions for product dosages and duration of use?*
- *Are you taking prescription or nonprescription medications intended for the same purpose as this herb?*

Popularity of herbs and phytomedicinals is increasing rapidly. For medical purposes, herbs are botanicals used to treat disease states, often of a chronic nature, or to attain or maintain improved health. Phytomedicinals are made by extracting herbs with various solvents to produce tinctures, fluid extracts, and extracts that permit concentration and standardization of the active principles.

Safety and Effectiveness

Most herbs and phytomedicinals are sold in the United States not as drugs but as dietary supplements. This reflects the fact that insufficient data concerning them have been submitted to the Food and Drug Administration (FDA) to permit that agency to classify them as safe and effective therapeutic agents. It does not necessarily mean that the herbs and phytomedicinals are unsafe or ineffective.

Ineffective Herbal Preparations

Herbal weight-loss preparations have become very popular but are not useful for this purpose. Most contain laxatives, such as senna, and diuretics, such as dandelion leaves, that produce temporary weight loss. Another popular ingredient is ephedra (ma huang), which acts as a central nervous system (CNS) stimulant but is not an effective anorectic agent and may cause serious side effects. Pharmacists should not recommend herbal weight-loss preparations.

Other conditions for which no effective botanical remedy is currently available include arthritis, cancer, human immunodeficiency virus (HIV), and acquired immunodeficiency syndrome (AIDS).

Editor's Note: This chapter is adapted from Varro E. Tyler and Steven Foster, "Herbs and Phytomedicinal Products," in Covington, T.R., ed., *Handbook of Nonprescription Drugs,* 11th edition. For a more extensive discussion of this topic, readers are encouraged to consult Chapter 35 of the *Handbook.*

Precautions

Because herbal dietary supplements are not approved drugs in the United States, information pertaining to their proper use and necessary cautionary warnings do not always appear on the label. Prospective users should make every effort to obtain accurate information about a product prior to purchasing it.

The FDA neither establishes nor enforces standards of quality for herbal products. One must rely on the reputation of the marketer for quality assurance. Products are often misbranded, and often the quantities of the ingredients are not listed. In mixtures containing large numbers of herbal constituents, quantities sufficient to render a therapeutic effect are often lacking. The consumer is best advised to purchase a preparation containing a specified amount of a standardized extract marketed by a reputable firm.

Other concerns about herbal consumption must include a general prohibition of use by pregnant or nursing mothers and by young children, especially infants. Many botanicals lack the necessary long-term toxicity testing to ensure safety during prolonged administration. Herbs used for therapeutic purposes are drugs, and proper dosage recommendations should be observed. Patients should be advised to seek advice from their pharmacist or physician before making any decisions concerning the use of these products.

Dosage Forms

One of the most common dosage forms is the coarsely comminuted botanical that is used to prepare an infusion (tea) or a decoction. This form is also used to prepare poultices for external application. More finely powdered herbs are either encapsulated or used to prepare compressed tablets. Herbs are also extracted with various solvents to produce liquid or solid phytomedicinals. Special preparations, such as nongelatin capsules that are not prepared from animal by-products, are sometimes encountered. Herbs derived from "organic" sources—that is, grown without synthetic chemical fertilizers or pesticides—are often advertised.

Digestive System Disorders

Ginger

Ginger is considered to be a carminative, an antiemetic, a cholagogue, and a positive inotrope. Dried ginger root has been shown to stimulate the gastrointestinal (GI) tract. Use is primarily indicated for atonic dyspepsia, colic, and the prophylactic relief of symptoms of motion sickness.

Given in amounts specified to prevent motion sickness, ginger has caused no reported side effects or toxic reactions. The herb should be avoided for treatment of postoperative nausea because it may prolong bleeding time and result in immunologic changes. Its use is also contraindicated in patients with gallstone pain and nausea associated with pregnancy.

The dosage is two 500-mg capsules taken 30 minutes prior to travel departure, followed by 1 or 2 more 500-mg capsule(s) taken as needed every 4 hours. The daily dose is 2–4 g of the drug or equivalent preparations.

Plantago Seed and Husk

Plantago or psyllium seeds are bulk-forming laxatives. Uses include treatment of chronic constipation and conditions necessitating soft stools, such as hemorrhoids, anal fissures, or rectal-anal surgery. The drug's efficacy in producing a modest but significant lowering of total cholesterol and low-density lipoprotein levels is recognized.

Rare allergic reactions have been reported. Its use is contraindicated in the presence of bowel and GI tract obstructions as well as diabetes mellitus.

The dose is 7.5 g (average 4–20 g per day), taken with at least 150 mL of water for each 5 g of drug, 30–60 minutes after a meal or the administration of other drugs.

Senna

Senna is used for the treatment of constipation. Patients may experience cramping discomfort in the GI tract. Use of stimulating laxatives should not continue beyond 1–2 weeks except under medical supervision. Chronic abuse or overdose can result in potassium loss, along with electrolyte and fluid imbalances. Senna is not recommended during pregnancy or lactation.

The dose is 2 g or appropriate formulations as needed.

Peppermint

Peppermint leaf and oil are in pharmaceutical use in the United States as flavoring agents. Peppermint has been reported to reduce symptoms of irritable bowel syndrome characterized by recurrent colicky abdominal pain, a feeling of distention, and variations in bowel habits with minimal attendant side effects. Peppermint leaf is recognized as a carminative and choleretic and has a direct spasmolytic effect on smooth muscles of the digestive tract. Peppermint leaf tea is used to treat dyspepsia, flatulence, and intestinal colic.

Peppermint tea is considered safe for normal individuals. Excessive use of the essential oil (0.3 g not enteric coated) may produce heartburn and relaxation of the lower esophageal sphincter. Peppermint leaf tea should be used with caution in infants and small children because of possible laryngeal and bronchial spasms from volatilized menthol. The oil may irritate mucous membranes.

The cut herb is used in hot infusions at an average daily dose of 1.5–3 g of the dried leaf. For relief of stomach upset, an infusion is made by pouring 160 mL of boiling water on 1–1.5 g of the herb, steeping for up to 10 minutes, and ingesting it up to three or four times daily. Each dose of enteric-coated peppermint oil is 0.2–0.4 mL, up to 0.6–1.2 mL per day.

Chamomile

The dried flower heads and volatile oil of chamomile have anti-inflammatory, spasmolytic, and antimicrobial activity. The flower preparations are used for GI spasms and GI tract inflammatory diseases. The drug is also used for peptic ulcers. An infusion (as a mouthwash) is used to treat inflammatory conditions of the oral cavity and gums.

Topical products are used for the treatment of skin and mucous membrane inflammations and bacterial skin diseases. Flower extracts have also proven useful in the treatment of eczema.

Only five cases of allergy attributed to German chamomile have been identified during the past century, which implies the drug's relative safety.

For GI ailments, tea (150 mL hot water over 3 g dried flower heads, steeped for 10 minutes) is drunk three to four times daily between meals.

Milk Thistle

Milk thistle preparations are considered hepatoprotectants. They are widely used in Europe in the prophylaxis and treatment of chronic hepatotoxicity. They have been especially useful in inflammatory liver disorders and cirrhosis of the liver.

Mild diarrhea has been reported in a small number of patients.

The average daily dose is 12–15 g of the seeds, corresponding to 200–420 mg per day of silymarin, or its equivalent in capsules or tablets, each containing 80–140 mg of silymarin in a concentrated extract.

Licorice

Licorice contains a triterpene glycoside, glycyrrhizin (glycyrrhizic acid) that is hydrolyzed glycyrrhetinic acid. Glycyrrhetinic acid has been found to inhibit two enzymes that are important for the metabolism of prostaglandins E and F_{2a}. The resulting increase in prostaglandins in the stomach produces a protective effect on gastric mucosa, thereby promoting the healing of gastric ulcers. Licorice is also used as an ingredient in antitussive and expectorant formulations.

Glycyrrhetinic acid also increases glucocorticoid concentrations in tissues responsive to mineralocorticoid, resulting in sodium retention, potassium excretion, and high blood pressure. The beneficial action and the side effects of glycyrrhetinic acid are inseparable; thus, the dose must be carefully controlled if the herb is to be used therapeutically.

Potassium loss may be increased by concurrent use of thiazide diuretics, resulting in an increased sensitivity to digitalis glycosides. Use of licorice is contraindicated in patients with liver cirrhosis, cholestatic liver disorders, hypertonia, and hypokalemia, as well as during pregnancy.

An average daily dose of 5–15 g of the finely cut or powdered root (calculated to contain 200–600 mg of glycyrrhizin) in infusions is recommended for the treatment of gastric/duodenal ulcers. Duration of this regimen should not exceed 4–6 weeks.

Kidney, Urinary Tract, and Prostate Disorders

Goldenrod

An aquaretic for use in irrigation therapy against lower urinary tract inflammation, goldenrod is also indicated for the prevention and treatment of urinary calculi and kidney stones.

Allergic cross-sensitivity to goldenrod can occur. The drug should be avoided in cases of known allergies to aster family members. It is also contraindicated in the presence of edema due to impaired heart or kidney function.

The herb is prepared as an infusion by pouring 240 mL boiling water over 3–5 g of the herb. Mean daily dose is 6–12 g.

Bearberry

The primary activity of bearberry is as an antibacterial for urinary tract infections (UTIs). Activation requires the urine pH to be alkaline. Administration should be in conjunction with a diet rich in foods capable of inducing alkalinuria (e.g., milk, tomatoes, potatoes, fruit, fruit juices).

A small percentage of patients may experience nausea and vomiting.

The dried cut or powdered herb is administered in a mean daily dose of 10 g (corresponding to 400–700 mg arbutin) macerated overnight in 150 mL of cold water. Use should be limited to 1 week or less.

Cranberry

Cranberry juice prevents the adhesion of *Escherichia coli* and other uropathogenic bacteria to the mucosal cells of the urinary tract. It is used to treat UTIs. It may also reduce the urinary odor of incontinent patients.

No precautions are noted.

As a UTI preventive, 90 mL of cranberry juice can be consumed daily; for UTI treatment, consumption should increase to 360–960 mL daily. Capsules containing dried cranberry and a dried, concentrated extract are available.

Saw Palmetto

Saw palmetto fruits and their preparations have antiandrogenic and anti-inflammatory activity and are used for the treatment of symptoms associated with benign prostatic hyperplasia (BPH). Placebo-controlled, double-blind studies of the use of saw palmetto extract carried out on more than 2000 BPH patients in Germany confirmed its effectiveness.

Stomach upset has been reported in rare instances.

The average daily dose is 1–2 g of the ground, dried fruits or 320 mg of a lipophilic fruit extract.

Respiratory Tract Disorders

Ephedra

The stem of ephedra (ma huang), contains a number of active compounds, including 1%–2% of an alkaloid mixture composed mainly of ephedrine and pseudoephedrine. Ephedra has been used to treat bronchial asthma and related conditions for at least 5000 years. Alkaloid-containing Asian species produce bronchodilation, vasoconstriction, and reductions in bronchial edema.

Ephedra should be avoided by patients with heart conditions, hypertension, diabetes, or thyroid disease. Overdose can result in nervousness, insomnia, and palpitation. Products containing ephedra herb, often spiked with ephedrine and/or pseudoephedrine, are used in weight-loss formulations, although there is no evidence to suggest that ephedra or its alkaloids are safe and effective in reducing weight or appetite. Because of reports of toxicity, FDA regulatory action on such products is anticipated. Several states restrict sales of ephedra because ephedrine is used in the manufacture of the illicit drugs methamphetamine and methcathinone.

Two grams of the herb is steeped in 240 mL of boiling water for 10 minutes (equivalent to 15–30 mg of ephedrine) and drunk as a tea.

Slippery Elm

Slippery elm bark is a mucilaginous demulcent, emollient, and nutrient. It is used to soothe irritated mucous membranes or ulcerations of the digestive tract as well as to relieve gastritis, colitis, and gastric or duodenal ulcers. The primary use in the United States is as a soothing demulcent for sore throat; it has received FDA approval for this purpose.

No precautions are noted.

Between 0.5 and 2 g of powdered bark steeped in 10 parts hot water (5–20 mL) are consumed as required. Commercially produced tablets and troches are available.

Horehound

Horehound is used as an expectorant, antitussive, and a cough suppressant. The herb is approved in Germany for supportive treatment of coughs and colds, and as a digestive aid and an appetite stimulant. The FDA has declared it ineffective as a nonprescription cough suppressant and expectorant.

No precautions are noted.

Two grams of the dried cut herb is steeped in 240 mL of boiling water, with a daily consumption of 0.75–1 L of the infusion. Horehound-flavored candy is used as a cough suppressant.

Cardiovascular System Disorders

Hawthorn

A member of the rose family, hawthorn is used in European phytomedical practice for treatment of diminished cardiac performance, heart conditions not requiring digitalis, mild and stable forms of angina pectoris, and mild forms of dysrhythmia. The flowering tops are used in sleep-inducing preparations.

No toxicity has been noted; however, given the nature of indications, hawthorn should be used only under medical supervision.

The European Scientific Cooperative for Phytotherapy has proposed a daily dosage of 3–4 g of the dried drug administered in 1-g doses in the form of an infusion.

Garlic

Garlic is considered antibacterial, antifungal, antithrombotic, and hypotensive; it activates fibrinolysis and is anti-inflammatory. Recent interest has focused on the use of garlic and its preparations for treatment of high blood pressure, atherosclerosis, hypoglycemia, digestive ailments, colds, flu, and bronchitis, as well as for its blood cholesterol– and triglyceride-lowering activity. Of all these activities, the best substantiated are those involving garlic's antihyperlipidemic properties.

Garlic may cause GI discomfort; rare allergic reactions are also reported.

The daily dosage is equivalent to 4–12 mg of alliin (2–5 mg of allicin) in appropriate formulations, 400–1200 mg of dried powder, or 2–5 g of the fresh bulb. Commercial products vary greatly in their chemical composition.

Ginkgo

The numerous pharmacologic and clinical studies of ginkgo leaf extract have demonstrated a positive effect in increasing vasodilation and the peripheral blood flow rate in capillary vessels and end arteries in various circulatory disorders. Among these are varicose conditions, post-thrombotic syndrome, chronic cerebral vascular insufficiency, short-term memory loss, cognitive disorders secondary to depression, dementia, tinnitus, vertigo, and obliterative arterial disease of the lower limbs.

Ginkgo leaf extract has been reported to produce minor reversible gastric disturbances. Rare side effects include headache, dizziness, and vertigo.

The daily dose is 120–160 mg of standardized ginkgo leaf extract.

Grapeseed and/or Pinebark

Grapeseed and pinebark extracts are used as antioxidants and to treat circulatory disorders such as hypoxia from atherosclerosis, inflammation, and cardiac or cerebral infarction. Much additional research is needed to ascertain efficacy.

No precautions are noted.

Tablets or capsules of 75–300 mg are ingested daily for up to 3 weeks, followed by a maintenance dose of 40–80 mg daily.

Nervous System Disorders

Valerian

Valerian is considered to be spasmolytic, mildly sedative, and a sleep aid. Valerian preparations are considered safe; however, additional controlled clinical trials are needed.

Two to three grams of the drug are generally taken one to three times per day.

St. John's Wort

St. John's wort is best classified as an antidepressant with anxiolytic, anti-inflammatory, and sedative effects. It apparently functions as a monoamine oxidase inhibitor, but CNS-stimulating effects have also been reported.

Light-skinned individuals are advised not to expose skin to direct sunlight after ingesting the herb because of a potential risk of photodermatitis.

In European phytomedicine, 2–4 g of herb (0.2–1.0 mg hypericin) is used, usually in the form of capsules.

Willow Bark

Willow bark contains phenolic glycosides, predominately salicylates and tremulacin. It has been used as an anti-inflammatory and analgesic for rheumatic and arthritic conditions, as an antipyretic in cases of the common cold or influenza, and as an astringent. The root bark has also been used to treat mild headaches and gout.

Salicylates reported in the crude bark of various species are highly variable. Products standardized on the basis of salicin content are not sold in the United States. Consumers contemplating use of a crude willow bark preparation as an analgesic or anti-inflammatory are advised to use aspirin or other appropriate nonsteroidal anti-inflammatory drugs.

Feverfew

Primary use of feverfew is as a prophylactic to reduce the frequency, severity, and duration of migraine headaches and to relieve associated symptoms such as nausea.

Some individuals may experience gastric discomfort following ingestion. Administration of fresh leaves has produced occasional mouth ulceration.

The average daily dose of the dried leaves with a minimum content of 0.2% parthenolide is 125 mg; the herb is usually consumed in tablet or capsule form.

Caffeine-Containing Plants

All caffeine-containing herbs are CNS stimulants. They are used alone to overcome drowsiness and in combination with nonprescription analgesics, which they potentiate. Caffeine-containing beverages have a weak diuretic activity of relatively short duration.

Caffeine-containing plants should be used with caution by persons with hypertension and related disorders.

The daily dose is equivalent to 100–200 mg of caffeine.

Metabolic and Endocrine Disorders

Black Cohosh

Black cohosh is used in European phytomedicine as an emmenagogue and for endocrine activity in the treatment of neurovisceral and psychic problems associated with menopause, premenstrual complaints, and dysmenorrhea. It is also used as a uterine antispasmodic.

GI disturbances have been reported in some patients. Use is contraindicated during pregnancy and lactation.

The dried rhizome is used in decoctions or tinctures (1:10, 60% ethanol), in amounts corresponding to a daily dosage of 40–200 mg. Duration of use should not exceed 6 months.

Chaste Tree Berry

Chaste tree has been used for centuries to treat menstrual difficulties. Germany allows use of preparations of this herb for menstrual disorders due to primary or secondary corpus luteum insufficiency, premenstrual syndrome, mastalgia, menopausal symptoms, and inadequate lactation.

Chaste tree preparations are contraindicated during pregnancy. Animal studies suggest the possibility of interference with dopamine-receptor antagonists.

Preparations include alcoholic extracts formulated to provide an average daily dose equivalent to 20 mg of the crude fruit, or 30–40 mg of the fruits in decoction.

Evening Primrose (Black Currant, Borage Seed) Oil

Studies suggest that evening primrose oil, which contains cis-gamma-linolenic acid (GLA) and *cis*-linoleic acid, may be of benefit to individuals unable to metabolize *cis*-linoleic acid in addition to persons whose diets are low in that acid. A number of trials have shown modest to insignificant improvement in symptoms associated with atopic eczema, especially relief from itching.

No precautions are noted.

Relevant clinical conditions for GLA supplementation, such as alcoholism and inflammation, may require doses of 600–6000 mg per day. For atopic eczema, dosage is four 250-mg capsules taken twice daily.

Arthritic and Musculoskeletal Disorders

All of the effective plant derivatives, mustard oil, methyl salicylate, etc, are covered in Chapter 5, "External Analgesic Products."

Disorders of the Skin, Mucous Membranes, and Gingiva

Witch Hazel

Witch hazel preparations are used topically to treat local inflammation of the skin and mucous membranes.

No precautions are noted.

Aloe Vera Gel

Fresh aloe gel is applied to first-degree burns and minor skin irritations. It has anti-inflammatory and emollient properties and enhances wound healing.

No precautions are noted.

Tea Tree Oil

The oil is considered bacteriostatic and germicidal. It has been used for treating boils, abscesses, sores, cuts, and abrasions, as well as wounds with pus discharge. It has been promoted for a number of other conditions, but its utility in many cases requires verification.

Tea tree oil may cause skin irritation or allergies in sensitive individuals.

The oil is applied topically in concentrations from 0.4% to 100%.

Goldenseal

Root preparations are used for their antimicrobial, astringent, and antihemorrhagic activities in the treatment of mucosal inflammation. The root is also used for the treatment of dyspepsia and gastritis. A modern folk use for goldenseal has been to mask illicit drugs in urinalysis tests. There is no scientific evidence to support this use.

The use of goldenseal is contraindicated during pregnancy.

The dosage is 0.5–1 g of the dried root or 2–4 mL of tincture (1:10, 60% ethanol) three times per day.

Melissa

The leaves of Melissa (primarily in tea form) have been used for their calmative, spasmolytic, and carminative activity and to treat functional GI symptoms. More recently, antibacterial and antiviral activities (on cold sores and genital herpes) have been confirmed.

No precautions are noted.

Performance and Endurance Enhancers

Ginseng

Ginseng has traditionally been characterized as an aphrodisiac and a tonic. Numerous conflicting pharmacologic and clinical benefits have been attributed to the root and its preparations. Ginseng is now designated as an adaptogen—an agent facilitating resistance to various kinds of stress. Additional clinical trials are needed to determine the degree of usefulness of this herb in specific conditions. Germany allows ginseng's use as a tonic to treat fatigue, diminished work capacity, and loss of concentration, in addition to its use as a general aid during convalescence.

Ginseng is generally considered safe.

The daily dosage is 1–2 g of root in appropriate formulations.

Eleuthero

Numerous biologic activities have been described for eleuthero root ethanolic extracts, including adaptogenic activity in cases of hyperthermia, electroshock-induced convulsions, gastric ulcers, and x-ray irradiation.

Well-designed trials are required to determine which of the claims of utility for eleuthero can be verified.

Side effects have been rarely reported.

The average daily dose is 2–3 g of the powdered or cut root in decoction.

Echinacea

Oral dosage forms of echinacea are used as nonspecific immunostimulants, especially as prophylactics at the first sign of cold and flu symptoms, for treatment of *Candida albicans* infections, and for other related conditions.

Topical preparations of *Echinacea purpurea* are used for treatment of wounds, eczema, burns, psoriasis, herpes simplex, etc. They are not available in the United States.

Echinacea products are contraindicated in patients with tuberculosis, leukosis, collagenosis, multiple sclerosis, and HIV infection and other autoimmune diseases.

Of the expressed fresh juice of *Echinacea purpurea,* the dose is 6–9 mL per day for not longer than 8 weeks. For *Echinacea pallida* root preparations, the average daily dose corresponds to 900 mg per day, often administered in the form of a tincture (1:5) prepared with 50% ethanol. Dosage of *Echinacea angustifolia* root in the form of capsules, tablets, or a tincture is 1 g, three times daily.

CHAPTER 36

Smoking Cessation Products

Questions to ask in patient assessment and counseling

- *Do you smoke? If so, how long have you smoked? How many cigarettes do you smoke per day?*
- *Have you ever tried to stop smoking? If so, which smoking cessation methods did you try? If not, are you ready to stop smoking now? Have you talked with your physician about your desire to stop smoking?*
- *Are you interested in trying nicotine polacrilex therapy or nicotine transdermal therapy? If so, do you understand how to use the product?*
- *Are you aware that you cannot use nicotine polacrilex or nicotine transdermal therapy if you continue to smoke cigarettes, pipes, or cigars; use snuff; chew tobacco; or use any other form of nicotine replacement therapy (i.e., prescription nicotine transdermal systems or nicotine nasal spray)?*
- *(If the patient is a woman) Are you pregnant or breast-feeding?*
- *Do you have heart disease or an irregular heartbeat, or have you had a recent heart attack? Do you have high blood pressure not controlled with medication?*
- *Do you have, or have you had, esophagitis or peptic ulcer disease?*
- *Do you have diabetes? If so, do you use insulin?*
- *Do you have mouth or jaw problems such as active temporomandibular joint disease?*
- *Do you take prescription medications to treat asthma or depression?*
- *Are you allergic to adhesive tape? Do you have any skin problems?*
- *What prescription or nonprescription medications are you taking?*

Cigarette smoking is the most prevalent modifiable risk factor for increased morbidity and mortality in the United States. To become a nonsmoker, the individual must overcome addiction to nicotine. Relapse can occur years after cessation of use. Maintaining cessation is very difficult for many individuals, and few smokers are successful in their first attempt.

Impact of Smoking on Health

Cardiovascular Morbidity

Nicotine affects the cardiovascular system by increasing the blood pressure, stimulating the heart rate, inducing electrocardiographic changes, exacerbating angina in coronary patients, and diminishing left ventricular performance in coronary patients.

Editor's Note: This chapter is adapted from Jack E. Fincham, "Smoking Cessation Products," in Covington, T.R., ed., *Handbook of Nonprescription Drugs,* 11th edition. For a more extensive discussion of smoking and its health consequences, readers are encouraged to consult Chapter 36 of the *Handbook.*

Cancer

Many types of cancer in active smokers have been linked to smoking, including bladder, breast, cervical, esophageal, kidney, laryngeal, lip, liver, lung, nasal, oral, pancreatic, pharyngeal, prostatic, skin, gastric, tongue, and tracheal. Several of the cancers (i.e., breast, cervical, lung) have been shown to occur also in passive smokers.

Respiratory Effects of Smoking

Lung diseases resulting from smoking and/or conditions affected by smoking include allergies, asthma, bronchitis, emphysema, persistent cough, and pneumonia. Smoking increases mucus secretion, cough, and sputum production and produces inflammation, ulceration, and squamous metaplasia in the smaller airways. These effects lead to fibrosis and airway narrowing.

The most common symptoms related to passive smoking are eye irritation, headache, cough, nasal irritation, wheezing, sore throat, and hoarseness.

Effects on Pregnancy

Smoking during pregnancy is harmful to the health of both mother and newborn. The adverse effects of smoking on pregnancy include miscarriages, full-term low birth-weights, perinatal deaths, birth defects, and preterm births. Sudden infant death syndrome has been linked to parental smoking behavior.

Other Diseases

Table 1 lists other diseases adversely affected by smoking.

Impact of Smoking on Drug Therapy

Many interactions between smoking and medications have been identified. The primary mechanism for many of these interactions appears to be induction of hepatic microsomal enzymes by compounds present in tobacco smoke. For example:

- *Analgesics*: decreased efficacy of acetaminophen and nonsteroidal anti-inflammatory drugs;

- *Anticoagulants (heparin, sodium warfarin)*: increased platelet activity, resulting in diminished efficacy of the anticoagulants;

- *Cardiovascular agents (beta-blockers, calcium-channel blockers, furosemide and other loop-type diuretics, thiazide diuretics)*: decreased activity of the drugs, making the underlying conditions more difficult to treat;

- *Estrogens (estrogen replacements for postmenopausal women, oral contraceptives containing estrogens)*: increased risk in female smokers for thromboembolic disorders;

- *H_2-receptor antagonists (cimetidine, famotidine, nizatidine, ranitidine)*: increased acid production in the gut, resulting in decreased or negated effect of the H_2-receptor antagonists;

- *Insulin*: decreased subcutaneous insulin absorption, possibly requiring an increase in insulin dosage;

- *Psychotropics (barbiturates, benzodiazepines, phenothiazines, and tricyclic antidepressants)*: decreased efficacy, delayed effects, or increased dose required;

- *Theophylline*: increased metabolism of theophylline, requiring increased doses; and

- *Vitamins*: decreased levels of vitamin C.

TABLE 1 Selected disease states adversely affected by smoking

Disease state	Effect of smoking
Allergies[a]	Exacerbated allergic symptoms
Angina pectoris[a]	Increased angina symptomatology; more frequent attacks
Cataracts (posterior subcapsular)	Increased incidence of cataracts and lens opacities in moderate to heavy smoking
Chronic obstructive pulmonary disease[a]	Increased incidence of bronchitis, emphysema, asthma, and other respiratory disorders; limited daily activities; decreased tolerance for exercise; decreased quality of life
Depression	Common factors (stress, anxiety, etc.) predispose individuals to both smoking and depressive symptomatology
Diabetes mellitus	Impaired glycemic control; increased gluconeogenesis
Gastrointestinal disease, infections, etc.	Increased incidence of peptic ulcer disease; delayed ulcer healing; increased susceptibility to *Helicobacter pylori* infection
Graves' disease	Greatly increased risk for Graves' ophthalmopathy
Hypertension[a] (in smokers)	Elevated blood pressure
Periodontal disease	Negative impact on oral health
Peripheral vascular disease	Increased incidence of deep vein thromboses; intermittent claudication

[a]Active and passive (i.e., those exposed to secondhand or sidestream smoke) smokers experience this effect.

Alternate therapy may be available for some patients who cannot stop smoking. For example, the ulcer patient could take sucralfate; it does not influence acid production but rather coats the site of ulceration with a spongy film, thus allowing the ulcerated lesion to heal. The continuance of smoking, however, will delay the healing. Patients with other conditions who stop smoking may need to adjust their medications (e.g., decrease theophylline or insulin dosages).

It is important for patients to be informed of these interactions because such awareness may increase their motivation to stop smoking.

Treatment

The response to nicotine withdrawal depends on how long the patient has smoked, how much he or she smokes, and other effects. Physiologic response to nicotine also varies from person to person. The recognition of this interindividual variation and the occurrence of withdrawal symptoms is the key to helping patients stop smoking. Successful programs address both the physical and psychologic aspects of nicotine addiction. No intervention will work optimally unless the smoker desires to stop smoking and maintain cessation.

Behavioral Interventions

Behavioral interventions used in smoking cessation therapies have included aversion therapy, educational programs, group therapy, hypnosis, and self-help literature. The success rate for each of these modalities has varied and is patient dependent. Some smokers can stop smoking through behavioral modification alone; however, the more highly addicted smoker usually needs pharmacologic assistance.

Nicotine Replacement Therapy

Three dosage forms of nicotine replacement are approved by the Food and Drug Administration (FDA): (1) nicotine transdermal systems (prescription and nonprescription forms), (2) nicotine nasal spray (prescription only), and (3) nicotine polacrilex (prescription and nonprescription). The initial intent of nicotine replacement therapy is to substitute pharmacologically dosed nicotine for smoked nicotine. By tapering doses, the patient is then gradually weaned from nicotine.

Although replacing nicotine from smoking with a pharmacologic source reduces the craving and withdrawal symptoms, the pharmacologic dose usually does not relieve these symptoms to the same degree as smoked nicotine. Any smoker who expects the same "smoking effect" from nicotine replacement products may be disappointed. Nicotine replacement therapy is designed to be used short term (6 months or less) to reduce the magnitude of the nicotine withdrawal syndrome experienced by smokers who stop "cold turkey." Nicotine replacement therapy should always be accompanied by behavioral and patient counseling.

There is controversy about the use of nicotine replacement therapy during pregnancy. Cigarette smoking is a preventable cause of fetal morbidity and mortality; however, the pharmacologic adjuncts to smoking cessation currently available are contraindicated during pregnancy.

Nicotine Polacrilex

Used correctly, nicotine polacrilex (Nicorette) has been shown to reduce withdrawal symptoms and increase cessation rates when compared with a placebo. Patients must understand how to use the resin dosage form (gum), how much to use per day, how long to use it, and how to stop use gradually. Strict patient compliance and cessation of product use are required if patients are to become free of nicotine use.

Dosage. Nicotine polacrilex is available in two package sizes: a starter kit containing 108 units and a supplemental package containing 48 units. Each package size is available in either the 2-mg or 4-mg dose. The 4-mg dosage packages are for individuals who smoke more than 24 cigarettes per day. Initial dosing is 12–24 units per day.

Usage Guidelines. The Nicorette package contains a cassette tape that provides instructions for use as well as a printed user's guide. Directions for use include the following:

■ Stop smoking completely when you begin using this product.

- Before using this product, read the user's guide. Use the product according to the directions provided.
- Do not eat or drink for 15 minutes before using this product or while using it.
- Use this product according to the following 12-week schedule:

    Weeks 1–6: One piece every 1–2 hours;

    Weeks 7–9: One piece every 2–4 hours;

    Weeks 10–12: Use one piece every 4–8 hours.

- Do not use more than 24 pieces a day.
- Stop using the product at the end of week 12. If you still feel the need for it, talk with your physician.

   Specific counseling tips on the proper use of nicotine polacrilex, in addition to the advice on the package label, include the following:

- Nicotine polacrilex is purposely made not to taste like ordinary chewing gum. It is a dose delivery device, not a chewing gum.
- It may take several days to adjust to the product's taste and the special manner in which it should be used.
- If acidic drinks (e.g., fruit juices, cola drinks, coffee) or foods (e.g., catsup, soy sauce, salsa, hot sauce) have been consumed, rinse the mouth with water before placing the gum in the mouth.
- To take advantage of the product's slow-release formula, use the bite-park-bite rotation method:

    Bite each piece slowly (10–15 times) until a peppery taste or tingling sensation occurs;

    When this sensation begins, place the gum between the upper or lower cheek and gums for approximately 1 minute;

    After the peppery taste fades, retrieve the dosing piece and repeat the process. (Keep the dosing piece in the mouth for approximately 30 minutes.)

    If biting the gum becomes tedious, push the gum from the outside of the cheek with a finger to expose a new surface of the gum to the saliva.

- Chewing the gum too quickly will result in an unpleasant taste caused by too much nicotine in the saliva and, if the nicotine is swallowed, may cause effects similar to those produced by excess smoking (e.g., nausea, irritation of the throat, hiccups, light-headedness).
- If jaw ache or belching occurs, combine the nicotine polacrilex gum with a small amount of sugar-free gum to soften the nicotine-containing gum and reduce the swallowing of air. Use the bite-park-bite rotation method with the gum mixture.
- Take the product on a scheduled basis.
- Follow the dosage regimen carefully and reduce the dosage at the recommended intervals.
- If a problem or severe symptoms develop, report them to a pharmacist or physician.
- Carry at least one full sleeve of nicotine polacrilex (12 doses per sleeve) at all times. Keep it in the same place where cigarettes were normally kept (e.g., shirt pocket or purse).
- Do not expose the product to extreme temperatures (e.g., do not place in a glove box or next to a source of heat).

■ Keep an extra sleeve of the product in the car, at work, and/or by the telephone.

■ Keep this product out of the reach of children and pets.

Parking the gum between the cheek and gum permits nicotine in the saliva to be absorbed into the bloodstream through the buccal mucosa. If the nicotine is swallowed with saliva or washed down when drinking a liquid, it will not be effective and may cause side effects such as heartburn, upset stomach, or hiccups. A basic pH is required for the nicotine to be properly released from the dosing piece into the saliva and then through the buccal mucosa. Thus, the consumption of acidic liquids must be avoided while the dosing piece is in the mouth.

Nicotine polacrilex is sugar free and, although somewhat sticky, suitable for use by many denture wearers. If additional gum is mixed with the nicotine polacrilex, a sugar-free gum should be used because sugar also produces acidity in the mouth and would hinder absorption of the nicotine.

Nicotine Transdermal Systems (NTS)

During 1991 and 1992, four forms of prescription nicotine transdermal systems were approved by the FDA for smoking cessation therapy. In 1996, two NTS products, Nicotrol and NicoDerm CQ, became available for nonprescription use.

NTS products use a controlled-release membrane which allows for the slow and steady absorption of nicotine through the skin. If an NTS is used, the patient must understand the purpose of the patches, their proper application, and the appropriate time to stop using them.

Dosage. The Nicotrol NTS is available in a 15-mg strength to be applied for 16 hours daily for 6 weeks. The NicoDerm CQ NTS is available in 7-, 14-, and 21-mg strengths. Heavy smokers (those smoking >10 cigarettes/day) should begin with the 21-mg strength daily for 6 weeks, followed by the 14-mg patch for two weeks, then the 7-mg patch for 2 weeks. Light smokers should begin with the 14-mg patch for 6 weeks, followed by the 7-mg patch for 2 weeks. NicoDerm CQ patches may be worn for 16 or 24 hours daily.

Usage Guidelines. The Nicotrol package contains "behavioral change" materials in the form of an audiotape, printed information, and a toll-free number. The NicoDerm CQ package contains a user's guide and a toll-free number that patients may call to enroll in a smoking cessation plan that includes newsletters and other mailings from the manufacturer.

Directions for use for both of these products include the following:

■ Stop smoking completely when you begin using this product.

■ Before using this product, read the user's guide and use the product according to the directions.

■ Remove backing from patch and apply the patch to clean, dry, hairless skin on upper arm or hip. Hold in place for 10 seconds. Wash hands.

■ Remove the used patch and apply a new patch to a different place on the skin at the same time every day.

■ For NicoDerm CQ:

If you crave cigarettes when you wake up, wear the patch for 24 hours.

If you begin to have vivid dreams or other disruptions of your sleep while wearing the patch 24 hours, try taking the patch off at bedtime (after about 16 hours of use) and putting on a new one upon arising the next day.

Precautions. All the warning statements that appear on product labeling for nicotine polacrilex also appear on product labeling for the nonprescription nicotine transdermal products, except for those relating to mouth, teeth, or jaw problems. Other precautions specific to the NTS include:

■ Keep this medication away from children and pets. Used patches have enough nicotine to poison children and pets. Fold sticky ends together and discard out of reach of children and pets.

■ Do not smoke, even when you are not wearing the patch. The nicotine in your skin will still be entering your bloodstream for several hours after you take the patch off.

■ Stop use and see your doctor if you the patch causes skin redness that does not go away after 4 days, if your skin swells, or if you get a rash.

About one third to one half of patients experience some local dermatological reaction (e.g., erythema, pruritus, edema, rash). Such reactions may not appear for several weeks.

Nicotine Nasal Spray

In 1996, the FDA approved nicotine nasal spray for use as a prescription smoking cessation therapy. The patient using this therapy must understand the purpose of the spray, its proper use, and the appropriate method of stopping its use.

The Pharmacist's Role in Smoking Cessation

Pharmacists should let their patients understand that they care enough about them to encourage them to stop smoking.

Counseling on the benefits of smoking cessation should be performed tactfully to current smokers, even those who profess not to want to stop smoking, at every pharmacist-patient encounter. Information about nicotine use should be noted on patient profiles. If a patient expresses a desire to stop nicotine use, pharmacists should advise them of available options.

The sale of tobacco products in pharmacies has been much debated and remains an ethical and individual decision for pharmacists. Making the pharmacy area a smoke-free area establishes a good example. Pharmacists can also set a good example by not using nicotine and by discouraging colleagues from doing so.

Patient Counseling

The success of any nicotine reduction therapy depends on behavioral change. The patient must truly desire to stop smoking and must alter habits and behaviors to accommodate a nicotine-free existence. Support from family, friends, and health care providers and proper counseling are important in achieving success with any smoking cessation therapy. Pharmacists can significantly improve patients' cessation rates by providing consultation on behavioral modification and encouraging patients to join a smoking cessation class.

After a patient completes a course of nicotine replacement therapy, the pharmacist must be prepared to continue to support the patient. The cessation rate can be improved through behavioral counseling. Pharmacists should help the patient understand the importance of avoiding behaviors that reinforced the urge to smoke, places or activities in which the individual previously smoked, and social and psychologic stimulators that influenced smoking.

Index

Index

The italic designations *f* and *t* that follow a page number indicate a figure or table.

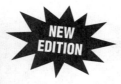
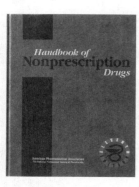

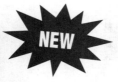

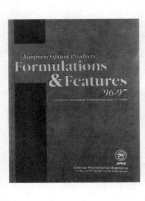

Nonprescription Products:
Formulations & Features*

Nonprescription Products: Formulations & Features presents detailed comparisons between more than 3,500 brand-name products in a convenient tabular format, and features:

■ **82 Product Category Tables,** with listings grouped by therapeutic use

■ **Timely Tables** on herbal and smoking cessation products as well as on hundreds of cold, cough, allergy, asthma, acid-peptic, diabetes care, and dermatologic products

■ **Alphabetical Index of Trade Names & Active Ingredients**

■ **Directory of OTC Manufacturers and Suppliers**

Order Code T217

APhA Member Price **$39.60**
Nonmember Price **$49.50**

ISBN 0-917330-78-1
1996; 447 pp.; softbound

*****Free with purchase of *Handbook of Nonprescription Drugs,* 11th Edition

Order Today! Call **800.878.0729** to place a credit card order.
APhA members, please have your ID number handy to receive member discounts.

Other APhA Publications

To order additional copies of *Nonprescription Products: Patient Assessment Handbook* or other quick-reference handbooks (below), call APhA Customer Service at 1-800-878-0729 or complete and return the adjacent postage-paid order form.

Pocket Guide to Evaluations of Drug Interactions, 1996–97 edition, by Frederic J. Zucchero, M.A.; Mark J. Hogan, Pharm.D.; and Christine D. Schultz, Pharm.D.

Contains 874 drug interaction monographs organized by drug class. Monographs provide eight concise pieces of information: title by generic names, significance rating, potential effects, patient management recommendations, findings from the literature, related drugs, mechanism for the interaction, and cross reference to *Evaluations of Drug Interactions.* 381 pages

Patient Counseling Handbook, 1995 edition, abstracted from *USP DI.*®

Concisely presents information for the health professional alongside information for the consumer. Covers approximately 3,000 drug products in monographs on 730 commonly prescribed drugs. Extensive index with generic and proprietary names, plus a handy patient counseling checklist. 932 pages

Drug Information Handbook,* 1996–97 edition, by Charles Lacy, Pharm.D.; Lora L. Armstrong, B.S.Pharm.; Naomi Ingrim, Pharm.D.; and Leonard L. Lance, B.S.Pharm.

Contains 994 monographs covering the most commonly prescribed medications. Each drug monograph presents up to 28 key points of information. Cross referencing helps the user rapidly locate brand names, generic names, and synonyms and related information in tables, charts, and graphs. 1,542 pages

Geriatric Dosage Handbook,* 1997–98 edition, by Todd P. Semla, Pharm.D.; Judith L. Beizer, Pharm.D.; and Martin D. Higbee, Pharm.D.

Contains monographs on 632 medications, emphasizing special geriatric considerations, dosing, changes in pharmacokinetics or pharmacodynamics, monitoring parameters, and adverse effects. 67 pages of clinical drug information relevant to the practice of geriatric pharmacotherapy are provided in useful charts, tables, and graphs. 833 pages

Pediatric Dosage Handbook,* 1997–98 edition, by Carol K. Taketomo, Pharm.D.; Jane Hurlburt Hodding, Pharm.D.; and Donna M. Kraus, Pharm.D.

Covers 592 pediatric medications. Written by pediatric pharmacists to be a practical, convenient guide to the use of medications in children, this book is a compilation of recommended pediatric doses, administration guidelines, food interactions, and extemporaneous preparations found in current literature. 894 pages

Infectious Diseases Handbook,* 1997–98 edition, by Carlos M. Isada, M.D.; Bernard L. Kasten, Jr., M.D.; Morton P. Goldman, Pharm.D.; Larry D. Gray, Ph.D.; and Judith A. Aberg, M.D.

Consists of four cross-referenced chapters: Disease Syndromes, Organisms, Laboratory Diagnosis, and Antimicrobial Therapy. 164 disease syndromes are cross referenced to 143 likely pathogens. 231 appropriate diagnostic testing procedures and 222 antimicrobial agents are presented in a consistent, concise format. 936 pages

*Available on CD ROM. Call 1-800-878-0729 for prices.